Nursing Research

Methods, Critical Appraisal, and Utilization

Second Edition

Geri LoBiondo-Wood, Ph.D., R.N.
Associate Professor and Chair, Parent/Child Nursing Program
University of Nebraska Medical Center
College of Nursing
Omaha, Nebraska

Judith Haber, Ph.D., R.N.
Director and Professor
Department of Nursing
College of Mount St. Vincent
Riverdale, New York

Illustrated

THE C. V. MOSBY COMPANY

St. Louis • Baltimore • Philadelphia • Toronto   1990

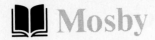

Editor Darlene Como
Developmental Editor Laurie Sparks
Project Managers Kathleen Teal, Patricia Tannian
Designer Candace Conner

Printed in the United States of America

The C.V. Mosby Company
11830 Westline Industrial Drive, St. Louis, Missouri 63146

Library of Congress Cataloging in Publication Data

Nursing research : methods, critical appraisal, and utilization /
  [edited by] Geri LoBiondo-Wood, Judith Haber. — 2nd ed.
    p. cm.
  Includes bibliographical references.
  ISBN 0-8016-3269-2
  1. Nursing — Research. I. LoBiondo-Wood, Geri. II. Haber,
Judith.
  [DNLM: 1. Nursing Research. WY 20.5 N9744]
RT81.5.N873 1990
610.73′072 — dc20
DNLM/DLC
for Library of Congress   89-13273
                                              CIP

GW/GW/D 9 8 7 6 5 4 3 2 1

Contributors

Ann Bello, M.A., R.N.
Associate Professor of Nursing
Norwalk Community College
Norwalk, Connecticut

Carolyn Oiler Boyd, Ed.D., R.N.
Associate Professor
Villanova University
Villanova, Pennsylvania

Betty Craft, M.P.N., R.N.
Assistant Professor
University of Nebraska Medical Center
College of Nursing
Omaha, Nebraska

Harriet R. Feldman, Ph.D., R.N.
Chairperson, Department of Nursing
Fairleigh Dickinson University
Rutherford, New Jersey

Margaret Grey, Dr. Ph., R.N.
Assistant Professor and Director of
    Primary Care Graduate Program
University of Pennsylvania
School of Nursing
Philadelphia, Pennsylvania

Judith Haber, Ph.D., R.N., C.S.
Director and Professor
Department of Nursing
College of Mount St. Vincent
Riverdale, New York

Judith A. Heermann, Ph.D., R.N.
Assistant Professor
University of Nebraska Medical Center
College of Nursing
Omaha, Nebraska

**Bettie S. Jackson, Ed.D.,
    R.N., F.A.A.N.**
Assistant Director of Nursing for Research
    and Quality Assurance
Moses Division
Montefiore Medical Center
Bronx, New York

Christine Kovner, Ph.D., R.N.
Associate Professor
Division of Nursing
New York University
New York, New York

Rona Levin, Ph.D., R.N.
Director, Division of Nursing
Felician College
Lodi, New Jersey

Geri LoBiondo-Wood, Ph.D., R.N.
Associate Professor and Chair,
    Parent/Child Nursing Program
University of Nebraska Medical Center
College of Nursing
Omaha, Nebraska

To our families
Pat and Brian and Lenny, Laurie, and Andrew

Foreword

Research is no longer within the purview of only those who conduct research seeking to develop nursing knowledge and to expand the scientific basis for nursing and nursing practice. Today, pressures internal and external to the profession require that all nurses be accountable not only for quality care, but also for providing important audiences with evidence that nursing does make a difference. To meet this requirement, nurses in a variety of roles, including student, educator, clinician, administrator, consultant, and entrepreneur, must be intelligent consumers of research results. *Nursing Research: Methods, Critical Appraisal, and Utilization* makes an important contribution in this regard.

When the first edition of this book was published in 1986, it was the first undergraduate textbook to systematically present the perspective of the nurse as a consumer of research. This perspective is expanded in the second edition as nurses are presented with a comprehensive introduction to the researcher role, the theories and principles of sound research practices, and a pragmatic account of the process of designing nursing research and testing and selecting instruments for the measurement of nursing variables in a variety of clinical and educational settings. The authors' experience in conducting research in a variety of nursing situations is evident in the selection of topics and examples; the content, strategies, and techniques have direct applicability for research utilization in diversified roles and settings. Thus students in basic nursing programs, as well as nurses who seek to expand their knowledge of research so they can judge the worth of research results for incorporation into their nursing practice, should have direct use for the book.

The authors begin their discussion assuming that most readers have little background in research, measurement, or statistics. They subsequently develop, explain in detail, and illustrate by example the concepts and principles that are operationally important to the content presented. The consumer perspective is evidenced in each chapter by the inclusion of (1) student-focused learning objectives and identification of key terms; (2) a pragmatic and detailed discussion of content specific to understanding the principles and practices addressed in the chapter; and (3) a set of critiquing criteria for judging the appropriateness and utility of the content presented when employed within the context of a research effort.

Throughout the book, attention is given to distinguishing between sometimes confused components of the research process and to introducing precision in the use of concepts and terms too often left ambiguous in other sources. Of particular value is the authors' focus on timely issues related to research roles; issues in the conduct of research; qualitative research approaches; ethical considerations, especially as they relate to animal experimentation; measurement and instrumentation; and the use of computers in research. The concluding chapters address research utilization and evaluation of the research effort, topics of particular salience for practicing nurses.

The authors are to be commended for assembling a comprehensive, thorough, and well-written research book that meets the unique needs of those who seek to benefit from the application of the results of the research efforts of others.

Carolyn F. Waltz, Ph.D., R.N., F.A.A.N.
Professor and Coordinator for Evaluation
School of Nursing
University of Maryland at Baltimore

Preface

The foundation of the second edition of this textbook continues to be the belief that nursing research is integral to all levels of nursing practice. All too often research is perceived as a complex process carried out in an ivory tower by expert nurse-scientists and having little or no relevance to the everyday practice of nursing. This dichotomous view of nursing research is not valid. Research is essential to the development of a unique scientific body of knowledge, a hallmark of any profession, and should be the foundation for shaping and guiding theory-based nursing practice.

Therefore all nurses need to understand, evaluate, and apply research. However, the kind of knowledge appropriate to different levels of education varies. There is a general consensus that the research role of the baccalaureate graduate calls for the skills of critical appraisal, that is, that the nurse should be a knowledgeable research consumer. Preparing students for this role involves developing their understanding of the research process, their appreciation of the role of the critiquer, and their ability to apply the critical appraisal process to research reports. An undergraduate course in nursing research should teach students how to understand, appraise, and apply research. The development of a basic level of competence in this area is essential for full integration of research into clinical practice. This is in contrast to the focus of a graduate level research course in which the emphasis is on carrying out research as well as understanding it.

The primary audience of this textbook remains undergraduate students who are concerned both with learning the steps of the research process and with learning how to critique published research literature. This book has also proved valuable as a secondary reference for students at the master's and doctoral levels who want a concise review of the basic steps of the research and critiquing processes. Furthermore, it is a relevant resource for practicing nurses. Its use of critiqued published research facilitates an understanding of how research can be used in clinical practice. The second edition of *Nursing Research: Methods, Critical Appraisal, and Utilization* prepares nursing students and practicing nurses to become knowledgeable nursing research consumers by emphasizing the following areas:

◇ Addressing the role of the nurse as a research consumer with the goal of increasing the appreciation of this role.
◇ Teaching the fundamentals of the research process and the critical appraisal process in a logical, systematic progression. This attitude toward research promotes a spirit of inquiry and encourages systematic thinking and judgment that will enable students and nurses to expand their knowledge base. This will be reflected in their increased application of the research literature to their clinical practice.
◇ Elevating the critiquing process to a position of importance comparable to that of

producing research. This enables students and nurses to make judgments regarding the relative utility and merit of a research project. Both consumers and producers of research need to be sophisticated appraisers of the state of the art. Moreover, before becoming a producer of research, the student needs to be a knowledgeable consumer. The goal is the stimulation of thoughtful practice that is both creative and innovative through the use of nursing research.

◇ Demystifying research, which is sometimes viewed as a complex process restricted to use by learned academicians. All practitioners of nursing should use research generated by academicians, but if the process remains mysterious, the majority of practitioners may feel incapable of understanding and using research findings.

The text is organized into two parts. Part I focuses on roles, approaches, and issues in nursing research. This part of the text provides an overview of the nurse's role as a research consumer. It introduces the sources of human knowledge, the characteristics of the scientific approach, and legal and ethical issues related to the conduct of research.

Part II focuses on the integration of the research and critiquing processes. Chapters 4 through 19 delineate each step of the research process, with clinical research studies used to illustrate each step. The interrelatedness of the steps is examined in relation to the total research process. Both qualitative and quantitative designs are presented. Critical thinking is stimulated by presentation of the potential strengths and weaknesses in each step of the process. These chapters include a section describing the critiquing process for each step, as well as lists of related Critiquing Criteria that are designed to stimulate a systematic and evaluative approach to research literature. Chapter 20 illustrates how the research process is used in and integrated with nursing practice. Chapter 21 presents a tabular summary of the Critiquing Criteria and uses it to evaluate several published research articles, including their applicability to practice.

Throughout the second edition numerous examples from published research studies are used. These examples operationalize the research process and illustrate how it unfolds in a research study. They are a critical link for the reinforcement of the research and critiquing processes.

The accompanying *Instructor's Manual* and *Testbank* complement the textbook and enhance the learning process.

The development of a scientific foundation for clinical nursing practice is the essential priority for nursing research in the future. The second edition of *Nursing Research: Methods, Critical Appraisal, and Utilization* will help students to develop a basic level of competence in understanding the steps of the research process that will enable them to critically analyze research studies and apply the findings in their clinical practice. To the extent that this goal is accomplished, nursing will have a cadre of practitioners who derive their practice from theory and research specific to nursing.

ACKNOWLEDGMENTS

No major undertaking is accomplished alone. There are those who contribute directly and those who contribute indirectly to the success of a project. We acknowledge with our warmest thanks the help and support of the following people:

⋄ Our students, particularly the nursing students at the University of Nebraska College of Nursing and Mount St. Vincent Department of Nursing, whose interest and lively curiosity sparked the idea for the revisions in the second edition.

⋄ Our contributors, whose expertise, cooperation, and punctuality made them a joy to have as colleagues.

⋄ Our editor Darlene Como, editorial assistant Barbara Carroll, and developmental editor Laurie Sparks, for their help with manuscript production and last minute details.

⋄ Our typists, Ann Gray and Betty Vinci, whose painstaking care with our sometimes disorderly manuscripts made the editorial process much smoother.

⋄ Our families, Pat and Brian Wood and Lenny, Laurie, and Andrew Haber, for their unending love, faith, understanding, and support throughout what is inevitably a consuming but exciting experience.

Geri LoBiondo-Wood
Judith Haber

Contents

PART I   NURSING RESEARCH: ROLES, APPROACHES, AND
         ISSUES

   1   The Role of Research in Nursing, 3
       GERI LOBIONDO-WOOD AND JUDITH HABER

   2   The Scientific Approach to the Research Process, 21
       HARRIET R. FELDMAN

   3   Legal and Ethical Issues, 37
       BETTIE S. JACKSON

PART II   THE RESEARCH PROCESS

   4   The Problem Statement, 59
       JUDITH HABER

   5   The Literature Review, 77
       MARGARET GREY

   6   The Theoretical Framework, 91
       HARRIET R. FELDMAN

   7   The Hypothesis, 109
       JUDITH HABER

   8   Introduction to Design, 127
       GERI LOBIONDO-WOOD

   9   Experimental and Quasiexperimental Designs, 147
       MARGARET GREY

  10   Nonexperimental Designs, 165
       GERI LOBIONDO-WOOD AND JUDITH HABER

  11   Qualitative Approaches to Research, 181
       CAROLYN OILER BOYD

  12   Additional Types of Research, 211
       GERI LOBIONDO-WOOD

13 **Data Collection Methods, 227**
MARGARET GREY

14 **Reliability and Validity, 247**
GERI LOBIONDO-WOOD AND JUDITH HABER

15 **Sampling, 267**
JUDITH HABER

16 **Descriptive Data Analysis, 291**
ANN BELLO

17 **Inferential Data Analysis, 311**
MARGARET GREY

18 **Computers in Research, 329**
CHRISTINE TASSONE KOVNER

19 **Analysis of the Findings, 345**
GERI LOBIONDO-WOOD

20 **Utilizing Nursing Research, 359**
RONA F. LEVIN

21 **Evaluating the Research Report, 381**
JUDITH A. HEERMANN AND BETTY J. CRAFT

GLOSSARY **415**

APPENDIX A **A Randomized Clinical Trial of Early Hospital Discharge and Home Follow-up of Very-Low-Birth-Weight Infants, 427**
DOROTHY BROOTEN, SAVITRI KUMAR,
LINDA P. BROWN, PRISCILLA BUTTS,
STEVEN A. FINKLER, SUSAN BAKEWELL-SACHS,
ANN GIBBONS, AND MARIA DELIVORIA-PAPADOPOULOS

APPENDIX B **Stress, Social Support, and Psychological Distress of Family Caregivers of the Elderly, 439**
VIRGINIA BAILLIE, JANE S. NORBECK, AND
LOU ELLEN A. BARNES

APPENDIX C **Comparisons of Rectal, Femoral, Axillary, and Skin-to-Mattress Temperatures in Stable Neonates, 453**
MARIAMMA T. KUNNEL, CECILLE O'BRIEN,
BARBARA HAZARD MUNRO, AND
BARBARA MEDOFF-COOPER

I

NURSING RESEARCH
Roles, Approaches, and Issues

1

The Role of Research in Nursing

Geri LoBiondo-Wood
Judith Haber

LEARNING OBJECTIVES

After reading this chapter the student should be able to do the following:

◇ State the significance of research to the practice of nursing.

◇ Identify the consumer of nursing research.

◇ Discuss the differences of trends within nursing research before and after 1950.

◇ Describe how research, education, and practice relate to each other.

◇ Evaluate the nurse's role in the research process as it relates to the nurse's level of educational preparation.

◇ Identify the future trends in nursing research.

◇ Formulate the priorities for nursing research for the remainder of the twentieth century.

KEY TERMS

applied research   consumer
basic research   critique
clinical research   research

As you begin to read the first chapter of this book you may be wondering, why on earth is a research course part of my nursing curriculum? You may be asking yourself, will this course help me pass the state boards when I graduate? You may also wonder, how will learning about **research** help me practice nursing in a better way? In answer to such questions, the research course you are taking will not specifically help you to pass your state boards. However, it may sharpen your critical thinking skills so that your ability to analyze the exam questions and potential answers is improved. More important, though, is the belief shared by many nurses that a knowledge of nursing research can have a significant effect on the depth and breadth of the professional practice of every nurse.

The purpose of this chapter is to introduce you to the significance and the historical evolution of nursing research and to highlight the multiple roles of the nurse in the research process. We will discuss the current status of research in nursing and then speculate on future directions for nursing research. We hope to engage you in a mutual learning process that begins with this chapter, a process that will clarify the role of the nurse in the research experience and the implications research has for nursing practice.

SIGNIFICANCE OF RESEARCH IN NURSING

The nursing profession has devoted great effort to developing the unique specialized body of knowledge used in the delivery of health care to clients. Indeed, having a specialized body of knowledge that is scientifically based is one of the hallmarks of a profession and is essential for fostering a sense of commitment and accountability to clients.

The current body of scientific knowledge can best be expanded through further research endeavors. But this expansion of knowledge has little meaning for the profession as a whole if it remains only in research journals or in the minds of the researchers. It must be part of the active repertoire of knowledge of those directly engaged in practice.

Today more than ever before nurses are required to be accountable for the quality of client care they deliver. In an era of consumerism and rising health care costs, clients are asking health professionals to document the effectiveness of their services. Essentially, they are asking nursing, "How do nursing services make a difference in my case?" Other groups, including insurance companies and governmental reimbursement agencies using prospective payment systems (PPSs) such as Medicare and Medicaid, are also requiring accountability for services provided.

Scientific investigations that are practice oriented can contribute significantly to validating the effectiveness of particular nursing measures and to improving the quality of client care. The findings of such studies provide a theory base for decision making about the delivery of nursing care. The nursing profession will be increasingly responsible for preparing its practitioners to be sophisticated producers of research and consumers of scientific literature; thus the new knowledge being generated can be evaluated and applied to nursing practice in a meaningful way.

The Commission on Nursing Research of the American Nurses' Association (ANA) (1981) has recognized the need for research skills at all levels of professional nursing. Scientific investigation promotes accountability, one of the hallmarks of a profession and a fundamental concept of the ANA Code of Conduct. There is a general consensus that the research role of the baccalaureate graduate calls for the skill of critical appraisal; that is, the nurse must be a knowledgeable **consumer** of research. The remainder of this text is devoted to helping you develop that expertise.

RESEARCH: THE LINK BETWEEN THEORY, EDUCATION, AND PRACTICE

Research is the link between theory, education, and practice. Mercer (1984) and Silva (1986) state that research is the process through which the knowledge base for nursing practice grows. Theory conceptualizes the abstract nature of the relationship among phenomena. Research, however, is the systematic, logical, and empirical inquiry into the possible relationships among particular phenomena. Educational settings provide a milieu where students can learn about the research process. In this setting they can also explore different theories and begin to evaluate them in light of research findings. Theoretical formulations supported by research findings may potentially become the foundations of theory-based practice in nursing.

At this point you might logically ask how the theory and research content of your course will relate to your nursing practice. The answer is twofold: it will help you to become a beginning producer of research; however, it must help you to become an intelligent *consumer* of research. A consumer uses, applies, and practices in an active manner. To be a knowledgeable consumer, a nurse must have a knowledge base about the relevant subject matter, the ability to discriminate and abstract information logically, and the ability to apply the knowledge that has been gained.

For example, nurses become knowledgeable consumers through educational processes and practical experience. The link between knowledgeably applying the nursing process and being a knowledgeable consumer is research. However, it is not necessary for nurses to conduct research studies to be able to appreciate and utilize research findings in practice. Rather, to be intelligent consumers, nurses must understand the research process and attain the critical evaluation skills needed to judge the merit and relevance of research findings before applying them in clinical practice and in caring for clients.

HISTORICAL PERSPECTIVE

Mid- and Late-Nineteenth Century

In the mid-nineteenth century, nursing as a formal discipline began to take root with the ideas and practices of Florence Nightingale. Her concepts have contributed to and are congruent with present values of nursing research. The promotion of health, prevention of disease, and care of the sick were central ideas of her system. Nightingale believed that the systematic collection and exploration of data were necessary for nursing. Her collection and analysis of data on the health status of British soldiers during the Crimean War led to a variety of reforms in health care (Palmer, 1977). Nightingale also noted the need for measuring outcomes of nursing and medical care (Nightingale, 1863). Other than Nightingale's work, there seems to have been little research during the early years of nursing's development. This may be in part because schools of nursing had just begun to be established in the United States, schools were unequal in ability to educate, and nursing leadership had just begun to develop.

Twentieth Century—Before 1950

Nursing research in the first half of the twentieth century focused mainly on nursing education, but some client- and technique-oriented research was evident. The early efforts in nursing education research were done by such leaders as Lavinia Dock (1900), Anne Goodrich (1932), Adelaide Nutting (1912, 1926), Isabel Hampton Robb (1906), and Lillian Wald (1915). Nutting's (1907) *The Education and Professional Position of Nurses* and Nutting and Dock's (1907) *A History of Nursing* were the earliest studies of nursing and nursing education. These pioneering works consist of documentation gathered for the purpose of reforming nursing education and establishing it as a viable profession.

The continued need for reform in nursing education was met by the Nursing and Nursing Education in the United States Landmark Study, known as the Goldmark Report (1923). Sponsored by the Rockefeller Foundation, the Committee on Nursing and Nursing Education was funded to survey on a national level the educational preparation of the faculty and the clinical experiences of the administrators, private duty nurses, public health nurses, and nursing students. The report identified multiple deficiencies and disparate educational backgrounds at all levels of nursing. This study, and others in the first half of the century, recommended reorganization of nursing education and, most important, its movement into the university setting.

Clinically oriented research slowly emerged in the early half of the century and mainly centered on the morbidity and mortality associated with such problems as pneumonia and contaminated milk (Carnegie, 1976). A few of these projects were instrumental in the development of client care protocols and the employment of nurses in community settings. An experimental project by Wald and Dock conducted in 1902 led to the employment of school nurses in the New York City school system and subsequently in other cities (Roberts, 1954). Although she did not perform formal research, Linda Richards, the first trained American nurse at Bellevue Hospital, was the first nurse to keep written documentation of client care. This documentation was used by the medical profession for their investigations (Carnegie, 1976).

In 1913 the Committee on Public Health Nursing of the National League of Nursing Education (NLNE) studied such concerns as infant mortality, blindness, and midwifery. The committee called for nursing to distinguish its role in the prevention of disease and the promotion of health through the knowledge and use of the scientific approach.

The 1920s saw the development and teaching of the earliest nursing research course because of the influence of Isabel M. Stewart (Henderson, 1977). A course titled "Comparative nursing practice," first taught by Smith and later by Henderson, introduced students to the scientific method of investigation. Students were encouraged to question all aspects of nursing care and to do laboratory experiments on such topics as measuring the oxygen content in an oxygen tent during a client's bed bath to assess whether it dropped below a therapeutic level. Also during this period, case studies appeared in the *American Journal of Nursing (AJN)*. These were used as a teaching tool for students and as a record of client progress (Gortner and Nahm, 1977). Scientific criteria were applied to assess the appropriateness of the methodology used (Gortner and Nahm, 1977).

Other practice-related research focused on improving nursing techniques (Clayton, 1927), handwashing procedures (Broadhurst et al., 1927), and thermometer disinfecting techniques (Ryan and Miller, 1932), among others. Clinical investigations similar to these and subsequent studies of nurses and nursing education were done through the first part of the century.

Social change and World War II affected all aspects of nursing, including research. There was an urgent need for more nurses; increased hospital admissions and military needs created a shortage of personnel. In 1943 the U.S. Cadet Nurses Corps was created after the Nurse Practice Act of 1943 was passed. The Corps provided assistance for nurses and after the war offered information that assisted in planning for nursing education. During the war, investigations focused on hospital environments, nursing status, nursing education, and nursing shortages.

After the war, nursing, like the rest of the world, began to reassess itself and its goals. In 1948 *Nursing for the Future* by Esther Lucille Brown was published. This was the culmination of a 3-year study funded by the Carnegie Foundation. This report reemphasized the inconsistencies in educational preparation and the need to move into the university setting, and it included an updated description of nursing practices. An outgrowth of Brown's report was a number of studies on nursing roles and needs. Also during the immediate postwar period many states carried out studies on nursing needs and resources (Simmons and Henderson, 1964).

Twentieth Century—After 1950

The 1950s saw the infancy stages of nursing research begin to develop and bloom. The developments of the 1950s laid the groundwork for nursing's current level of research skill. Nursing schools at the undergraduate and graduate levels were growing in number, and graduate programs were including courses related to research. The worth and benefit of research was appreciated by nursing leadership and was beginning to filter to the various levels of nursing. This period saw the inception of the *Journal of Nursing Research*, which was dedicated to the promotion of research in nursing. In 1955 the American Nurses' Foundation was chartered as a center for research; the audience for its publications consisted of receivers and administrators of research monies. Also at the national level of the ANA a standing Committee on Research and Studies was formed in 1954. This committee was charged with planning, promoting, and guiding research and studies relating to the functions of the Association (See, 1977). A secondary function of the Committee was to collect and unify nursing information that could be used to advise the ANA Board regarding periodic inventories of nurses. Concurrently in 1955 the Commonwealth Fund endowed the National League of Nursing (NLN) with monies for the support of research education and training. Throughout the 1950s these organizations and others, such as the U.S. Public Health Service, put forth funds and personnel to study the characteristics of nursing members and students; the supply, organization, and distribution of nursing services; and job satisfaction.

The first nursing unit for practice-oriented research was set up at the Walter Reed Army Institute of Research. This unit was geared toward chemical research. Even though research during this period was focused on nurses and their characteristics, the fields of psychiatric nursing and maternal-child health care received monies from federal grants to develop nursing content and educational programs at the master's and doctoral levels. Grants were also conferred on individuals who studied the social context of psychiatric facilities and its influence on relations between staff and clients (Greenblatt et al., 1955; Stanton and Schwartz, 1954) and the role of the nurse with single mothers (Donnell and Glick, 1954).

In the late 1950s nursing studies began to address clinical problems. In a guest editorial featured in *Nursing Research* (1956), Virginia Henderson commented that studies about nurses outnumber clinical studies 10 to 1. She stated that "the responsibility for designing its methods is often cited as an essential characteristic of a profession" (p. 99).

Thus in the 1960s there began a reordering of research priorities and a targeting of practice-oriented research. These priorities were supported by the American Nurses' Foundation and other major nursing organizations. However, even with this support, research did not flourish. This may be partly attributed to the lack of educational preparation of nurses in research. Where research education did exist, nurses had not yet developed sufficient expertise in research design and methodology to teach their own research courses. So nurses were, until very recently, dependent on others from related disciplines such as psychology, education, and sociology, who had this expertise to teach these courses. Today this is not usually the case.

Consistent with this need for guidance, many of the studies during the 1950s and 1960s were coinvestigated by individuals from the social sciences and medicine. Another reason for the paucity of research was the small number of nurses with baccalaureate and higher degrees. Although enrollment in these programs had increased by 1960, fewer than 2% of the employed registered nurses held master's degrees and fewer than 7% held baccalaureate degrees (ANA, 1960).

During the 1960s, studies on nurses and nursing continued, but at the same time the pioneers in the development of nursing theories and models, such as Ida Jean Orlando (1961), Hildegarde Peplau (1952), and Ernestine Wiedenbach (1964), called for the development of nursing practice based on theory. Although their theories and those of others have only begun to be tested, the early development of those theories has spurred nurses into a more critical level of thinking regarding nursing practice.

Collaborative efforts in the 1960s on practice-oriented research led to follow-up research by Diers and Leonard (1966) and Dumas and Leonard (1963). These studies done at Yale University explored the effects of nurse-patient teaching and communication on such events as hospitalization, surgery, and the labor experience. Another classic study, the culmination of 8 years of work by Glaser and Strauss (1965), explored various aspects of thanatology among dying patients and their caretakers.

A review of the nursing research studies published during the 1960s reveals that clinical studies were beginning to predominate. These studies investigated a wide gamut of nursing care issues such as infection control, alcoholism, and sensory deprivation. Lydia Hall (1963) published the results of a 5-year study that looked at alternatives to hospitalization for a select group of elderly clients. This study gave rise to a totally nurse-run care facility, the Loeb Center in New York City, which is still in operation and run by nurses today.

The rich history of nursing was also recognized during the 1960s. Nursing archives at Boston University's Mugar Library were established through a federally funded grant with the goal of promoting nursing research. In 1967 the First Nursing Research Conference of the ANA was held. A group of nurses and nursing faculty gathered to report on research and **critique** the findings presented.

The opening of the 1970s saw the publication of the National Commission for the Study of Nursing and Nursing Education Report or the Lysaught Report (1970). This report, conducted with the support of the ANA, NLN, and other private foundations, surveyed nursing practice and education. It offered the conclusion that more practice-oriented and education-oriented research was necessary and these data must be applied to the improvement of educational organizations and curricula. The call for clinically oriented study was becoming a reality. Carnegie (1976) noted that the majority of research published in the nursing journals was clinically oriented.

The 1970s also saw new growth in the number of master's and doctoral programs for nursing. These programs, along with the ANA, NLN, Sigma Theta Tau, and the Western Interstate Council for Higher Education in Nursing, clearly supported nurses learning the research process as well as producing research that could be used to enhance care quality. In the 1970s newer journals such as *Advances in Nursing Sciences, Research in Nursing and Health,* and *The Western Journal of Nursing Research* were established that promoted the generation of nursing theory and research.

The 1980s

The 1980s were an exciting and productive decade for research in nursing. The 1980s have seen extended growth among upper-level programs in nursing, especially at the doctoral level. By 1989 there were 47 doctoral programs in nursing in the United States, and more than 5000 of the doctorally prepared nurses held their doctorate in nursing. Consistent with the increased numbers of nurses with advanced training, there has also been increased federal funding and support not only in universities but also in practice settings for research. Many centers for nursing research exist in educational settings and in hospitals. A number of these centers have programs joining education and practice that provide support and guidance for research efforts.

Mechanisms for communicating research have also increased. A number of journals and reviews such as *Annual Review of Nursing Research, Scholarly Inquiry for Nursing Practice,* and *Applied Nursing Research* have come into existence in order to provide additional forums for communicating research. Most nursing organizations also have research sections that serve to foster the conduct and use of research.

Public Law 99-158, which was enacted in 1985, allowed for the establishment of the National Center for Nursing Research (NCNR). Established in 1986, NCNR provides funding programs that focus on studies related to health care outcomes. The NCNR program areas are organized in three broad categories: (1) health promotion/disease prevention, (2) acute and chronic illness, and (3) nursing systems/special programs (Hinshaw, 1988a). The National Advisory Council of the NCNR in 1988 identified seven nursing research priorities. The areas include (1) low birth weight—mothers and infants, (2) patients, partners, and families with human immunodeficiency virus, (3) long-term care, (4) symptom management, (5) information systems, (6) health promotion, and (7) technology dependency across the life span.

The efforts of the 1980s have been aimed at the refinement and development of research and the utilization of research findings in clinical practice. The developments and strides in the area of research made in the 1980s suggest that nursing is ready to rise to the societal and professional demands that will confront the discipline in the 1990s.

THE ROLES OF THE NURSE IN THE RESEARCH PROCESS

There are many roles for nurses in research. One of the marks of success in nursing research is the delineation of research activities geared for nurses prepared in different types of educational programs (Fawcett, 1984a; McBride, 1988).

Graduates of associate degree nursing programs should demonstrate an awareness of the value or relevance of research in nursing. They may assist in identifying problem areas in nursing practice within an established structured format, and they may assist in data collection activities (ANA, 1989).

Nurses with a baccalaureate education must be intelligent consumers of research; that is, they must understand each step of the research process and its relationship to every other step. Such understanding must be linked with a clear idea about the standards of satisfactory research. This comprehension is necessary when critically reading and understanding research reports and thereby determining the validity and merit of reported studies. Through critical appraisal skills that use specific criteria to judge all aspects of the research, a professional nurse interprets, evaluates, and determines the credibility of research findings. The nurse discriminates between an idea that is interesting but requires further investigation before implementation in practice, and findings that have sufficient support to be considered for utilization (Batey, 1982; Massey and Loomis, 1988).

In this context, understanding the research process and acquiring critical appraisal skills open a broad realm of information that can contribute to the professional nurse's body of knowledge and that can be applied judiciously to practice in the interest of providing scientifically based client care (Batey, 1982; Duffy, 1987). Thus the role of the baccalaureate graduate in the research process is primarily that of a knowledgeable consumer, a role that promotes the integration of research and clinical practice.

Lest anyone think that this is an unimportant role, let us assure you that it is not. Fawcett (1984b) states that we are all aware of those who assert that research is the bailiwick of "ivory tower" investigators. She goes on to state, however, that it is the average clinical practitioner who is ultimately responsible for utilization of the findings of nursing and other health-related research in clinical practice. To appropriately use such research findings, nurses must understand and critically appraise them. Thus if nursing as a profession is ever to have a genuine theory-based practice, it will be in large part up to nurses in their role as consumers of research to accomplish this task.

Baccalaureate graduates also have a responsibility to identify nursing problems that need to be investigated and to participate in the implementation of scientific studies (ANA, 1989). It is often clinicians who generate research ideas or questions from hunches, gut-level feelings, intuition, or observations of clients or nursing care. These ideas are often the seeds of further research investigations. For example, a nurse working on a psychiatric unit observed that a certain percentage of discharged clients were readmitted to the unit within 2 months of discharge. She noted that there were differences in the discharge procedure and wanted to find out if the type of aftercare treatment made a difference in the readmission rate. Of particular interest was the variation related to whether the client was connected to the aftercare therapist or facility before discharge and how this influenced the readmission rate. The presence and support of an expert nurse-researcher in the clinical setting can often provide leadership and direction for staff nurses in the systematic investigation of such an idea in an on-site clinical research project. Systematic collection of data about a clinical problem contributes to the refinement and extension of nursing practice.

Baccalaureate graduates may also participate in research projects as a member of an interdisciplinary or intradisciplinary research team. The nurse may participate in one or more phases of such a project. For example, a staff nurse may work on a clinical research unit where a particular type of nursing care is part of an established research protocol. In such a situation the nurse administers the care according to the format described in the protocol. The nurse may also be involved in the collection and recording of data relevant to the administration of and client response to the nursing care.

As members of a profession, it is also incumbent on baccalaureate graduates to share research findings with colleagues. This may involve collaborative dissemination of the findings of a study that you have participated in for an article or for a research or clinical conference. Or it may involve sharing with colleagues the findings of a research report that you have critiqued and have found to have merit and potential applicability in your practice.

Nurses who are educationally prepared at the master's and doctoral levels must also be sophisticated consumers of research. However, they are also being prepared to conduct research as either a coinvestigator or primary investigator.

At the master's level, nurses can analyze and reformulate nursing problems so that scientific knowledge and methods can be used to find solutions. They enhance the quality and relevance of nursing research by providing clinical expertise about problems and by providing knowledge about the way that clinical services are delivered. They facilitate the investigation of clinical problems by providing a climate conducive to conducting research. This includes collaborating with others in investigations and enhancing nursing's access to clients and data. At the master's level, nurses conduct research investigations for the purpose of monitoring the quality of the practice of nursing in a clinical setting. They assist others in applying scientific knowledge in nursing practice (ANA, 1989).

Doctorally prepared nurses have the greatest amount of expertise in appraising, designing, and conducting research. They develop theoretical explanations of phenomena relevant to nursing. They develop methods of scientific inquiry and use analytical and empirical methods to discover ways to modify or extend existing knowledge so that it is relevant to nursing. Three types of research are conducted by doctorally prepared nurses: **basic research, applied research,** and **clinical research.** Table 1-1 provides a definition and example of each type of research. In addition to their role as producers of research, doctorally prepared nurses also act as role models and mentors who guide, stimulate, and encourage other nurses who are developing their research skills. They also collaborate with and serve as consultants to educational or health care institutions or agencies in their research endeavors.

The most important implication of the delineation of research activities according to educational preparation is the necessity of having a collaborative research relationship within the nursing profession. Not all nurses must or should conduct research. However, all nurses can play some part in the research process. Nurses at all educational levels, whether they are consumers or producers of research or both, need to view the research process as something of *integral value* to the growing professionalism in nursing.

Professionals need to take the time to read research studies and to evaluate them using the standards congruent with scientific research. The critiquing process is used to identify the strengths and weaknesses of each study. Nurses should keep in mind

Table 1-1 Types of Nursing Research

Type of research	Definition	Example
Basic research	Theoretical or pure research that generates, tests, and expands theories that describe, explain, or predict the phenomenon of interest to the discipline without regard to its later use (Silva, 1986)	Butcher and Parkers' (1988) study of pleasant guided imagery is related to testing manifestations of the principle of resonancy, a postulate of Rogers' Science of Unitary Human Beings
Applied research	"Answers questions related to the applicability of basic theories in practical situations" (Donaldson and Crowley, 1978); tests the practical limits of descriptive theories but does not examine the efficacy of actions taken by practitioners	Baillie, Norbeck, and Barnes' (1988) study of the relationship between stress, social support, and psychological distress of caregivers to families of the elderly tested the applicability of the stress-buffering model of social support in these caregivers
Clinical research	Examines the effects of nursing processes on health status and examines the effects of actual implementation of knowledge in clinical practice settings (Fawcett, 1984b)	Munro, Creamer, Haggerty, and Cooper (1988) studied the differential effect of relaxation therapy on rehabilitation (blood pressure, heart rate, aerobic conditioning level, and psychosocial functioning) of patients after myocardial infarction

that no study is perfect; whereas the limitations should be recognized, nurses may extrapolate from the study whatever is sound and relevant to be considered for potential use in clinical practice.

FUTURE DIRECTIONS IN NURSING RESEARCH

In a complex health-oriented society such as ours that is increasingly responsive to consumer concerns related to the cost, quality, availability, and accessibility of health care, it is of paramount importance to define the future direction of nursing research and establish research priorities (Hinshaw, 1988b; 1988c).

There is unanimous agreement among nursing leaders that the essential priority for nursing research in the future will continue to be the extension of the scientific knowledge base for nursing practice (Mercer, 1984; Lindemann, 1984; Fawcett, 1984b; Phillips, 1988). This priority will definitely have implications for nursing education and nursing administration.

An increasing number of nurses who have significant expertise in appraising, designing, and conducting research will continue to emerge within the profession. They will be at the forefront of the ongoing refinement of our scientific knowledge base for nursing practice.

Nursing researchers will have increasing methodological expertise. They will be more knowledgeable about computer technology as it applies to the research process. There will be a greater emphasis on measurement issues such as the development of tools that accurately measure clinical phenomena. The increasing focus on the need to utilize multiple measures to accurately assess clinical phenomena will also be apparent. Related to the need to accurately measure clinical phenomena will be the development of noninvasive methods to measure physiological parameters of interest in high-technology settings. This may well be another aspect of utilizing multiple measures to assess particular clinical phenomena. The development of qualitative measures will also expand as this mode of inquiry becomes a more frequently used research methodology.

Nurses who are prepared to direct the conduct of research will head an expanding number of nursing research departments in clinical settings. They in turn will involve the nursing staff in generating and conducting research projects as well as critically evaluating existing research investigations. An expanded number of centers for nursing research will be established in university settings as faculty members become qualified to run them (Pollock, 1986).

The collaborative relationship between educational and practice settings will continue to intensify. Faculty members from universities will increasingly be invited to work collaboratively with nursing research departments or directly with nursing staff members in hospitals or agencies.

Staff members from clinical settings such as hospitals and other health care agencies will collaborate with students or faculty, or both in the university setting to share clinical ideas, observations, and research endeavors. Joint appointments between educational and clinical settings will increase. These will maximize the sharing of expertise in all areas of the research process in the interest of improving the quality of care for the object of our mutual concern, the client. The net result will be expanded intradisciplinary collaboration. Nurses will also be in a stronger position to engage in interdisciplinary research with members of other professions.

Another trend will be the proliferation of cluster studies, multiple site investigations of clinical problems. Hinshaw (1988b) states that the accumulation of evidence supporting or negating an existing theory will help define the base of nursing practice. Clinical consortia will help delineate the common and unique aspects of client care for the various health professions.

Replication of research studies will become a valuable component of building the theory base for nursing practice. Hinshaw (1988b) states that the adoption of research findings in practice with their potential risks and benefits, including the cost of implementation, should be based on a series of replicated studies.

The emphasis of research studies will be related to clinical issues and problems. The Commission on Nursing Research of the ANA (1981) has stated that the preeminent goal of scientific inquiry by nurses is the ongoing development of knowledge for use in the practice of nursing. Consequently, priority should be given to nursing research that would generate knowledge to guide practice in the following areas:

◇ Promoting health
◇ Preventing health problems
◇ Decreasing the negative impact of health problems on coping abilities, productivity, and life satisfaction
◇ Ensuring that the care needs of vulnerable groups such as the aged are met through appropriate strategies
◇ Designing and developing health care systems that are cost-effective in meeting the nursing needs of the population
◇ Promoting health, well-being, and competency for personal health in all age groups

Nurses with graduate research preparation will be conducting research studies to accomplish these goals. Baccalaureate graduates will be critically appraising the research literature to examine the findings of clinical studies for potential incorporation into theory-based nursing practice. Examples of research consistent with the priorities given earlier include the following:

◇ Identifying determinants of wellness and health functioning in individuals and families, and identifying factors predictive of successful coping with chronic illness
◇ Identifying phenomena that negatively influence the course of recovery and that may be alleviated by nursing practice, such as anorexia, pain, sleep deprivation, and nutritional deficiencies
◇ Developing and testing strategies that facilitate the individual's health-enhancing behaviors such as altering nutrition; reducing stressful responses associated with medical management of surgical patients; providing more effective management of high-risk populations such as families with an impaired child; and enhancing the care of clients culturally different from the majority, clients with special problems such as teenagers, and underserved client groups such as the poor
◇ Designing and assessing, in terms of cost and effectiveness, models for delivering nursing care strategies found to be effective in clinical studies

By the year 2000 the population will include an increased proportion of children and elderly who are chronically ill or disabled. The health problems of mothers and infants will provide a renewed concern for dealing effectively with the rising maternal-infant mortality rate. People who have sustained life-threatening illnesses will live with new life-sustaining technology that will create new demands for self-care and family support. Cancer, heart disease, arthritis, chronic pulmonary disease, diabetes, and Alzheimer's disease are prevalent during middle and later life and will command large proportions of the available health resources. Mental health problems will result from rapid technological and social change. Alcohol and drug abuse will be responsible for significant health care expenses. The impact of human immunodeficiency virus (HIV) on individuals, families, and communities dealing with the crisis of acquired immune deficiency syndrome will continue to have a major effect on the health care delivery system. Increasingly, the settings where client care is provided for individuals and families will be homes, schools, workplaces, and ambulatory care centers.

In light of the priority given to clinical research issues, the funding of investigations will be increasingly in the area of clinical research projects. This is not to say that other types of research investigations such as those utilizing historical, philosophical, or evaluative designs are not important. As nurses define their practice, become eligible for third-party reimbursement, and are held more accountable for the quality and cost-effectiveness of their practice, they will have to engage in more evaluative outcome studies. In fact, nursing research will be used increasingly to affect health policy that guides the delivery of health care. Providing accurate data bases from systematic evaluation of nursing care intervention or from innovative programs is a necessary forerunner to nursing's ability to influence health policy at the level of nursing practice, the health care environment, or regional/national concerns and issues (Aiken, 1981).

It is apparent from the previous discussion that the future directions of nursing research will focus on the scientific validation of nursing practice. Both consumers and producers of research will engage in a unified effort to accomplish this priority.

SUMMARY

Nursing research provides the basis for expanding the unique body of scientific knowledge that forms the foundation of nursing practice. Research is the link between education theory and practice. Nurses become knowledgeable consumers of research through educational processes and practical experience. As consumers of research, nurses must have a basic understanding of the research process as well as critical appraisal skills that provide a standard for evaluating the strengths and weaknesses of research studies before applying them in clinical practice.

A historical perspective of nursing research traces its origins to Florence Nightingale. Moving forward to the first half of the twentieth century, nursing research focused mainly on studies related to nursing education. However, some clinical studies related to nursing care were evident. Nursing research blossomed in the second half of the twentieth century; graduate programs in nursing expanded, research journals began to emerge, the ANA formed a research committee, and funding for graduate education and nursing research increased dramatically. Basic, applied, and clinical research studies were carried out by an increasing number of nurse researchers.

Nurses at all levels of educational preparation have a responsibility to participate in the research process. The role of the baccalaureate graduate has been delineated as one of knowledgeable consumer of research. Nurses prepared at the master's and doctoral levels must be sophisticated consumers but will also be producers of research studies. A collaborative research relationship within the nursing profession will extend and refine the scientific body of knowledge that provides the grounding for theory-based practice.

The future of nursing research will continue to be the extension of the scientific knowledge base for nursing expertise in appraising, designing, and conducting research and will provide leadership in both academic and clinical settings. Collaborative research relationships between education and service will multiply. Cluster research studies and replication of studies will have increased value.

The emphasis of research studies will be related to clinical issues and problems. Priority will be given to research studies focusing on health promotion, the deminution of the negative impact of health problems, the ensuring of care for the health needs of vulnerable groups such as the aged, and the development of cost-effective health care systems. The recipients of health care will increasingly be mothers, children, and elderly people with chronic health problems. Alcohol- and drug-related problems will increase. The incidence of acquired immune deficiency syndrome will also increase. The settings where clients will receive care will be homes, workplaces, schools, and ambulatory care centers.

Both consumers and producers of research will engage in a collaborative effort to further the growth of nursing research and accomplish the research priorities of the profession.

References

Aiken L.H. (1981). *Health policy and nursing practice,* New York, McGraw-Hill Book Co.

American Nurses' Association. (1960). *Facts about nursing,* New York, pp. 109-116.

American Nurses' Association. (1981). Guidelines for the investigative function of nurses, Kansas City, Mo., pp. 2-3.

American Nurses' Association. (1989). Commission on Nursing Research: preparation of nurses for participation in research, Kansas City, Mo.

Baillie, V., Norbeck, J.S., and Barnes, L.E.A. (1988). Stress, social support, and psychological distress of family caregivers of the elderly, *Nursing Research,* **37**:217-222.

Batey, M.V. (1982). Research: A component of undergraduate education. In *Evaluating research preparation in baccalaureate nursing education: national conference for nurse educators,* Ames, University of Iowa College of Nursing.

Broadhurst, J., and others, (1927). Hand brush suggestions for visiting nurses, *Public Health Nursing,* **19**:487-489.

Brown, E.L. (1948). *Nursing for the future,* New York, Russell Sage Foundation.

Butcher, H.K., and Parker, N.I. (1988). Guided imagery within Rogers' Science of Unitary Human Beings: an experimental study, *Nursing Science Quarterly,* **1**:103-110.

Carnegie, E. (1976). *Historical perspectives of nursing research,* Nursing Archive, Special Collections, Boston, Boston University.

Clayton, S.L. (1927). Standardizing nursing techniques, its advantages and disadvantages, *American Journal of Nursing,* **27**:939-943.

Committee on Nursing and Nursing Education in the United States, Josephine Goldmark, sec. (1923). New York, Macmillan Inc.

Diers, D., and Leonard, R.C. (1966). Interaction analysis in nursing research, *Nursing Research,* **15**:225-228.

Dock, L.L. (1900). What we may expect from the law, *American Journal of Nursing,* **1**:8-12.

Donaldson, S.K., and Crowley, D.M. (1978). The discipline of nursing, *Nursing Outlook,* **26**:113-120.

Donnell, H., and Glick, S.J. (1954). The nurse and the unwed mother. *Nursing Outlook,* **2**:249-251.

Duffy, M.E. (1987). The research process in baccalaureate nursing education: a ten-year review, *Image,* Summer, **19**:87-91.

Dumas, R.G., and Leonard, R.C. (1963). The effect of nursing on the incidence of postoperative vomiting. *Nursing Research,* **12:**12-15.

Fawcett, J. (1984a). Another look at utilization of nursing research, *Image,* Spring, **16:**59-61.

Fawcett, J. (1984b). Hallmarks of success in nursing research, *Advances in Nursing Science,* **1:**1-11.

Glaser, B.G., and Strauss, A.L. (1965). *Awareness of dying* (Observations series), Chicago, Aldine Publishing Co.

Goodrich, A. (1932). *The social and ethical significance of nursing: a series of addresses,* New York, The Macmillan Co.

Gortner, S.R., and Nahm, H. (1977). An overview of nursing research in the United States, *Nursing Research,* **26:**10-33.

Greenblatt, M., and others. (1955). *From custodial to therapeutic patient care in mental hospitals,* New York, Russell Sage Foundation.

Hall, L.E. (1963). A center for nursing, *Nursing Outlook,* **11:**805-806.

Henderson, V. (1956). Research in nursing practice—when (editorial), *Nursing Research,* **4:**99.

Henderson, V. (1977). We've "come a long way," but what of the direction? (guest editorial), *Nursing Research,* **26:**163-164.

Hinshaw, A.S. (1988a). The new National Center for Nursing Research: patient care research program, *Applied Nursing Research,* **1:**2-4.

Hinshaw, A.S. (1988b). The national center for nursing research: challenges and initiatives, *Nursing Outlook,* **36:**21-24.

Hinshaw, A.S. (1988c). Using research to shape health policy, *Nursing Outlook,* **36:**21-24.

Larson, E. (1981). Nursing research outside academia: a panel presentation, *Image,* October, **13:**75-77.

Lindemann, C. (1984). Dissemination of nursing research, *Image,* Spring, **16:**57-58.

Massey, J., and Loomis, M. (1988). When should nurses use research findings? *Applied Nursing Research,* **1:**32-40.

McBride, A.B. (1988). Making research an activity for all nurses, *Reflections,* **14:**2.

Mercer, R.T. (1984). Nursing research: the bridge to excellence in practice, *Image,* Spring, **16:**47-50.

Munro, B.H., Creamer, A.M., Haggerty, M.R., and Cooper, F.S. (1988). Effect of relaxation therapy on post-myocardial infarction patients' rehabilitation, *Nursing Research,* **37:**231-235.

National Commission for the Study of Nursing and Nursing Education. (1970). *An abstract for action,* New York, McGraw-Hill Book Co.

Nightingale, F. (1863). *Notes on hospitals,* London, Longman Group.

Nutting, M.A., and Dock, L.L. (1907-1912). *A history of nursing,* 4 vols., New York, G.P. Putnam's Sons.

Nutting, M.A. (1912). Educational status of nursing, U.S. Bureau of Education, Bull. no. 7, Washington, D.C., U.S. Government Printing Office.

Nutting, M.A. (1926). *A second economic basis for schools of nursing and other addresses,* New York, G.P. Putnam's Sons.

Orlando, I.J. (1961). *The dynamic nurse-patient relationship,* New York, G.P. Putnam's Sons.

Palmer, I. (1977). Florence Nightingale: reformer, reactionary, researcher, *Nursing Research,* **26:** 84-89.

Peplau, H.E. (1952). *Interpersonal relations in nursing: a conceptual frame of reference for psychodynamic nursing,* New York, G.P. Putnam's Sons.

Phillips, J.R. (1988). The reality of nursing research, *Nursing Science Quarterly,* **1:**48-49.

Pollock, S. (1986). Top-ranked schools of nursing: network of scholars, *Image,* Summer, **18:**58-60.

Robb, I.H. (1906). *Nursing: its principles and practice for hospitals and private use,* 3rd ed., Cleveland, E.C. Koeckert.

Roberts, M.M. (1954). *American nursing: history and interpretation,* New York, Macmillan Inc.

Ryan, V., and Miller, V.B. (1932). Disinfection of clinical thermometers: bacteriological study and estimated costs. *American Journal of Nursing,* **32:**197-206.

See, E.M. (1977). The ANA and research in nursing. *Nursing Research,* **26:**165-176.

Silva, M.C. (1986). Research testing nursing theory: state of the art, *Advances in Nursing Science,* **9:**1-11.

Simmons, L.W., and Henderson, V. (1964). *Nursing research: a survey and assessment,* New York, Appleton-Century-Crofts.

Stanton, A.H., and Schwartz, M.A. (1954). *The mental hospital: a study of institutional participation in psychiatric illness and treatment,* New York, Basic Books, Inc.

Wald, L.D. (1915). *House on Henry Street,* New York, Henry Holt & Co.

Wiedenbach, E. (1964). *Clinical nursing: a helping art,* New York, Springer Publishing Co., Inc.

2

The Scientific Approach to the Research Process

Harriet R. Feldman

LEARNING OBJECTIVES

After reading this chapter the student should be able to do the following:

◇ Describe the relationship between philosophy and science.

◇ Identify the major sources of human knowledge.

◇ Contrast the strengths and weaknesses of the major sources of human knowledge.

◇ Compare the inductive and deductive methods of logical reasoning.

◇ Identify the characteristics of the scientific approach as they relate to the research process.

◇ Define theory.

◇ Describe the points of critical appraisal used to examine the relationship between theory and method.

KEY TERMS

assumption	inductive reasoning
control	objectivity
deductive reasoning	research
generalization	scientific approach
hypothesis	theory

THE PHILOSOPHY OF SCIENCE

Philosophers and scientists pursue a common goal of working toward the expansion of knowledge. Their approaches to understanding reality, however, are different. For example, the philosopher uses intuition, reasoning, contemplation, and introspection to examine "the purpose of human life, the nature of being and reality, and the theory and the limits of knowledge" (Silva, 1977, p. 60). On the other hand, the scientist observes, verifies, constructs operational definitions, tests hypotheses, and conducts experiments to derive scientific laws and interpret reality. Another contrast is in the kinds of questions philosophers and scientists ask. Philosophy deals with *metaphysical* questions: What is knowledge? Are people inherently good or bad? Science deals with *empirical* questions: How are X and Y related? Does the application of ice result in reduced muscle swelling?

The development of *nursing knowledge* depends on both philosophy and science. For example, an individual's philosophy of human behavior, health, and client care will guide the intent and direction of a research effort. If a researcher thinks that health behaviors are influenced by the amount of information clients have, it is likely that investigations of that researcher will focus on the effects of different teaching strategies on specific client outcomes, for example, blood sugar levels in a patient with diabetes. In addition, through logic and reasoning the researcher/scientist can organize, formulate, and verify ideas and relationships. This provides the framework for studying the problem. For example, Martinson (1978) states,

> Before making observations, the investigator must decide what she is going to observe and where she will make these observations. She must have already articulated in her own mind why she is selecting certain factors for observation and rejecting others. Prior to making such decisions, she must formulate some ideas regarding her study. These ideas, whether in the form of vague hunches or clearly formulated propositions, will serve as a guide in determining what questions are to be addressed by the research and which procedures and tools are to be used in searching for the answers (p. 155).

The research consumer can also employ these processes to critically appraise the content, methods, and utility of research projects in light of moral and ethical standards. For example, you might ask the following questions: Does the theoretical rationale reflect a philosophical view of reality as a cause-and-effect relationship or as an interactional relationship? On what basis are sample delimitations made? Why were identified study variables selected? What are the propositions and how were they derived? Do subject selection and data collection procedures adhere to accepted moral and ethical guidelines? To follow through on the previously cited example, how would an investigator determine what type of clients to include in this study? Would clients with brittle (unstable) diabetes be appropriate study subjects or would a more stable sample of clients provide a better basis for evaluating the teaching strategy in relation to the outcome of blood sugar level? What content area(s) would be emphasized in the teaching; that is, what knowledge is essential to impart to a client with diabetes that, if learned and applied, can ultimately produce the desired effect of lowered blood sugar? What theoretical reason is there for making a connection between knowledge and behavior?

Science can be viewed from at least two perspectives: as a body of theoretical knowledge (Andreoli and Thompson, 1977; Johnson, 1974) or as a method or process of inquiry (Beckwith and Miller, 1976; Newman, 1979). The body-of-knowledge perspective is very specifically concerned with interrelated *facts, principles, laws,* and *theories* and not with random or unrelated data. The method or process of inquiry is the medium for systematically collecting, quantifying, and evaluating data. It is useful to include both perspectives when defining science.

This chapter will examine the sources or origins of human knowledge and the components of the **scientific approach** that guide the process of inquiry. In addition, the relationship between **theory** and method will be discussed.

SOURCES OF HUMAN KNOWLEDGE

Ideas are generated in many ways. Some sources of knowledge are highly structured and are generally bound by defined rules of process or method. Examples include scientific inquiry, critical thinking, and logical reasoning. Other sources are less structured and have few defined rules; they include empathy, intuition, trial-and-error experience, and meditation. As a research consumer it is important for you to know how information is approached in a research or scientific context. Therefore several of these sources of knowledge, intuition, trial and error, tradition and authority, and logical reasoning, will be discussed.

Intuition

Webster's (1983) defines intuition as "immediate knowing or learning of something without the conscious use of reasoning; instantaneous apprehension" (p. 964). Intuition is a frequently used method of problem solving. It can operate in one of two ways, for example, as a form of inference where intuition closely resembles sensory perception or as an extrasensory experience independent of sensory input. Vaughan (1979) says, "Whatever the explanation or belief about it, intuition is widely acknowledged as being essential to problem solving and creativity in many different forms" (p. 150).

Intuitive leaps in science and the arts, made by such people as Einstein and Beethoven, have led to great contributions to humanity. The following situation illustrates an intuitive leap, or an "ah ha." Each time I taught a course in change theories and strategies, I listed the stages of the change process. A few years ago a student enthusiastically blurted out, "That's the same as the nursing process," and another student said, "It's also like the research process." Each of these students expressed an insight and consequently that insight helped them have a clearer understanding of the change process. How many times have *you* unsuccessfully sought a solution to a problem, only to awaken in the middle of the night with a creative answer? Some of you may even keep writing materials or a tape recorder near your bed to catch the insights while they are fresh!

In the case of research pursuits, intuition also plays a role. Whereas intuition is not a sufficient means to approach information in a research context, it can serve as a guiding and creative adjunct. Often it is an initial "hunch," "gut feeling," or inference that leads many investigators to the examination of anticipated relationships. Furthermore the logical process of inquiry is often complemented by intuitive insights that bring depth and breadth to the total research experience. For example, you sense a pervasive attitude of anxiety on the part of parents of clients who are treated in a particular well-baby clinic. You are curious as to whether this is typical or atypical, so you visit a second well-baby clinic in the next town. Although the physical attributes and type of clientele are similar, intuitively you sense a difference in these settings. You decide to investigate what makes these two seemingly similar clinic settings different.

When research reports are reviewed, the use of intuition in beginning and throughout the research process may or may not be apparent. Sometimes the introductory section of a research report identifies how the investigators first became aware of the problem they studied. Authors do not always include this information in the introduction, nor do they necessarily document insights that arose along the way.

Trial-and-error experience

An early approach to problem solving uses the process of elimination. When a problem is identified, a solution is attempted. Depending on whether or not the solution works, you either adopt the trial solution or try another one. When the second solution fails, you keep trying, eliminating one solution after another until the problem is solved. For example, you may try five or six approaches to promoting the healing of a decubitus ulcer before you find the one that works for a particular client. Moving on to another client with a similar problem, the solution you found for the first client may not work, and so you proceed with other trials until you achieve success. This can be a very inefficient method of problem solving in terms of both time and energy, because it may take a very long time to find a successful solution. In addition, that solution may have already been determined by someone else. You may wonder how to find out if a solution has been found and how the trial-and-error method can be short-circuited. There are alternatives; for example, you can review the literature pertinent to that problem to see what solutions exist or you can ask a consultant about possible solutions.

In your role as consumer you will be evaluating research methodology to see if the approach to solving the problem, as compared to testing the **hypothesis,** is appropriate to the study. You would ask if the hypothesis directly answers the research problem, if other possibilities were considered, and if the data collection instruments are valid and reliable. Given that the rationale for and the method of hypothesis testing are theoretically sound, it is logical to conclude that trial and error was not the approach used.

Tradition and authority

Often we are tricked into believing that something is right or acceptable because it is backed by tradition and authority. Although it is important to look at tradition and listen to what those in authority are saying, both of these sources of human knowledge must be critically evaluated in light of other sources of available data, for example, related literature and experts in the field. As a research consumer you have a responsibility to examine the validity and utility of knowledge derived from these sources. This is accomplished by questioning, identifying, and synthesizing all available data sources and noting the data that clearly and logically support valid solutions.

When trial-and-error experiences lead to problem resolution, a ready source of known solutions becomes available. That resource pool forms the basis for tradition or precedent. As we become more invested in those traditional solutions, they take on an air of authority. The ritual of temperature taking is an example in nursing of this evolution of problem solving from trial and error to authority. In many instances nurses have come to accept over time that individuals require temperature readings every 4 hours simply because they are admitted to an acute care facility. The initial rationale for this procedure has been long forgotten, and more current investigations have refuted this practice. In fact, some hospitals have discontinued this temperature-taking routine after doing research on the subject. Another example is the procedure used for charting information about clients. Tradition has often dictated the charting procedure(s) used in each health care institution, and although newer methods of charting may have been shown to better communicate critical information among health care professionals, the institution continues to follow what it sees as "tried and true."

Another example of how tradition and authority have guided practice relates to tracheotomy care. Traditionally the use of sterile technique in tracheotomy care has been advocated and in many cases mandated. The rationale for this approach certainly seems sound and authoritative. Harris (1981), however, reported no statistically significant differences between sterile and clean techniques in her study of patients with tracheotomies. In fact, the trend toward infection was greater in the sterile versus clean procedure group.

As a research consumer you must question tradition and authority. The more you challenge the kind of practice that evolved solely by precedent, the sooner nursing will advance in its development of a scientific basis for practice.

Logical reasoning

The two major methods of logical reasoning are inductive and deductive. As you tackle daily problems you often utilize these approaches without realizing that you do. **Inductive reasoning** involves the observation of a particular set of instances that belongs to and can be identified as part of a larger set. This reasoning moves from the particular to the general. On the other hand, **deductive reasoning** uses two or more variables or related statements that, when combined, form the basis for a concluding assertion of a relationship between the variables or the statements. This reasoning moves from the general to the particular.

Inductive reasoning

As stated above, inductive reasoning moves from the particular to the general. A **generalization** is developed from specific observations. For example, Freud gathered a great deal of information by listening to his clients report their dreams; he then made generalizations about the symbolism he identified. As a nurse, you may observe that many of the children you care for behave in a particular way and may conclude that the unfamiliar setting of the hospital is very stressful to those children. Unfortunately, as one individual who must observe a limited number of patients, your conclusion cannot be generalized to the claim that the hospital setting is stressful for *all* children. Another example is the observation that an increasing number of newborns in the nursery are developing a rash on their backs. You conclude that there is a problem with the method of laundering the sheets on which the newborns lie. Your conclusion cannot be generalized to the claim that the laundromat is using harsh detergents on *all* their sheets.

A third example of inductive reasoning is the study conducted by Brooten, Kumar, Brown, Butts, Finkler, Bakewell-Sachs, Gibbons, and Delivoria-Papadopoulos (1986). Based on their findings, both from their practice and through a search of the literature, (1) that prolonged hospitalization of very-low-birth-weight infants can have an adverse effect on the babies' physical and mental health, (2) that "formalized home care services are almost completely lacking after these infants are discharged" (p. 934), and (3) that the rate of rehospitalization for very-low-birth-weight infants is much higher than that for normal-birth-weight infants, Brooten et al. (1986) decided to try follow-up care in the home by a perinatal nurse specialist to determine if this approach affected the safety, efficacy, and cost savings of early discharge from the hospital of very-low-birth-weight infants.

The pitfall of generalization is one you as a research consumer should look for when you critique **research;** for example, did the investigator overgeneralize? The following questions elaborate on this point: If the study focused on a laboratory population, was the generalization extended to include a clinical population? If the study involved clients who had hysterectomies, was the generalization extended to all ethnic groups?

In summary, the inductive approach begins with an observation or some other way of obtaining information and leads to a predicted conclusion or hypothesis (see Chapter 7). In cases where conclusions are arrived at by use of specific or limited data, the generalization of results can be erroneous. "The only valid conclusion which can be drawn is that a particular relationship existed in a particular situation at a particular point in time, and that further studies are required to test or control for rival hypotheses that may have been instrumental in determining the results" (Downs and Newman, 1977, p. 11).

Deductive reasoning

Deductive reasoning moves from the general to the particular. A specific hypothesis can be deduced from a theory that serves as a more general statement or from a network of interrelated phenomena. Observations and predictions can be made from deduction. Rather than a source of new information, deductive reasoning can serve as an approach to unveiling existing relationships. For example, if we know that theory R is true, we could anticipate what outcomes and behaviors are logically expected. Here are two examples of how a nurse can use deductive reasoning.

1. Since you know certain physiological changes take place in bedridden clients as a result of continuous or uneven pressure to bony prominences, you could deduce that pressure-relieving methods will decrease the incidence and intensity of decubitus ulcers.

2. The gate control theory of pain identifies the interaction of motivational, affective, and sensory processing that modulates the perception of and response to pain. Therefore such factors as anxiety, attention, age, culture, meaning of the present pain experience, and pathophysiological findings are associated with the pain experience. Since anxiety and the pain sensation tend to reinforce each other, thereby increasing the intensity of the pain experience, you could deduce that anxiety-reducing measures (for example, empathic interaction, a back rub, an explanation to the client, and promptness in the administration of pain medication) will result in decreased pain.

3. Social support can be viewed as "a characteristic of the social situation that buffers the effect of stress on the health of the individual" (Northouse, 1988). In other words, social support helps the individual to see an event as less stressful so he or she can cope with it more effectively. An example of a stressful situation that can affect the health of an individual is breast cancer. Given what is known about social support and its effects on stress and health, a researcher studying the adjustment of women to mastectomy might deduce that patients with breast cancer who receive social support after mastectomy will have fewer adjustment problems than those who do not receive social support.

As with inductive reasoning, there may be inherent problems in the deductive approach. First, not all deductions can be verified, particularly in the case where the measurement methods are poor or underdeveloped. Second, a deduction that is based on a tentative premise may result in a conclusion that is logically valid, yet unsound. Finally, an unsound conclusion may be assumed sound, especially if it seems reasonable. If a systematic, scientific approach is used to test a hypothesis deduced from a theory, the conclusion is more likely to be sound and have utility.

Scientific approach

The scientific approach offers a logical, orderly, and objective means of idea generation. By combining several components (for example, logic and reasoning, order and **control,** and empiricism and generalization), a rather sophisticated system of inquiry has been developed. This system has limitations, such as moral and ethical problems, measurement and control problems associated with nursing and social science research, and the general difficulty related to studying human beings; however, it has been found to be more useful and predictive than other sources of human knowledge such as intuition, trial and error, or tradition and authority.

The example of tracheotomy care (see Tradition and Authority in this chapter) illustrates the scientific approach as a more advanced method of acquiring knowledge. The traditional approach of use of sterile technique for tracheotomy care has been advocated as the most appropriate to eliminate infection. This means that each time tracheotomy care is provided, sterile gloves and other equipment are used, at high costs, both in materials and labor. Despite the fact that this procedure has been followed, a certain number of people still acquire infections. One could not predict that if sterile technique were followed, an infection would not occur. In conducting research on tracheotomy care Harris (1981-82) found that the results of use of sterile technique were not statistically different from results when clean technique was used. From her findings you can conclude that both techniques are useful. Use of the scientific approach enabled Harris (1981-82) to make a prediction about alternative techniques for tracheotomy care, a prediction that would have been difficult if not impossible to make had primary sources of knowledge been tradition and authority, trial and error, or intuition.

As a research consumer you will be evaluating reported studies in terms of the investigators' adherence to the scientific approach. Questions you may ask are as follows: What controls were in effect for this study; that is, what were the delimitations? What research method was used, for example, descriptive, experimental, or quasiexperimental? How was the sample selected and was it representative of the defined population? What steps were taken to control extraneous variables? Overall, was the approach carried out in a logical, orderly, objective fashion?

A more in-depth discussion of the characteristics of the scientific approach will help clarify these components. Table 2-1 compares the scientific method used for the natural sciences with the research process of the social sciences and with the nursing process commonly followed in the delivery of nursing care. These approaches attest to the logical and systematic process involved in knowledge acquisition. They are parallel, scientific approaches involving problem identification and description, predictions, methods to support or refute predictions, results, and some statement about results (i.e., interpretation, generalization, and evaluation). The language used for the various steps is unique to each discipline.

Components of the scientific approach

Kerlinger (1986) defines scientific research as the "systematic, controlled, empirical, and critical investigation of hypothetical propositions about the presumed relations among natural phenomena" (p. 11). This definition reflects a complex process. For the scientific approach to yield results that are minimally biased in all aspects (that is, sample selection, theoretical rationale, methodology, tools of analysis, and conclusions), the investigator must pursue an orderly and precise method of inquiry. The following is an examination of the major components of this approach.

Order and control. As a systematic method of problem solving, the scientific approach requires order, that is, the use of clearly delineated, *ordered steps.* For example,

Table 2-1 Systematic Ways of Acquiring Knowledge

Scientific method	Research process	Nursing process
State the problem	Formulate and delimit the problem	Gather information
Gather the facts (collect and organize data)	Review the related literature	Classify data
Devise experiments to also gather facts	Develop a theoretical framework	Make inferences about the problem
Test the hypotheses	Identify the variables	Make a nursing diagnosis
Make the generalizations or deductions	Formulate the hypotheses	Develop a plan of care
Check the truth of the generalization or deduction against reality by means of more experiments and fact gathering	Select a research design	Implement the plan of care
	Collect the data	Evaluate interventions
	Analyze the data	
	Interpret the results	
	Communicate the findings	

you would not develop a hypothesis until a thorough search of the literature had been conducted. Similarly, you would not draw conclusions before you statistically analyze the collected data. This predetermined system or process guides the research so that you have greater confidence in your predictions and outcomes. When reviewing a research report, you should look for the investigator's approach to the problem, study methods, data analysis, and conclusions. Ask yourself if the steps are ordered appropriately and if there is continuity in terms of the focus of the content. Is the conclusion based on actual findings? Is the hypothesis developed from the theoretical rationale?

Control involves holding the conditions of the study constant so there is confidence that the outcome of the study is due to the experimental intervention and not some other influencing factor(s). Whereas control is almost impossible to achieve totally, it is an important facet of the scientific approach (see Chapter 8). To isolate and study specific variables, it is necessary to control as much as possible these extraneous, influencing factors; to control such events and conditions, it is essential to know what they are. For example, it is known that pain perception is influenced by age, sex, culture, and other factors. In examining the relationship between self-esteem and pain perception, the investigator must specify which age group, sex, and culture will be delimited, that is, included and excluded. An alternate approach would be to select a large sample that reflects a variety of ages, sexes, and cultures (see Chapter 15). Then the data would be analyzed as a total sample and for each of the influencing factors. This would yield information about the strength of each factor in terms of study outcomes. In your role as research consumer you should determine if the sample is representative of the defined population or if there was bias in the selection process.

You should ask how and why the subjects were chosen, whether or not there was support of sample delimitations, and what steps were taken in the procedure for data collection to control the extraneous variables.

Empiricism. Empiricism is the **objectivity** component of the scientific approach, that is, the reality foundation for investigations. Observations are made and verified on the basis of actual information instead of the personal beliefs or biases of the researcher. In addition, other investigators are able to evaluate and replicate or repeat the empirical inquiry process. Documented evidence of empiricism in research will include objective, appropriate, and stable instruments for data collection, unbiased selection of subjects, and data collection methods and settings that are valid representations of reality. You should evaluate the investigator's use of valid and reliable instruments and unbiased sampling procedures, as well as the controls and setting used in the process of data collection (see Chapters 13 to 15).

Generalization. One goal of science is to provide understanding of relationships among phenomena to allow generalization (predict future outcomes and relationships). Focusing on isolated events would not make it possible to "explain a wide variety of phenomena in a manner that consistently holds and therefore is not tentative" (Chinn and Jacobs, 1987, p. 71). The following example will clarify the intent of generalization.

If a nurse-scientist were studying maternal attachment behaviors, there would be more interest in understanding what general factors influence these behaviors (for example, skin-to-skin contact [Curry, 1982]) than in "Jane Doe's" specific experience with maternal attachment. Similarly, if a nurse-scientist were studying the psychological well-being of caregivers to families of impaired elderly patients, it would be more helpful to have a general understanding of the effects of such factors as stress and social support on psychological distress (Baillie, Norbeck, and Barnes, 1988) than of one caregiver's experience with an impaired elderly individual. Although understanding individuals is important, a more substantive contribution to science can be made from a broad range of empirical data that have been subjected to repeated investigations.

Another example relates to the study of progressive muscle relaxation (PMR) and pain. It would be more useful to determine effectiveness of PMR with several different types of chronic pain conditions rather than the experience of one individual with arthritis. Whereas it is important to understand an individual's experience with PMR, knowledge about a variety of conditions that could benefit from PMR as an intervention for pain would have wider application.

Questions that elicit information about generalization include the following: When and to whom do the conclusions apply? What are the limits and scope of the findings, for example, in terms of extraneous factors and sample delimitations? Does the investigator generalize beyond the population on which the study was based?

Theory. A *theory* can be defined as a process of organizing reality into systematically identified relationships among variables to explain and make predictions about phenomena. Through empirical observations and research, theories are developed and tested, and generalizations evolve. As a component of the scientific approach, a theory provides a framework for testing hypotheses. It also guides decision making with regard to definition of variables and subsequent interpretation of results. The following examples are intended to clarify this definition.

King's theory of goal attainment was derived from the interpersonal system component of her Interacting Systems Conceptual Framework. This theory proposes that "nurse and client interactions are characterized by verbal and nonverbal communication, in which information is exchanged and interpreted; by transactions, in which values, needs, and wants of each member of the dyad are shared; by perceptions of nurse and client and the situation; by self in role of client and self in role of nurse; and by stressors influencing each person and the situation in time and space" (King, 1981, p. 144). Some hypotheses (King, 1986, p. 206) derived from the propositions (relationship statements) of this theory are as follows:

◇ Goal attainment will be greater in patients who participate in mutual goal setting than in patients who do not participate
◇ Mutual goal setting will increase the morale of elderly patients
◇ Goal attainment decreases stress and anxiety
◇ Goal attainment increases patients' learning and coping abilities in nursing situations

Three theories developed from Orem's Self-Care Conceptual Framework are the theory of self-care deficit, the theory of self-care, and the theory of nursing systems (Orem, 1985). The theory of self-care proposes that "self-care and care of dependent family members are learned behaviors that purposely regulate human structural integrity, functioning, and human development" (Orem, 1985, p. 36). The theory states that "mature or maturing persons contribute to the regulation of their own functioning and development and to the prevention, control or amelioration of disease and injury and their effects by performing, within the context of their day-to-day living, learned actions directed to themselves or their environments that are known or assumed to have regulatory value with respect to human functioning and development" (Orem and Taylor, 1986, p. 44). One proposition of the theory of self-care is that "the individual's abilities to engage in self-care or dependent care are conditioned by age, developmental state, life experience, sociocultural orientation, health, and available resources" (Orem, 1985, p. 35). Hypothesis testing of the propositions of Orem's Framework is in the early stages of development.

Individual theories of the four adaptive modes of the Roy Adaptation Model (that is, physiological, self-concept, role function, and interdependence) have been developed. A proposition taken from the theory of interdependence states, "Adequacy of seeking nurturance and nurturing positively influences interdependence" (Roy and Roberts, 1981, p. 277). A hypothesis developed from the theory of independence is "If the nurse provides time and space for private family visits, the patient will demonstrate more appropriate attention-seeking behavior" (Roy and Roberts, 1981, p. 280).

A more detailed discussion of the theoretical framework is provided in Chapter 6. Some of the questions to ask as a research consumer are as follows:

Is the theoretical rationale explicitly stated? Are the hypotheses explicitly substantiated; that is, do they clearly arise from the theory? Are the definitions of variables clear, and do they adequately reflect the theory? Are the results interpreted in relation to the theory?

Assumptions about reality and causality (determinism). **Assumptions** are basic principles assumed to be true without need for scientific proof. For example, it has been assumed that people will have pain during their lives, people are mortal, "infants are born with unique, individual characteristics that affect the development of maternal attachment" (Curry, 1982, p. 74), and "both nurse-practitioners and physicians identify and manage health problems of their patients (Chen et al., 1982, p. 164). The first two assumptions are broad and apply to human beings in general; the last two are part of the foundations of specific theories. As a final example, Rogers (1970) espouses a particular view of human beings as more than and different from the sum of their parts. This underlying assumption is one of several that form the basis for testing relationships by use of Rogers' conceptual framework.

Assumptions that guide the scientific approach are that there is an objective reality independent of an individual's perceptions, the world is real, and nature has order, regularity, and consistency. Another assumption relates to determinism, which has to do with causality of phenomena. Events and situations are assumed to have causes. For example, cancer may be the result of several phenomena, such as smoking and certain chemicals and pollutants, and the inflammatory response occurs as a result of certain conditions. This traditional assumption of cause-and-effect relationships, which has guided many of the activities of scientists, has been challenged in favor of assumptions about mutual and simultaneous interactions among phenomena (Rogers, 1970), from which changed phenomena evolve.

Assumptions are not always stated in an obvious way. They may be implicit rather than explicit, and this is a question you should ask. You should also identify what the assumptions are, if they reflect a specific value orientation, and whether or not there are inconsistencies between assumptions.

THE RELATIONSHIP BETWEEN THEORY AND METHOD

As stated earlier, relationships are examined by testing hypotheses that are based on propositions (see Chapter 6) derived from a theoretical framework. That examination takes place under the aegis of order and control, empiricism, assumptions, theory, and generalization. To validate relational statements, an overall design or method must be implemented. That method must also operate in a systematic, controlled way to ensure that "the empirical indicators for the conceptual relationship specified by the theory are valid" (Chinn and Jacobs, 1987, p. 109). A variety of designs can be used to address the problem under study; however, there must be consistency between the hypothesis or relational statement and the type of design used. Fig. 2-1 illustrates the components or "links" of the research process that connect theory with method. There must also be consistency between each of these important links.

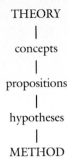

Fig. 2-1 Links between theory and method.

Chapter 8 focuses on the meaning, purposes, and issues related to research design. Suffice it to say at this point that, as a research consumer, you should evaluate the study concepts and how they are defined, the underlying propositions that support hypothesis development, and the overall design and procedure of hypothesis testing (including the setting, instrumentation, conformity to established criteria for implementing the specific design, data collection procedure, and control of extraneous factors) to make sure that there is a coherent, consistent relationship between theory and method.

SUMMARY

This chapter serves as an introduction to the sources of human knowledge and characteristics of the scientific approach as they relate to the research process. The relationship between philosophy and science underlies the nursing research effort, a focus of which is the development of nursing knowledge. The philosophical view of the researcher guides the intent and direction of a research project.

There are many sources of human knowledge. Some sources are relatively unstructured (for example, intuition and trial-and-error approaches); other sources are highly structured (for example, the scientific approach, including inductive and deductive methods of logical reasoning). Both sources play a role in the research process, although the scientific approach is the most advanced and objective of these methods of inquiry.

The scientific approach is a complex process that is systematic and controlled. As an empirical approach it yields results that are minimally biased in all aspects. Additionally, since a goal of science is to provide understanding of relationships among phenomena, a more formal process of inquiry makes it possible to explain a wide variety of phenomena and at the same time to make predictions or generalizations about future outcomes and relationships.

Theories help organize reality by systematically identifying relations among variables. Through empirical observations and research, theories are developed and tested. Theories also provide a framework for testing hypotheses (that is, statements about relationships) and form the basis for determining the overall design or method of a study. Fundamental to the testing of relationships are the underlying assumptions or the basic principles that are assumed to be true and that need no scientific proof. These assumptions guide the research effort in much the same way as the researcher's philosophical views of human behavior and health.

As research consumers, nurses are called on to judge the soundness of the research approach used, including why and how ideas were generated and related, how hypotheses were derived, what method or design was used, and what assumptions and generalizations were made.

References

Andreoli, K., and Thompson, C. (1977). The nature of science in nursing, *Image,* **9**:32-37.

Beckwith, J., and Miller, L. (1976). Behind the mask of objective science, *The Sciences,* **16**: 16-19.

Baillie, V., Norbeck, J., and Barnes, L. (1988). Stress, social support, and psychological distress of family caregivers of the elderly, *Nursing Research,* **37**:217-222.

Brooten, D., Kumar, S., Brown, L., Butts, P., Finkler, S., Bakewell-Sachs, S., Gibbons, A., and Delivoria-Papadopulos, M. (1986). A randomized clinical trial of early hospital discharge and home follow up of very-low-birth-weight infants, *The New England Journal of Medicine,* **15**:934-938.

Chinn, P., and Jacobs, M. (1987). *Theory and nursing: a systematic approach,* St. Louis, The C.V. Mosby Co.

Chen, S., Barkauskas, V., and Chen, E. (1982). Health problems encountered by nurse practitioners and physicians, *Nursing Research,* **31**:163-169.

Curry, M. (1982). Maternal attachment behavior and the mother's self-concept: the effect of early skin-to-skin contact, *Nursing Research,* **31**:73-78.

Downs, F.S., and Newman, M.A. (1977). *A sourcebook of nursing research,* 2nd ed., Philadelphia, F.A. Davis Co.

Harris, R.B. (1981-82). Clean versus sterile suctioning and inner cannula tracheotomy cleaning technique in relation to level of infection in first week post-operative head and neck surgical patients, *PRN: The Adelphi Report.*

Johnson, D. (1974). Development of theory: a requisite for nursing as a primary health profession, *Nursing Research,* **23**:372-377.

Kerlinger, F.N. (1986). *Foundations of behavioral research,* 3rd ed., New York, Holt, Rinehart & Winston, Inc.

King, T. (1981). *A theory for nursing: systems, concepts, process,* New York, John Wiley & Sons.

King, T. (1986). King's theory of goal attainment. In P. Winstead-Fry, ed.: *Case studies in nursing theory,* New York, National League for Nursing, pp. 197-312.

Martinson, I. (1978). Why research in nursing? In N.L. Chaska, ed.: *The nursing profession: views through the mist,* New York, McGraw-Hill Book Co.

Newman, M. (1979). *Theory development in nursing,* Philadelphia, F.A. Davis Co.

Northouse, L. (1988). Social support in patients' and husbands' adjustment to breast cancer, *Nursing Research,* **37**:91-95.

Orem, D. (1985). *Nursing: concepts of practice,* 3rd ed., New York, McGraw-Hill Book Co.

Orem, D., and Taylor, S. (1986). Orem's general theory of nursing. In P. Winstead-Fry, ed.: *Case studies in nursing theory,* New York, National League for Nursing, pp. 37-71.

Rogers, M. (1970). *An introduction to the theoretical basis of nursing,* Philadelphia, F.A. Davis Co.

Roy, C., and Roberts, S. (1981). *Theory construction in nursing: an adaptation model,* Englewood Cliffs, N.J., Prentice-Hall.

Silva, M. (1977). Philosophy, science, theory: interrelationships and implications for nursing research, *Image,* **9**:59-63.

Vaughan, F. (1979). *Awakening intuition,* Garden City, N.Y., Anchor Books.

Webster's new universal unabridged dictionary, deluxe 2nd ed. (1983). Ohio, Dorset & Baber.

Additional Readings

Benoliel, J. (1977). The interaction between theory and research, *Nursing Outlook,* **25**:108-113.

Broome, M.E., Lillis, P.P., and Smith, M.C. (1989). Pain interventions with children: a meta-analysis of research, *Nursing Research,* **38**:154-158.

Fawcett, J. (1989). *Analysis and evaluation of conceptual models of nursing,* 2nd ed., Philadelphia, F.A. Davis Co.

Greene, J. (1979). Science, nursing and nursing science: a conceptual analysis, *Advances in Nursing Science,* **2**:57-64.

Hinds, P.S. (1989). Method triangulation to index change in clinical phenomena, *The Western Journal of Nursing Research,* **11**:440-447.

Hyman, R.B., Feldman, H.R., Harris, R.B., Levin, R.F., and Mallory, G.B. (1989). The effects of relaxation training on clinical symptoms: a meta-analysis, *Nursing Research,* **38**:216-220.

Reynolds, P. (1971). *A primer in theory construction,* Indianapolis, Bobbs-Merrill/Educational Publishing.

Ruchlis, H. (1963). *Discovering scientific method,* New York, Harper & Row, Publishers.

3

Legal and Ethical Issues

Bettie S. Jackson

LEARNING OBJECTIVES

After reading this chapter the student should be able to do the following:

◇ Describe the historical background that led to the development of ethical guidelines for the use of human subjects in research.

◇ Identify the essential elements of an informed consent form.

◇ Evaluate the adequacy of an informed consent form.

◇ Discuss the nurse's role in ensuring that Food and Drug Administration guidelines for testing of medical devices are followed.

◇ Describe the institutional review board's role in the research review process.

◇ Describe the nurse's role as client advocate in research situations.

◇ Identify research situations, specifically populations of subjects, that require special consideration when research involving them is considered.

◇ Appreciate animal rights in research situations.

> ## KEY TERMS
>
> animal rights   informed consent
> anonymity   institutional review board
> confidentiality   product testing
> ethics

Listen, Martin. I am aware that the technique of experimenting on humans without their consent is against any traditional concept of medical ethics. But I believe the results justify the methods. Seventeen young women have unknowingly sacrificed their lives. That is true. But it has been for the betterment of society and the future guarantee of the defense superiority of the United States. From the point of view of each subject, it is a great sacrifice. From the point of view of two hundred million Americans, it is a very small one. Think of how many young women willfully take their lives each year, or how many people kill themselves on the highways, and to what end? Here these seventeen women have added something to society, and they have been treated with compassion. (From Cook, R. [1981]. *Brain,* New York, Signet, p. 292).

"When people rely on rules to protect them from harm, they are not interested in pieces of paper but in the conduct of the people who are supposed to be governed by the rules" (Hanks, 1984b, p. 1). It is not just the rules and regulations that deal with the involvement of human subjects in research that ensures that research will be conducted legally and ethically. Researchers themselves and those who provide care to patients who also happen to be research subjects must be fully commited to the tenets of informed consent and clients' rights. The principle of "the ends justify the means" must never be tolerated.

This chapter deals with the legal and ethical considerations that must be made before, during, and after the conduct of research. Caregivers of research subjects and researchers should take every precaution to protect people who are study subjects from physical or mental harm or discomfort. It is not always clear what constitutes harm or discomfort. This chapter will trace the historical development of the concept of **informed consent.** It will discuss the systems that have been established to oversee the rights of people who are potential and actual research subjects. Research on special groups of potential subjects (i.e., elderly, incompetent, and animals) will be discussed. The nurse as client advocate, whether she or he functions in her role as researcher or caregiver, will also be addressed.

ETHICAL AND LEGAL CONSIDERATIONS IN RESEARCH

Developments in the field of biostatistics over the last 80 years have enabled scientists to combine their new knowledge with analytical means to evaluate the effects of their interventions. For example, advanced statistics and computers have made it possible to analyze the outcomes of therapies in control and experimental groups to determine if any differences are statistically significant. These powerful analytical abilities enabled researchers to experiment on subjects as never before.

Ethical and legal considerations as they regard research received attention only beginning with the post-World War II Nuremberg Military Tribunal. This Tribunal's prosecution of Karl Brandt and others represented the first major effort of the law to cope with problems of modern biomedical research. Before the Tribunal could measure the activities of the defendants, a set of basic principles of *ethical, moral, and legal concepts* for the conduct of acceptable experiments had to be written as the standard (Creighton, 1977, p. 337). The following are among the 10 rules included in the Nuremberg Code; these rules are still used today:

1. Voluntary consent of the human subject is essential.
2. The experiments should be so designed and based on the results of animal experimentation and knowledge of the natural history of the disease or other problems that the anticipated results will justify the experiment.
3. The degree of risk to be taken should never exceed that determined by the humanitarian importance of the problem to be solved.
4. Through all stages of the experiment the highest degree of skill and care should be required of those who conduct or engage in the experiment, and the experiment should be conducted by only scientifically qualified persons.*
5. During the course of the experiment the human subject should be at liberty to bring the experiment to an end.
6. The scientist in charge must be prepared to terminate the experiment at any stage if he has probable cause to believe that continuation of the experiment is likely to result in injury, disability, or death to the experimental subject.†

Informed consent

Informed consent is the legal principle that, at least in theory, governs the client's acceptance or rejection of individual medical interventions designed to diagnose an illness or treat the client; it is also the doctrine that determines and regulates

---

* It would be inappropriate for a nurse-midwife to conduct research on clients with cancer. If pregnant study subjects have cancer, then special consultation regarding the aspects of cancer as they relate to the research study should be sought. A researcher is often required to submit a curriculum vitae to the appropriate research review board so that the expertise of the researcher in the field under study can be determined.

† Several years ago I coauthored an article on the LeVeen shunt (Seybert, P.L., Gordon, K., and Jackson, B.S. [1979]. The LeVeen shunt: new hope for ascites patients, *Nursing '79,* 9[1]:24-31). Dr. LeVeen wrote the authors to compliment them on the article but also to comment on his research. At the time clients with ascites were randomly assigned to one of two groups, those who received medical management and those who received surgical implantation of the LeVeen shunt. It was clear to the researchers partway into the study that the group receiving surgical intervention was faring much better. The experiment was terminated before the number of subjects originally planned had been accessed. It would have been unethical and perhaps illegal (that is, malpractice or failure to provide the acceptable standard of care) to continue the experiment.

participation in research (Dubler, 1987, p. 545). The Code of Federal Regulations (Dubler, p. 545) states in the section on general requirements that the "legally effective informed consent of the subject or the subject's legally authorized representative is a precondition to research. Voluntary agreement to participate or not participate, based on adequate knowledge and understanding, is essential." However, informed consent goes beyond just this point. To safeguard the basic human right of self-determination, free and informed consent is expected to include the following: an explanation of the study and the procedures to be followed and their purposes; a description of associated physical and mental crises or discomforts, any invasion of privacy, and any threat to dignity; and the methods used to protect **anonymity** and ensure **confidentiality.** The client should also be informed of alternate courses of treatment available (ANA Commission on Nursing Research, 1975; Gargano, 1978, p. 167).

Although quite simplistically the tenets of informed consent make good sense and seem easy to follow, and everyone should, could, and does follow them, that has not in fact been the case. Before the 1970s there is essentially no mention of informed consent in the nursing research texts. The federal guidelines for research in human subjects that will be discussed in this chapter were not developed until the mid-1970s, and in fact, unethical research took place in the United States even in the 1960s and 1970s. Some of the most atrocious and hence memorable are worth mentioning as sad reminders of our own tarnished research heritage, in addition to the more difficult conundrums encountered when research involving human subjects was undertaken.

In the 1965 case of Hyman vs. The Jewish Chronic Disease Hospital, New York, it was revealed that aged and senile clients were given live cancer cells to study their rejection responses. Informed consent was not obtained. Fraud and deceit had been used in dealing with subjects. The two physicians involved were placed on probation for 1 year. They claimed that they did not wish to evoke emotional reactions or refusals to participate by informing the subjects of the nature of the study.

In the infamous Milledgeville, Georgia, case exposed in 1969, the opinion of a clinical psychiatrist was not obtained before investigational drugs were given to mentally disabled children, and there was no explicit review or institutional approval of the program before it was implemented.

It must be emphasized here, and it will be repeated later, that researchers themselves must not take the privilege, nor are they vested with the privilege, of determining such things as risk/benefit ratios and who is or is not competent to give consent. From their expertise they may suggest such things, but then an objective panel of experts from the professional and public communities must review these plans before the research is conducted.

This final example draws from the 1973 suit of the infamous Tuskegee (Alabama) syphilis study. For 40 years the United States Public Health Service conducted a study of two groups of black male subjects. One group consisted of those who had untreated syphilis and the second group consisted of about half as many who were judged free of the disease. During the study no treatment for syphilis was provided. Withholding treatment remained part of the study even after penicillin became generally available in the 1950s. Steps were even taken to keep the subjects from obtaining it. The charge that low-income and poorly educated people are used for research is hard to deny in this case.

Whereas it seems clear that these three cases were clinical research studies, what constitutes *research versus clinical evaluation* is not always clear. When the formalities of the research review process should be pursued may seem be vague at times. Although it is advisable to err in the direction of conservatism and seek out a formal, objective review of the plan for informed consent, this is not always done. Sometimes the reason is naiveté, which is less an acceptable excuse as time goes on, and sometimes the reason is the investigator's unilateral determination that to do so would be less than expeditious.

Marsha D.M. Fowler (1988, p. 354), a consulting nurse-ethicist, calls for an international code of **ethics** for nursing research. She raises many ethical questions that nurses around the world need to address; these include the following:

1. To whom is the nurse-researcher primarily responsible?
2. Is the good of the client ever subservient to the acquisition of nursing knowledge?
3. Do legal and ethical responsibilities for nursing research differ or conflict?
4. At what point must a nurse stop a specific nursing research project?
5. When must a nurse intervene to halt a specific medical research project?
6. Are there conditions under which a nurse should not include a specific subject in a study, even though consent has been secured?

Product testing

Nurses are often approached by manufacturers to test products on clients. Moore (1984) points out that all nurses should be aware of the Food and Drug Administration guidelines and regulations for *testing of medical devices* before they initiate any form of clinical testing. Medical devices are classified under Section 513 in the Federal Food, Drug and Cosmetic Act according to the extent of control necessary to ensure safety and effectiveness of each device. The following classes are defined:

Class I: General Controls. Included in Class I are devices whose safety and effectiveness can be reasonably guaranteed by the general controls of the Good Manufacturing Practices Regulations. The Regulations part of the act ensures that manufacturers will follow specific guidelines for packaging, storing, and providing specific product instructions. An example of Class I devices is ostomy supplies.

Class II: Performance Standards. General controls are insufficient in this case to ensure safety and efficacy of the product, and the manufacturer must provide this assurance in the form of information. Devices included here are cardiac pacemakers, sutures, surgical metallic mesh, and biopsy needs.

Class III: Premarket Approval. This class includes devices whose safety and effectiveness are insufficiently ensured by general controls and for which performance standards are insufficient to ensure safety and effectiveness. These products are represented to be life-sustaining or life-supporting, are implanted into the body, or present a potential, unreasonable risk of illness or injury to the client. Devices in this class are required to have approved applications for premarket approval. Extensive laboratory, animal, and human studies, which often require 2 to 3 years to complete, are required for Class III devices. Examples include heart valves, bone cements, contact lenses, and implantable devices left in the body for 30 days or longer.

It is important that nurses be aware of their own institution's policies for **product testing.** The class of the drug will obviously make a difference in the institution's reaction. If a nurse suspects that, for example, a Class II device is being tested in an ad hoc or unauthorized manner and without client consent, she should discuss this with her supervisor and other appropriate authorities.

Unauthorized research

It is not unusual for ad hoc or informal and *unauthorized research* to take place. Although it may seem to be harmless, again it is not the purview of the investigator to make that determination. Nurses must carefully avoid being involved in ad hoc research for a number of reasons:

1. These treatments or methods of care are usually not monitored as closely for untoward effects, hence exposing the client to unwarranted risk.
2. Clients' rights to informed consent in clinical trials are not protected.
3. The success or failure of these unrecorded trials contributes nothing to the organized scientific knowledge of the efficacy or complications of the treatment.
4. The lack of independent quality supervision allows deviations from the adopted experimental program that may eliminate the program's effectiveness (Hanks, 1984).

Additional considerations of an ethical nature need to be addressed. Generally speaking, the public trusts caregivers, especially nurses and physicians. It is sometimes necessary for the caregiver to assume the awkward role of asking the client to become a research subject. Risks might be inherent in the research that do not exist in the care. Even when these risks are clearly identified, and they must be, is the caregiver comfortable in posing those risks? Is the caregiver convinced that the benefits outweigh the risks? Will the client feel comfortable in refusing to participate in the caregiver's research, while continuing to require care? Has it been made clear to the client, as it must be, that refusal to participate or withdrawal from the study is an option at any time without consequence or compromise to care received or to the client's relationship to the institution? What if harm occurs? Will the research cost the client additional money, is it warranted, and has the client been apprised, as must be done?

Numbers of books and articles have been written on this subject. They are introduced here to illustrate that the legal and ethical concepts behind research and informed consent are rarely clear-cut. The nurse researcher or the nurse who is involved in any way with a research project must raise cogent self-directed questions when evaluating the ethics and legal points of research.

FEDERAL GUIDELINES REGARDING ETHICAL AND LEGAL CONSIDERATIONS AS THEY PERTAIN TO RESEARCH INVOLVING HUMAN SUBJECTS

Institutional review boards

The National Research Act (P.L. 93-348) was passed on July 12, 1974. The subject was **institutional review boards** (IRBs) Ethics Guidance Program. Quite simply, it requires that any agency such as a hospital or school applying for a grant or contract for any project or program that involves the conduct of biomedical or behavioral research involving human subjects must submit with its application assurances that it has established a board or IRB to review the research and protect the rights of the human subjects of such research.

At agencies where no federal grants or contracts have been awarded, there is usually a review mechanism resembling the IRB system.

The IRB must have at least five members of various backgrounds to promote complete and adequate project review. The members must be qualified through their expertise and experience and reflect a racial and cultural diversity. The IRB must be made up of both men and women, and more than one profession must be represented. The IRB must have one member whose concerns are primarily nonscientific (i.e., lawyer, clergy, ethicist). At least one member must be from outside the agency.

The IRB's function is to review research and report any serious or continuing noncompliance by investigators. The IRB has the authority to approve research, require modifications, or disapprove research activities. A researcher must receive some form of IRB approval, such as expedited, exempt, or emergency-compassionate, or full review before beginning to conduct research.

To approve research, the IRB must determine the following Code of Federal Regulations has been satisfied:

1. The risks to subjects are minimized.
2. The risks to subjects are reasonable in relation to anticipated benefits.
3. The selection of the subjects is equitable.
4. Informed consent, in one of several possible forms, must be sought from each prospective subject or the subject's legally authorized representative.
5. The informed consent form must be properly documented.
6. Where appropriate, the research plan makes adequate provision for monitoring the data collected to ensure the subject's safety.
7. Where appropriate, there are adequate provisions to protect the privacy of subjects and the confidentiality of data.
8. Where some or all of the subjects are likely to be vulnerable to coercion or undue influence, as are persons with acute or severe physical or mental illness or persons who are economically or educationally disadvantaged, appropriate additional safeguards are included.

IRBs have the authority to suspend or terminate approval of research that is not conducted in accordance with IRB requirements or that has been associated with unexpected serious harm to subjects.

IRBs have a mechanism for reviewing research in an expedited manner when there is minimal risk to research subjects. Once again, it is worth mentioning that the researcher may determine that a project involves minimal risk, but the IRB makes the final determination and research may not be undertaken until that determination has been made. An expedited review usually shortens the review process. A full list of research categories eligible for expedited review is available from any IRB office and includes the following: (1) the collection of hair and nail clippings in a nondisfiguring manner; (2) the collection of excreta and external secretions including sweat; (3) the recording of data from subjects 18 years of age or older, by means of noninvasive procedures routinely employed in clinical practice; (4) voice recordings; and (5) the study of existing data, documents, records, pathological specimens, or diagnostic data. An expedited review does not exempt the researcher from obtaining informed consent.

The *Federal Register* contains updated information on federal guidelines for research involving human subjects. Every researcher should consult with an agency's research office to ensure that the application being prepared adheres to the most current requirements. A nurse involved in research, such as caring for research subjects, may consult the agency's research office to determine if research is being conducted according to the most up-to-date regulations.

Guidelines for informed consent

There have already been a number of references to informed consent in this chapter. This section deals with what informed consent is and what constitutes an acceptable informed consent form.

No investigator may involve a human being as a research subject before obtaining the legally effective informed consent of the subject or the legally authorized representative. Prospective subjects must have time to decide if they want to participate, and the investigator must not coerce the subject into participating. The language of the consent form must be understandable. According to the Code of Federal Regulations the subject should never be asked to waive his rights or release the investigator or the institution from liability for negligence.

The following are basic elements of informed consent:

1. A statement that the study involves research, an explanation of the purposes of the research, a delineation of the expected duration of the subject's participation, a description of the procedures to be followed, and identification of any procedures that are experimental
2. A description of any reasonably foreseeable risks or discomforts to the subject
3. A description of any benefits to the subject or to others that may reasonably be expected from the research
4. A disclosure of appropriate alternative procedures or courses of treatment, if any, that might be advantageous to the subject
5. A statement describing the extent, if any, to which the confidentiality of the records identifying the subject will be maintained

6. For research involving more than minimal risk, an explanation as to whether any medical treatments are available if injury occurs and, if so, what they consist of, or where further information may be obtained
7. An explanation of whom to contact for answers to pertinent questions about the research and research subjects' rights, and whom to contact in the event of a research-related injury to the subject
8. A statement that participation is voluntary, that refusal to participate will not involve any penalty or loss of benefits to which the subject is otherwise entitled, and that the subject may discontinue participation at any time without penalty or loss of otherwise entitled benefits

Anonymity and confidentiality

Assurance of anonymity and confidentiality in research is usually conveyed in writing. This is sometimes difficult in unique research situations that capture the public's attention, for example, Dr. Barney Clark, first recipient of an artificial heart. *Anonymity* is the protection of the participant in a study so that even the researcher cannot link the subject with the information provided. Often one will see written on an informed consent form a statement to the effect that data are pooled; hence it is impossible to identify one research subject from an aggregate. This also makes it impossible for a subject to withdraw from a study once data have been pooled. *Confidentiality* is slightly different from anonymity and protects the participants in a study so that their individual identities will not be linked to the information that they provided and will not be publicly divulged.

There are exceptions to these guidelines and situations in which the IRB might grant waivers or amend its process or guidelines. The researcher is advised to consult with the IRB in individual and unusual circumstances. The boxed material on pp. 46 and 47 provides a specific example of informed consent.

Generally the signed informed consent form is given to the subject. The researcher may also wish to keep a copy. Some research, such as retrospective chart audit, may not require informed consent. Or in some cases, where minimal risk is involved, the investigator may only have to provide the subject with an information sheet. The IRB will help advise on these matters and make the final determination as to the most appropriate documentation format.

Special legal and ethical considerations in research

This section serves as an overview to ethical and legal considerations that must be taken when particularly *vulnerable and/or incompetent populations* are identified as potential research subjects. Researchers are advised to consult their agency's IRB for the most recent federal and state rules and guidelines when considering research involving the elderly, children, the mentally ill, prisoners, the deceased, the unborn, and students. In addition, researchers should consult the IRB before planning research that potentially involves an oversubscribed research population, such as organ transplant clients or "captive" and convenient populations such as students.

Informed Consent

The Caldwell Medical Center
Code No. _____

I understand that I am being treated with the drug *cis*-platin, which may cause the unpleasant side effects of nausea and vomiting. Treatment to control these side effects includes using various medications, reducing the intake of food and fluids before chemotherapy, maintaining a quiet environment, and accepting support from others. In addition, I understand that using various coping strategies is helpful to persons in similar situations.

I understand that the purpose of this study is to help clients learn some coping techniques and evaluate how their use affects the occurrence of nausea and vomiting after *cis*-platin is administered. If I agree to participate in this research study, I understand that I will be randomly assigned to one of the following three nursing treatment programs:

1. I will meet with one of the investigators before I receive my chemotherapy. We will discuss my experience and the methods that other clients and I have found helpful.

or

2. I will meet with one of the investigators before I receive my chemotherapy. I will follow directions for practicing a technique that produces, under my own control, a state of altered consciousness called *self-hypnosis*. I will be asked to practice this technique during and after receiving my chemotherapy. I will be expected to practice this technique daily so that I may learn to use it without being directed by another person.

or

3. I will be given the customary nursing care that is rendered to every client taking the drugs that I am receiving.

In addition, if necessary, I will receive only the medication Reglan to control nausea and vomiting.

I understand that in no case will I receive less than the customary standard and expected level of nursing care that I am already receiving.

I understand that if I am selected to be in Group 2, a simple test to determine my susceptibility to this technique will be performed. Most people are susceptible, but if I am not and I wish to continue in the study, I will be randomly assigned to one of the two remaining groups.

I understand that this research study has been discussed with my physician and that he is aware of my participation. The treatments prescribed to control the side effects of nausea and vomiting will not be altered if I participate in this study.

Informed Consent — cont'd

I understand that a nurse investigator will be in my room while my chemotherapy is ending and for 4 hours after the treatment. I understand that nursing care will be provided by the nurses on the unit and not by the nurse-investigator. The research nurse will be taking notes on my reactions to the chemotherapy. Once an hour she will ask me to rate my nausea. I can expect that this will take only a few minutes of my time and that, if I am sleeping, I will not be awakened.

I have been told that this routine will be followed for three courses of chemotherapy, during three separate hospitalizations.

I understand that the benefits from this treatment are that I may experience less nausea and vomiting or fewer of the feelings of being sick to my stomach that often occur with *cis*-platin. There are no side effects or risks from my participation.

My participation is voluntary and I may choose to not participate or to withdraw at any time without jeopardizing my future treatment.

My identity will not be revealed in any way. My name will be encoded so that I will remain anonymous.

I also understand that if I believe I have sustained an injury as a result of participating in this research study, I may contact the investigators, Ms. B. J. Simon at 608-0011 or B. A. Smith at 124-6142, or the Office of the Institutional Review Board at 124-2500 so that I can review the matter and identify the medical resources that may be available to me.

I understand the following statements:

1. The Caldwell Medical Center will furnish whatever emergency medical care that the medical staff of this hospital determine to be necessary.

2. I will be responsible for the cost of such emergency care personally, through my medical insurance, or by another form of coverage.

3. No monetary compensation for wages lost as a result of an injury will be paid to me by The Caldwell Medical Center.

4. I will receive a copy of this consent form.

_____   _____
Date   Patient

_____   _____
Witness   Investigator

The Institutional Review Board of the Caldwell Medical Center has approved the solicitation of subjects for participation in this research proposal.

It should be emphasized that special populations do not preclude the research being done; extra precautions must be taken, however, to protect subjects' rights.

Davis (1981a) reminds us that a society can be judged by the way it treats its most vulnerable people—a point worth remembering in research that involves the elderly. In addition, Davis continues a cogent argument, "To insure continuing progress in pediatric research and practice, experimentation is necessary. If the consent requirement is taken seriously to the point of excluding research in children, then children themselves will be the ultimate sufferers" (1981b, p. 247).

Mitchell cites the classic 1965 Darling case in which physicians and nurses were found negligent in the care of a teenager who lost his leg because of poor cast application and observation. "In addition to serving as advocates for the psychologic as well as physical welfare of children, nurses are legally accountable for protecting children's rights and reporting inappropriate actions of other health professionals" (Mitchell, 1984, p. 9).

Mitchell discussed the concept of *assent* versus *consent* in regard to pediatric research. Assent contains three fundamental elements: a basic understanding of what the child will be expected to do and what will be done to the child, a comprehension of the basic purpose of the research, and an ability to express a preference regarding participation. In contrast to assent, consent requires a relatively advanced level of cognitive ability. Informed consent reflects competency standards requiring abstract appreciation and reasoning regarding the information provided. The issue of assent versus consent is an interesting one when one determines at what age children can make meaningful decisions about participating in research. According to the work by Piaget regarding cognitive ability, children at age 6 years and older can give assent. Whereas children at age 14 years and older are not legally authorized to give sole consent unless they are emancipated minors, they can make such decisions as capably as adults (Mitchell, 1984).

Federal regulations require parental permission whenever a child is involved in research, except in specific cases, for example, child abuse or mature minors at minimal risk. If the research involves more than minimal risk and does not offer direct benefit to the individual child, both parents must give permission. When an individual reaches maturity (at 18 years of age in cases of research), he may render his own consent. He may do so at a younger age if he has been legally declared an emancipated minor. Questions regarding this should be addressed to the IRB or research administration office and not left to the discrimination of the researcher to answer.

No vulnerable population may be singled out for study for simple convenience. For example, prisoners may not be studied simply because they are an available and convenient group. Prisoners may be studied if the study pertains to, for example, the effects and processes of incarceration. Students are often convenient groups of subjects for research. They must not be singled out as research subjects because of convenience, but the research questions must have some bearing on their status as students.

Dubler (1987) writes cogently as an advocate for the vulnerable elderly who are increasingly dependent and have declining cognitive ability. She states that they are precisely the class of persons who were historically and are potentially vulnerable to abuse and for whom the law must struggle to fashion specific protections (p. 545). The issue of legal competence is often raised. There is no issue if the potential subject can supply legally effective informed consent. Competence is not a clearly "black or white" situation. The complexity of the study may affect ability to consent to participate. For example, a patient may be able to consent to participate in a simple observation study but not in a phase 1 drug trial.

Dubler quotes federal regulations when she states that IRBs must determine whether the involvement of institutionalized individuals in the research would be exploitative, and the burden should be on the investigator to show that it is appropriate to involve such subjects in research.

The issue often arises regarding the necessity of requiring the elderly to provide consent. Dubler (personal communication) refers to Research Regulation 46.116, which provides that requirements for some or all of the elements of informed consent may be waived for the following:

1. The research involves no more than minimal risk to the subjects.
2. The waiver or alteration will not adversely affect the rights and welfare of the subjects.
3. The research could not practicably be carried out without the waiver or alteration.
4. Whenever appropriate, the subjects will be provided with additional pertinent information after participation.

Researchers and caregivers involved in research with vulnerable people are well advised to seek advice from appropriate IRBs, clinicians, lawyers, ethicists, and others.

The concept of ethics in research is dynamic and ever changing. Just as informed consent itself in research was defined in the 1970s, the 1980s have witnessed some interesting, yet perplexing issues, two of which deserve mention here.

Periodically, the public becomes aware of the unethical conduct of medical research. Any number of unethical practices may have been commited, including illegal, unethical recruitment of subjects and falsification of data for purposes of self-aggrandizement. The risks are many, including harming research subjects or basing clinical practice on false data. Nurses, as advocates of patient welfare and professional practice, should be aware that, albeit hopefully rare, there are occasions when misconduct by the researcher is observed or suspected. In such cases nurses are advised to escalate their concerns in order to ensure matters receive appropriate attention and review.

Of equal importance is the issue of basing practice on reports that appear in journals, where subsequent research and reports on those subjects change the scientific basis for practice. Journals may print corrections or further research in follow-up reports that are buried, obscure, or underreported. Lawrence K. Altman (1988), a physician, stated, "Such shortcomings are critically important because the thousands of journals that cover a range of specialties are the central reservoir of scientific knowledge. They are the standard references for crediting discoveries and determining treatments." It is incumbent on the nurse as patient advocate to keep up-to-date on scientific reports related to nursing practice and adjust practice as directed by ever-evolving research findings.

With the plague of acquired immune deficiency syndrome (AIDS) in the 1980s, considerable research on victims of AIDS, those at risk, and others has been undertaken. A number of ethical questions have arisen, including the potential "overuse" of people with AIDS in research and whether those with seropositive tests for human immunodeficiency virus should be so informed. The most current policy on the latter states:

> It is the policy of the Public Health Service (PHS) that when HIV testing is conducted or supported by PHS, individuals whose test results are associated with personal identifiers must be informed of their own test results and provided with the opportunity to receive appropriate counseling. This policy applies to all intramural and to all extramural PHS activities including both research and service activities, domestic and foreign. Individuals may not be given the option "not to know" the result, either at the time of consenting to be tested or thereafter. This policy does not apply to testing situations in which subjects consent to be tested but specimen results cannot be linked to individual subjects by anyone other than the subjects themselves. The PHS encourages testing facilities to advise test subjects to obtain test results and to abstain from risk behaviors (Department of Health and Human Services, May 1988).

Principles of informed consent and other legal/ethical matters in regard to research are ever changing. Nurses are urged to keep apprised of the most current thinking on these issues.

Once again, it is advisable to consult with the IRB as early as possible in research proposal development to avoid designing a study that is not feasible in terms of human use.

Reviewing research involving the use of human subjects

It is customary today when presenting a research report at a meeting or in a publication to comment that "before the research was conducted, the project was reviewed by the IRB and the following plans (which are then described) were approved for the use of human subjects." It is likely that a paper will not be accepted for publication without such a discussion. It is often brief, no more than two or three sentences, but it tells the reader that the ethical and legal guidelines that have been discussed throughout this chapter have been applied in the conduct of that particular project. This also makes it almost impossible to report on informal, ad hoc research, as has been described earlier. In addition, the public's trust in nurses as client advocates in their researcher role will be reaffirmed if the concept of human rights is discussed as a basic tenet preempting any scientific investigation.

It should be apparent from the preceding sections that whereas the need for guidelines for the use of human subjects in research is quite evident, and the principles themselves are clear, in many instances the nurse must use her best judgment, both as a client advocate and as a researcher, in evaluating the ethical nature of a research project. In any research situation the basic guiding principle of protecting the client must always apply. When conflicts arise the nurse must feel free to raise suitable questions and have access to appropriate resources. These resources may include the nursing supervisor, the director of nursing research, and the chairperson of the IRB. The nurse should pursue her answers to her questions about the clients as research subjects and her role in the project until she is satisfied that the client's rights and her rights as a professional nurse are protected.

LEGAL/ETHICAL ASPECTS OF ANIMAL EXPERIMENTATION

The federal laws that have been written to protect the rights of animals in research emanate from an interesting history regarding attitudes toward animals and the value man places on them. Animal activists (The Animal Liberation Front) and antivivisectionist societies gained considerable public attention starting in the 1970s. Of interest, however, is the fact that the oldest piece of legislation controlling animal experimentation goes back to 1876 in the United Kingdom. With the increase in the use of animals in research after World War II, a number of states passed legislation, called *pound seizure laws,* that allowed and even mandated the release of unclaimed animals from pounds to laboratories. The first pound seizure law was enacted in 1949, and it took until 1972 for the first law of that type to be repealed. In 1966 in the United States the first Laboratory Animal Welfare Act was passed. The act did not deal with what we consider today to be some of the most salient issues related to animal experimentation (for example, pain management), and amendments continued to be passed to address these concerns. The 1970 Act provided for the establishment of an Institutional Animal Care and Use Committee, one member of which must be a veterinarian. The U.S. Department of Agriculture oversees compliance with animal welfare acts and holds institutions' administration accountable for compliance.

In 1985 the President signed P.L. 99-198, which contains "Improved Standards for the Laboratory Animals' Act." Provisions in the series of acts and amendments to acts pertaining to animal experimentation include, but are by no means limited to, the following (PHS Policy on Humane Care, 1985):

1. The transportation, care, and use of animals should be in accordance with the Animal Welfare Act (7 U.S.C. 2131 et. seq.) and other applicable Federal laws, guidelines, and policies.
2. Procedures involving animals should be designed and performed with due consideration of their relevance to human or animal health, the advancement of knowledge, or the good of society.
3. The animals selected for a procedure should be of an appropriate species and quality, and the minimum number should be required to obtain valid results. Methods such as mathematical models, computer simulation, and in vitro biological systems should be considered.
4. Proper use of animals, including the avoidance or minimization of discomfort, distress, and pain, when consistent with sound scientific practices,

is imperative. Unless the contrary is established, investigators should consider that procedures that cause pain or distress in human beings may cause pain or distress in other animals.

5. Procedures with animals that may cause more than momentary or slight pain or distress should be performed with appropriate sedation, analgesia, or anesthesia. Surgical or other painful procedures should not be performed on unanesthetized animals paralyzed by chemical agents.

6. Animals that would otherwise suffer severe or chronic pain or distress that cannot be relieved should be painlessly killed at the end of the procedure or, if appropriate, during the procedure.

7. The living conditions of animals should be appropriate for their species and contribute to their health and comfort. Normally, the housing, feeding, and care of all animals used for biomedical purposes must be directed by a veterinarian or other scientist trained and experienced in the proper care, handling, and use of the species being maintained or studied. In any case, veterinary care shall be provided as indicated.

8. Investigators and other personnel shall be appropriately qualified for and experienced in conducting procedures on living animals. Adequate arrangements shall be made for their in-service training, including the proper and humane care and use of laboratory animals.

9. Where exceptions are required in relation to the provisions of these Principles, the decisions should not rest with the investigators directly concerned but should be made, with due regarding to Principle 2, by an appropriate review group such as an institutional animal research committee. Such exceptions should not be made solely for the purposes of teaching or demonstration.

This section serves only as an introduction to the concept of legal/ethical issues related to animal experimentation. Principles of protection of **animal rights** in research have evolved over time. Animals, unlike human beings, cannot give informed consent, but other conditions related to their welfare must be not ignored. Nurses who encounter the use of animals in research should be alert to their rights. Nurses who wish to read further on this subject may find the references at the end of this chapter of interest.

THE NURSE AS RESEARCHER AND PATIENT ADVOCATE

This section addresses the concept of the *nurse as client advocate* in the role as caregiver or researcher.

The American Nurses' Association (ANA) Commission on Nursing Research affirmed the profession's obligation to support the advancement of scientific knowledge. The ANA supports two sets of human rights in this regard. One set is concerned with the rights of qualified nurses to engage in research and to have access to resources necessary for implementing scientific investigations. The second set deals with the rights of all persons who are recipients of health care services or who are participants in research performed by investigators whose studies impinge on the care provided by nurses.

The relationship of trust between client and nurse is an essential element of the professional code of ethics. This trust between client-subject and investigator requires that the researcher assume a special obligation to safeguard the subject. The nurse as researcher or caregiver must assure the client of the following:

1. The subject's rights will not be violated without his voluntary and informed consent.
2. No risk, discomfort, invasion of privacy, or threat to dignity beyond that initially stated in describing the subject's role in the study will be imposed without further permission being obtained.
3. The subject is assured that if he does not wish to participate in the study, neither will he be subjected to harrassment nor will the quality of his care be influenced by this decision (ANA Commission on Nursing Research, 1975).

Upon employment, a nurse should ask about what is expected of her regarding research. Will she be required to collect data or provide medicines or treatments in double-blind studies? Is she free not to participate? Are written protocols as reference available? Has the IRB ruled on each protocol? Is she free to decline to participate without jeopardizing her position?

The *ANA Human Rights Guidelines for Nurses* (1975) state "conditions of employment in settings in which clinical and/or other research is in progress need to be spelled out in detail for all potential workers. As a corollary, it follows that anyone employed in work that carries the potential of risk to others needs to be advised as to the types of risks involved, the ways of recognizing when risk is present, and the proper actions to take to counteract harmful effects and unnecessary danger."

Ignorance and naiveté vis-à-vis ethical and legal guidelines for the conduct of research must never be an excuse for a nurse's failure to be a client advocate in research situations.

SUMMARY

Since the National Research Act was passed in 1974, the federal government has taken special precautions to protect the rights of human research subjects. Institutional review boards were established at agencies conducting research in order to review all proposed research involving human subjects before its initiation. Ethical and legal guidelines are the underlying principles by which researchers design protocols and IRBs review them. No investigator may unilaterally determine the risk/benefit ratios inherent in that investigator's project and then conduct it without IRB approval. In addition, ignorance of ethical and legal guidelines directing the conduct of human research is no excuse for not following the proper review system.

This chapter reviews the evolution of the concept of informed consent as it was borne out of the Nuremberg Tribunals after World War II. The concept of informed consent in research is discussed, and examples from relatively recent research in the United States, which by current standards would be considered unethical, are given.

The point is emphasized throughout the chapter that the researcher cannot and must not take sole responsibility for determining whether research is ethical and beneficial.

As put forth in the National Research Act of 1974, IRBs were mandated in all institutions receiving federal funds. It is the IRB that objectively reviews research proposals for the involvement of human subjects and evaluates the risk/benefit ratio.

Guidelines for adequate informed consent are listed and examples are given. Special considerations (i.e., children, the elderly, and the incompetent) are discussed.

Finally, the concept of the nurse as caregiver and researcher is discussed. Nurses are first and foremost client advocates. They must always work to ensure that client's rights have been ethically and legally considered before clients' participation in research.

References

Altman, L.K. (May 31, 1988). A flaw in the research process: uncorrected errors in journals, Medical Science, *The New York Times.*

ANA Commission on Nursing Research. (1975). *Human rights guidelines for nurses in clinical and other research,* Kansas City, Mo.

Code of Federal Regulations, 45 CFR 46, Protection of Human Subjects, OPRR Reports, revised March 8, 1983.

Cook, R. (1981). *Brain,* New York, Signet.

Creighton, H. (1977). Legal concerns of nursing research, *Nursing Research,* **266:**337-340.

Davis, A. (1981a). Ethical consideration in gerontological nursing research, *Geriatric Nursing,* **2:**269-272.

Davis, A. (1981b). Ethical issues in nursing research, *The Western Journal of Nursing Research,* **3:**247-248.

Department of Health and Human Services. (May 1988). Policy on informing those tested about HIV sero status.

Dubler, N.N. (1987). Legal judgments and informed consent in geriatric research, *Journal of the American Geriatric Society,* **35:**545-549.

Fowler, M.D.M. (1988). Ethical issues in nursing research: a call for an International Code of Ethics for nursing research, *The Western Journal of Nursing Research,* **10:**352-355.

Gargano, W.J. (1978). Cancer nursing and the law: informed consent, Part II, *Cancer Nursing,* **1:**167-168.

Hanks, G.E. (1984a). The dangers of ad hoc protocols, *Journal of Clinical Oncology,* **2:** 1177-1178.

Hanks, G.E. (1984b). *Implementing human research regulations,* Second biennial report on the adequacy and uniformity of federal rules and policies, and of their implementation, for the protection of human subjects, President's Commission for the Study of Ethical Problems in Medicine and Biomedical and Behavioral Research, March 1983.

Mitchell, K. (1984). Protecting children's rights during research, *Pediatric Nursing,* **10:**9-10.

Moore, L. (1984). Conducting clinical trials, *Journal of Enterostomal Therapy,* **11:**229-232.

Public Health Service policy on human care in use of lab animals by awardee institution. In NIH guide for grants and contracts, vol. 14, No. 8, June 25, 1985.

Additional Readings

Appelbaum, P.S., and Roth, L.H. (1982). Competency to consent to research, *Archives of General Psychiatry,* **39:**951-958.

Davis, A.J. (1989). Clinical nurses' ethical decision making in situations of informed consent, *Advances in Nursing Science,* **11:**63-69.

Goldberg, R.J. (1984). Disclosure of information to adult cancer clients: issues and update, *Journal of Clinical Oncology,* **2:**948-955.

Jameton, A., and Fowler, M. (1989). Ethical inquiry in the concept of research, *Advances in Nursing Science,* **11:**1-24.

Levine, R.J. (1983). Research involving children: an interpretation of the new regulations, *IRB: A Review of Human Subjects Research,* **5:**1-5.

May, K. Antle. (1979). The nurse as researcher: impediment to informed consent? *Nursing Outlook,* **27:**36-39.

Orlans, F.B., Simmonds, R.C., and Dodds, W.J. (1987). Effective animal care and use committees, *Laboratory Animal Science.*

Robinson, G. and Merav, A. (1976). Informed consent: recall by clients tested postoperatively, *The Annals of Thoracic Surgery,* **22:**209-212.

Rowan, A.H. (1984). *Of mice, models and men: a critical evaluation of animal research,* Albany, N.Y., State University of New York Press.

Tuffery, A.A., ed. (1987). *Laboratory animals: an introduction for new experimenters,* New York, Wiley-Interscience.

Wilcox, R., Gerber, R.M., and DeWalt, E. (1977). Clinical research in nursing homes, *Nursing Outlook,* **25:**255-257.

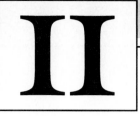

THE RESEARCH PROCESS

The following chapters will introduce you to the systematic and orderly conduction of the research process and its relationship to the establishment of nursing theory, practice, and education based on research studies. Understanding the step-by-step process that researchers use will assist you in judging the soundness of research investigations. As you proceed through the chapters, research terminology pertinent to each step will be identified and exemplified. The steps of the research process generally proceed in the order outlined in the text but may vary depending on the nature of the research problem. It is important to remember that a researcher may vary the order of the steps slightly, but the steps must still be addressed in an orderly and systematic manner.

4

The Problem Statement

Judith Haber

LEARNING OBJECTIVES

After reading this chapter the student will be able to do the following:

⬦ Describe the relationship of the problem statement to the other components of the research process.

⬦ Describe the process of identifying and refining a research problem.

⬦ Identify the criteria for determining the significance of a research problem.

⬦ Identify the characteristics of a research problem.

⬦ Formulate a problem statement.

⬦ Identify the criteria for critiquing a problem statement.

⬦ Apply the critiquing criteria to the evaluation of a problem statement in a research report.

KEY TERMS

dependent variable   testability
independent variable   theory
population   variable
problem statement

Formulating a **problem statement** is one of the key steps in the research process. It is the starting point of any research study. But selecting and defining the problem is often a difficult task, particularly for those who are just becoming acquainted with the research process. The task is difficult for several reasons. One reason is the bewildering array of possible topics to study, even in just one area. There are so many aspects of a topic to study that it is difficult to choose just one. Another reason is that a beginning researcher often lacks familiarity with the previous research studies done in a specific area. Yet another difficulty is selecting a problem to study if the beginning researcher is unsure of what the research process entails and what constitutes a researchable problem.

The research consumer will often not see a formal statement of the problem included in research reports or articles because of space constraints in such publications. Nevertheless it is equally important for both the consumer and the producer of research to understand the importance of a problem statement as the foundation of a research study, as well as the process leading to its development. The ability to critique a problem statement is as important as the ability to formulate such a statement. Both the beginning researcher and the research consumer must have a working knowledge of what a problem statement is, the standards for writing one, and a set of guidelines for its evaluation.

This chapter introduces the ways that researchers formulate a problem statement and the research consumer's criteria for evaluating the merit of a problem statement.

EXPLORING A PROBLEM AREA

The researcher spends a great deal of time selecting a problem for study. This process should not be hurried, because it is the crux of the research project and provides an orderly direction for the remainder of the endeavor. This phase of the research process involves both thoughtful reflection and creativity to arrive at a problem that is specific, significant, interesting, and researchable.

Students may wonder where ideas for research studies come from. They may be uncertain about how a topic is selected and may feel that their inexperience hampers their ability to develop or assess an appropriate problem for study. It is reassuring to find that a problem or topic is not pulled from "thin air." A research problem should indicate that practical experience, a critical appraisal of the scientific literature, or an interest in an untested **theory** has provided the basis for the germination of a research idea. Table 4-1 illustrates how each of the preceding areas can influence the generation of ideas for a research problem.

Table 4-1 How Practical Experience, Scientific Literature, and Untested Theory Influence the Development of a Research Idea

Area	Influence	Example
Practical experience	Clinical practice provides a wealth of experience from which research problems can be derived. The nurse may observe the occurrence of a particular event or pattern and become curious about why it occurs as well as its relationship to other factors in the client's environment.	A nurse working on an oncology unit observes that certain clients appear to have a delayed grief reaction after being diagnosed as having a recurring malignancy. They seem to mourn ineffectively and often end up angry or hopeless. On the other hand, other clients appear to go through the stages of grieving in a systematic way and usually emerge with a more positive philosophical attitude. The nurse notes the differences in the two groups of clients and speculates about other factors that might contribute to this difference, such as open family communication patterns.
Critical appraisal of the scientific literature	The critical appraisal of research studies that appear in journals may indirectly suggest a problem area by stimulating the reader's thinking. The nurse may observe a conflict or inconsistency in the findings of several related research studies and wonder which findings are most valid.	A nurse working on a medical-surgical unit reads two research articles on methods for promoting wound healing in decubitus ulcers. Both studies propose similar theoretical rationales for the method of treatment, yet both propose different treatment protocols. One study reports significant findings and the other does not. The nurse thinks, "There is a conflict in this literature. How do I evaluate the discrepancy in these findings?"

Continued.

Table 4-1 **How Practical Experience, Scientific Literature, and Untested Theory Influence the Development of a Research Idea—cont'd**

Area	Influence	Example
Gaps in the literature	A research idea may be suggested by a research report that offers other areas for future study. Research ideas can be generated by research reports that suggest the value of replicating a particular study to extend or refine the existing scientific knowledge base.	A nurse working on an obstetrical unit observes that both the birthing chair and the delivery table are used for vaginal deliveries. However, there is disagreement between staff members about which delivery method has the most beneficial effect on the duration of the second stage of labor, on maternal blood loss, and on fetal outcome. However, when the literature is reviewed relative to this topic, no research studies in this area are uncovered that would provide a scientific basis for determining which method is most effective.
Interest in untested theory	Verification of an untested nursing theory provides a relatively uncharted territory from which research problems can be derived. Inasmuch as theories themselves are not tested, a researcher may think about investigating a particular concept or set of concepts related to a particular nursing theory. The deductive process would be used to generate the research problem. The researcher would pose questions such as, "If this theory is correct, what kind of behavior would I expect to observe in particular clients and under which conditions?" *or* "If this theory is valid, what kind of supporting evidence would I find?"	A nurse researcher utilizes Orem's self-care model (which views the person as a self-care agent) as the basis of a research study designed to verify particular aspects of this theory. A study is designed to investigate the effect of informational intervention about knowledge of chemotherapy on self-care behaviors of patients with cancer. Orem's theory provides the conceptual framework for the study.

REFINING THE PROBLEM STATEMENT

The problem statement should reflect a refinement of the researcher's thinking. The evaluator of a research study should be able to discern that the researcher has done the following:
1. Defined a specific problem area
2. Reviewed the relevant scientific literature
3. Examined the problem's potential significance to nursing
4. Pragmatically examined the feasibility of studying the research problem

Defining the problem area

Defining a problem area or topic is essentially a creative process. Unfortunately the evaluator of a research study is not privy to this process, since it occurred during the study's conceptualization. And, often, the final problem statement does not appear in the research article. Since that is the case, let me provide you with a glimpse of what the process of defining a problem area may be like for a researcher.

The researcher may have started with a list of general topics such as mother-infant relationships, family communication patterns, factors contributing to pain, or stress-reduction strategies for patients with heart disease who are at high risk of myocardial infarctions. General areas of interest are narrowed and defined so that the topic is more specific and circumscribed. A good research problem must have a specific focus. Having a narrowly defined problem does not mean that the topic is trivial or insignificant.

Consultation with teachers, advisors, or colleagues may provide valuable feedback that helps the beginning researcher to focus on a specific problem area. For example, the researcher may have told a faculty advisor that the area of interest was families' relationships with elderly relatives. The advisor may have said, "What is it about the topic that specifically interests you?" Such a conversation may have initiated a chain of thought that resulted in a decision to explore stress in family caregivers of the elderly. This example illustrates how a broad area of interest (family relationships with elderly relatives) was narrowed to a specific research topic (stress in family caregivers of the elderly).

Beginning the literature review

The literature review should reveal that the scientific literature relevant to the problem area has been critically examined (see Chapter 5). In the previous example of stress in family caregivers of the elderly, the researcher may have conducted a preliminary review of books and journals for theories and research studies regarding factors apparently critical to the families caring for an elderly relative. These factors should be potentially relevant, of interest, and measurable. Possible relevant factors mentioned in the literature would include any emotional, social, physical, and financial difficulties associated with caregiving. Other **variables,** such as demographic characteristics of caregivers and of elders, characteristics of the caregiving situation, and social support, that mediate the effect of caregiver stress must also be considered. This information could then be used by the researcher to further define the research problem. At this point the researcher could write the following tentative problem statement: *What is the effect of stress and social support on the psychological distress of family caregivers of the elderly?* Although the problem statement is not yet in its final form, the reader can envision the interrelatedness between the initial definition of the problem area, the literature review, and the refined problem statement. The person reading a research report examines the end product of this formulation process and thus should have an appreciation for this time-consuming effort.

Significance

Before proceeding to a final formulation of the problem statement, it is crucial for the researcher to have examined the problem's potential significance to nursing. The research problem should have the potential for contributing to and extending the scientific body of nursing knowledge. The problem does not have to be of prize-winning caliber to be significant. However, it should meet the following criteria:

◇ Clients, nurses, the medical community in general, and society will potentially benefit from the knowledge derived from this study.

◇ The results will be applicable for nursing practice, education, or administration.

◇ The results will be theoretically relevant.

◇ The findings will lend support to untested theoretical assumptions, challenge an existing theory, or clarify a conflict in the literature.

◇ The findings will potentially formulate or alter nursing practices or policies.

If the research problem has not met any of these criteria, it would be wise to extensively revise the problem or discard it. For example, in the previously cited problem statement the significance of the problem includes these facts:

◇ The number of elderly in the population will more than double in the next 40 years.

◇ A decline in federally funded programs for the elderly will place further demands on families for caregiving responsibilities.

◇ The toll of caregiving on families can be high.

◇ Previous research studies have been largely exploratory and atheoretical, which make it difficult to draw conclusions from diverse findings.

Feasibility

The feasibility of a research problem needs to be pragmatically examined. Regardless of how significant or researchable a problem may be, pragmatic considerations such as time; the availability of subjects, facilities, equipment, and money; the experience of the researcher; and any ethical considerations may cause the researcher to decide that the problem is inappropriate because it lacks feasibility (see Chapters 3 and 8).

THE FINAL PROBLEM STATEMENT

A problem may be written in a declarative form as illustrated in Table 4-2 or in an interrogative form. Stating a problem in an interrogative form, as illustrated in Table 4-3, is often advantageous, because research problems posed in question form invite answers. Other experts propose that the problem statement that is presented in declarative form provide clear direction for the research study. A good problem statement exhibits the following four characteristics:

◇ It clearly and unambiguously identifies the variables under consideration
◇ It clearly expresses the variables' relationship to each other
◇ It specifies the nature of the population being studied
◇ It implies the possibility of empirical testing

Since each of these elements is crucial to the formulation of a satisfactory problem statement, we will discuss the above criteria in greater detail.

The variables

When concepts are operationalized, they are usually called variables. Researchers call the properties that they study variables. Such properties take on different values. Thus a *variable* is, as the name suggests, something that varies. Properties that differ from each other, such as age, weight, height, religion, and ethnicity, are examples of variables. Researchers attempt to understand how and why differences in one *variable* are related to differences in another variable. For example, a researcher may be concerned about the variable of cervical cancer in young women. It is a variable because not all young women have cervical cancer. A researcher may also be interested in what other factors can be linked to cervical cancer. It has been discovered that use of diethylstilbestrol (DES) during pregnancy appears to be related to cervical cancer in daughters. Thus DES use is also a variable, since not every mother has taken DES.

When speaking of relationships between variables, the researcher is essentially asking, "Is X related to Y? What is the effect of X on Y? How are X_1 and X_2 related to Y?" The researcher is asking a question about the relationship between one or more **independent variables** and a **dependent variable.***

An *independent variable,* usually symbolized by X, is the *antecedent* or the variable that has the presumed effect on the dependent variable. In experimental research studies the independent variable is manipulated by the researcher. For example, a nurse may study how different intramuscular injection sites affect the client's perception of pain. The researcher may manipulate the independent variable — intramuscular injection sites — by using different injection sites (see Chapter 9). In nonexperimental research the independent variable is not manipulated and is assumed to have occurred naturally before or during the study. For example, the researcher may be studying the relationship between the level of anxiety and the

---

* In cases where there are more than one independent or dependent variables, subscripts are used to indicate the number of variables under consideration.

Table 4-2 **Problem Statements in Declarative Form**

Research focus	Problem statement
Music and postoperative pain and anxiety	The effect of music on postoperative pain and anxiety is unknown (Mullooly et al., 1988).
Relaxation and physical and psychosocial outcomes in patients after myocardial infarction	The physical and psychosocial effects of relaxation techniques on patients' rehabilitation after myocardial infarction have not been demonstrated (Munro et al., 1988).
Influence of feeding methods on transcutaneous oxygen pressure and temperature in small preterm infants	The effects of bottle-feeding and breast-feeding on transcutaneous oxygen pressure in small preterm infants have not been compared (Meier, 1988).

Table 4-3 **Problem Statements in Interrogative Form**

Research focus	Problem statement
Effects of educational interventions in diabetes care	What is the magnitude of the effect of patient teaching in adults with diabetes (Brown, 1988)?
Physical restraint of the hospitalized elderly; perceptions of patients and nurses	What are the differences between patients' and primary nurses' perceptions of responses, effects, coping strategies, and alternatives to physical restraint (Strumpf and Evans, 1988)?
Disruption of circadian rhythm and surgical recovery	What is the relation between fluctuations in core temperature and timing and rhythmic variations in locomotor activity after surgery in an animal model (Farr et al., 1988)?

perception of pain. The independent variable—the level of anxiety—is not manipulated; it is just presumed to occur and is observed and measured as it naturally happens (see Chapter 10).

The *dependent variable,* represented by Y, is often referred to as the *consequence* or the presumed effect that varies with a change in the independent variable. The dependent variable is not manipulated. It is observed and assumed to vary with changes in the independent variable. Predictions are made *from* the independent variable *to* the dependent variable. It is the dependent variable that the researcher is interested in understanding, explaining, or predicting. For example, it might be assumed that the perception of pain—the dependent variable—will vary with changes in the level of anxiety—the independent variable. In this case we are trying to explain the perception of pain in relation to the level of anxiety.

Although variability in the dependent variable is assumed to depend on changes in the independent variable, that does not imply that there is a causal relationship between X and Y or that changes in variable X cause variable Y to change. Let us look at an example where nurses' attitudes toward rape were studied. The researcher discovered that older nurses had a more negative attitude about rape than had younger nurses. The researcher did not conclude that the nurses' attitudes toward rape were *caused* by their age, but at the same time it is apparent that there is a directional relationship between age and attitudes about rape. That is, as the nurses' age increases, their attitudes about rape become more negative. This example highlights the fact that causal relationships are not necessarily implied by the independent and dependent variables. Rather, only a relational statement with possible directionality is proposed.

Although one independent and one dependent variable are used in the examples just given, there is no restriction on the number of variables that can be included in a problem statement. However, remember that problems should not be unnecessarily complex or unwieldy, particularly in beginning research efforts. Problem statements that include more than one independent or dependent variable are generally broken down into subproblems that are more concise.

Finally, it should be noted that variables are not inherently independent or dependent. A variable that is classified as independent in one study may be considered dependent in another study. For example, a nurse may review an article about personality factors that are predictive of alcoholism. In this case alcoholism is the dependent variable. When another article about the relationship between alcoholism and marital conflict is reviewed, alcoholism is the independent variable. Whether a variable is independent or dependent is a function of the role it plays in a particular study.

Population

The nature of the **population** being studied needs to be specified in the problem statement. If the scope of the problem has been narrowed to a specific focus and the variables have been clearly identified, the nature of the population will be evident to the reader of a research report. For example, a problem statement that poses the question "Is there a relationship between rooming-in by mothers and preschool childrens' adjustment to hospitalization?" suggests that the population under consideration includes mothers and their hospitalized preschool children. It is also implied that some of the mothers will have had rooming-in, in contrast to other mothers who have not. The researcher or the reader will have an initial idea of the composition of the study population from the outset (see Chapter 15).

Testability

The statement of the research problem must imply that the problem is testable, that is, measurable by either qualitative or quantitative methods. For example, the problem statement "Should nurses work with dying clients?" is incorrectly stated for a variety of reasons; one reason is that it is not testable. It represents a value statement rather

Table 4-4 **Components of the Problem Statement and Related Criteria**

Variables	Population	Testability
Independent variable: perceived caregiver stress and social support Dependent variable: psychological distress	Family caregivers of the elderly	Differential effect of perceived stress and social support on psychological distress

than a relational problem statement. A scientific or relational problem must propose a relationship between an independent and a dependent variable and do this in such a way that it indicates that the variables of the relationship can somehow be measured.

Many interesting and important questions are not valid research problems, because they are not amenable to testing.

The question "Should nurses work with dying clients?" could be revised from a philosophical question to a research question that implies **testability.** Two examples of the revised problem statement might be the following:

⋄ Is there a relationship between nurses' attitudes toward dying clients and the quality of nursing care?

⋄ What is the effect of nurses' attitudes about death and dying on empathic communication with terminally ill clients?

These examples illustrate the relationship between the variables, identify the independent and dependent variables, and imply the testability of the research problem.

Now that the elements of the formal problem statement have been presented in greater detail, this information can be integrated by formulating a formal problem statement about stress in families caring for an elderly relative. Earlier in this chapter the following unrefined problem statement was formulated: *What is the effect of stress and social support on the psychological distress of family caregivers of the elderly?* This problem statement was originally derived from a general area of interest—family relationships with elderly relatives. The topic was more specifically defined by delineating a particular problem area—stress in families caring for an elderly relative. The problem crystalized still further after a preliminary literature review and emerged in the unrefined form just given. With the four criteria inherent in a satisfactory problem statement, it is now possible to propose a refined or formal problem statement, that is, one that specifically states the problem in question form and specifies the relationship between the key variables in the study, the population being studied, and the empirical testability of the problem. Congruent with these four criteria, the following problem statement can then be formulated: *What is the effect of perceived caregiver stress and social support on the psychological distress of family caregivers of the elderly* (Baillie, Norbeck, and Barnes, 1988)? Table 4-4 identifies the components of this problem statement as they relate to and are congruent with the four problem statement criteria.

Table 4-5 Examples of Unrefined and Refined Problem Statements

Type of design suggested	Unrefined problem statement	Critique of problem statement	Refined problem statement
Nonexperimental	Do nurses' attitudes toward clients with acquired immune deficiency syndrome (AIDS) affect the emotional state of the client?	Not a concise relational statement Testability is not implied	Is there a relationship between the nurse's attitude toward AIDS and the emotional status of the AIDS client?
Experimental	How does client teaching influence maternal anxiety in primiparas after discharge?	Not a concise relational statement Testability is not implied Variables are not clear	The relationship between the amount of client teaching and the level of anxiety in primiparas after discharge is unknown.
Experimental	To measure the effectiveness of health teaching for hospitalized clients with heart disease in a group setting	Population is not specific	Research has not demonstrated the effect of postcardiac group health teaching on health behaviors of patients after an initial myocardial infarction.
Experimental	Does positioning have an effect on the occurrence of contractures in unconscious clients?	Variables are not clear	What is the difference in the incidence of contractures in comatose clients in relation to frequency of repositioning?
Experimental	How do nurse-run client education classes impact on the housebound elderly?	Not a relational statement Population is not defined adequately Variables are not clearly defined Testability is not implied	The effect of nurse-administered educational rehabilitation programs on independent behavior in chronically ill housebound elderly clients has not been determined.

Continued.

Table 4-5 provides additional examples of unrefined and refined problem statements. It is important to note that the process of moving from the general topic area to the unrefined problem and finally to the refined, formal problem statement often involves several intermediate steps.

Table 4-5 **Examples of Unrefined and Refined Problem Statements — cont'd**

Type of design suggested	Unrefined problem statement	Critique of problem statement	Refined problem statement
Nonexperimental	How does the mother's feeling of well-being during pregnancy affect how the mother attaches to her baby?	Not a concise relational statement Variables are not clearly defined	Is there a relationship between the physical symptoms of pregnancy and maternal-fetal attachment in primigravidas?
Experimental	Do patients need sexual counseling after hysterectomies?	Not a relational statement Variables are not clearly specified Testability is not implied	Research has not demonstrated the relationship between sexual counseling and the postoperative adjustment of patients after hysterectomy.
Nonexperimental	How does assertiveness relate to feelings of power in depressed women?	Not a clear relational statement Variables are not clearly specified	Is there a relationship between assertive behavior and the perception of power in depressed women?

DIFFERENTIATING THE PROBLEM STATEMENT FROM THE PURPOSE

A formal problem statement is not included in most current research articles. What is more commonly used is a statement of purpose. As such, it is important for the research consumer to be clear about the difference between these two components of the research process.

As stated earlier, a research problem is a question for which an answer or solution is to be described, explained, or predicted. The problem is associated with the purpose of the study, but it is not identical. The *purpose* of the study is the specific aim or goal of the study, the task to be accomplished, not the problem to be solved. For example, a nurse working with rehabilitation clients with bladder dysfunction may be disturbed by the high incidence of urinary tract infections. The nurse may wonder "What is the optimum frequency of changing urinary drainage bags in clients with bladder dysfunction to reduce the incidence of urinary tract infections?" If this nurse were to design a study, its purpose might be to determine the difference in effect between a 1-week and a 4-week change schedule for the urinary drainage bag on the incidence of urinary tract infections in clients with bladder dysfunction.

CRITIQUING THE PROBLEM STATEMENT

The box on p. 72 offers critiquing criteria pertinent to the material discussed in this chapter.

Once the basics of developing a problem statement have been learned, a transition can be made from the development of a research problem to the critical appraisal of a research problem.

Several criteria for evaluating this initial phase of the research process — the problem statement — can be derived from the preceding discussion. Such criteria provide valid guidelines for critiquing this phase of the research process, regardless of whether the nurse is evaluating the potential merit of a researchable problem or is critically evaluating a published research study that is potentially applicable in practice. Since this text focuses on the nurse as a critical consumer of research, the following discussion will pertain primarily to the evaluation of the problem statement in a research report.

Since the problem statement represents the basis for the study, it is essential that it be introduced at the beginning of the research report. This will indicate the focus and direction of the study to the readers, who will then be in a position to evaluate whether the rest of the study logically flows from its base. Often the author will begin by identifying the general problem area that originally represented some vague discontent or question regarding an unsolved problem. The experiential and scientific background that led to the specific problem is briefly summarized, and the purpose of the study, is identified. Finally, the formal problem statement and any related subproblems are proposed.

The purpose of the introductory summary of the experiential and scientific background is to provide the reader with a glimpse of how the author thought about the research problem's development. The introduction to the research problem places the study within an appropriate conceptual framework and sets the stage for the unfolding of the study. This introductory section should also include the significance of the study, that is, why the investigator is doing the study. For example, the significance may be to solve a problem encountered in the clinical area and thereby improve client care, or to resolve a conflict in the literature regarding a clinical issue, or to provide data supporting an innovative form of nursing intervention that is cost-effective.

In reality, the reader will often find that the research problem is not clearly stated at the conclusion of this section. In fact, in some cases it is only hinted at, and the reader is challenged to identify the problem under consideration. In other cases the problem statement is embedded in the introductory text or purpose statement. To some extent, this will depend on the style of the particular journal. Nevertheless the evaluator must remember that the main problem statement should be clearly delineated in the introductory section even if the subproblems are not.

After the quality of the problem statement has been evaluated, the reader looks for the presence of four key elements that were described and illustrated in an earlier section of this chapter. They are the following:

1. Is the problem stated clearly and unambiguously in question form?
2. Does the problem statement express a relationship between two or more variables, or at least between an independent and dependent variable?

Critiquing Criteria

1. Was the problem introduced promptly?
2. Is the problem stated clearly and unambiguously in declarative or question form?
3. Does the problem statement express a relationship between two or more variables, or at least between an independent and a dependent variable?
4. Does the problem statement specify the nature of the population being studied?
5. Does the problem statement imply the possibility of empirical testability?
6. Has the problem been substantiated with adequate experiential and scientific background material?
7. Has the problem been placed within the context of an appropriate conceptual framework?
8. Has the significance of the problem been identified?
9. Have pragmatic issues, such as feasibility, been addressed?

3. Does the problem statement specify the nature of the population being studied?
4. Does the problem statement imply the possibility of empirical testing?

The reader will use these four elements as criteria for judging the soundness of a stated research problem. It is likely that if the problem is unclear in terms of the variables, the population, and the implications for testability, the remainder of the study is going to falter. For example, a research study contained introductory material on anxiety in general, anxiety as it relates to the perioperative period, and the potentially beneficial influence of nursing care in relation to anxiety reduction. The author concluded that the purpose of the study was to determine whether or not selected measures of client anxiety could be shown to differ when different approaches to nursing care were used during the perioperative period. The author did not go on to state the research problems. A restatement of the problem in question form might be the following:

$$(Y_1) \qquad\qquad (X_1, X_2, X_3)$$

What is the difference in client anxiety level in relation to different approaches to nursing care during the perioperative period?

If this process is clarified at the outset of a research study, all that follows in terms of the design can be logically developed. The reader will have a clear idea of what the report should convey and can evaluate knowledgeably the material that follows.

Conclusion

The care that a researcher takes when formulating and stating a problem is often representative of the thoroughness of the overall design and conceptualization of the study. A methodically developed problem that is concisely and clearly stated provides both the researcher and the evaluator of the research with a firm foundation to depart from when conducting or critically appraising a research study. This may be a time-consuming and often frustrating endeavor for the researcher. But in the final analysis, the product, as evaluated by the consumer, has most often been worth the struggle.

SUMMARY

Formulating a problem statement is one of the key procedures in the research process. It is the starting point of any research study. A great deal of time is spent in selecting an appropriate problem for study. Practical experience, a critical appraisal of the scientific literature, or an interest in an ungrounded theory provides the basis for the germination of a research idea.

The research problem is refined through a process that proceeds from the identification of a general idea of interest to the definition of a more specific and circumscribed topic. A preliminary literature review reveals related factors that appear critical to the research topic of interest and aids in further definition of the research problem. The significance of the research problem must be identified in terms of its potential contribution to clients, nurses, the medical community in general, and society. Applicability of the problem for nursing practice as well as its theoretical relevance must be established. The findings should also have the potential for formulating or altering nursing practices or policies.

The feasibility of a research problem must be examined in light of pragmatic considerations such as time; availability of subjects, money, facilities, and equipment; experience of the researcher; and ethical issues.

The final problem statement consists of an interrogative statement about the relationship between two or more variables. The problem statement clearly identifies the relationship between the independent and dependent variables. It specifies the nature of the population being studied. The problem statement implies the possibility of empirical testing.

The critiquing process provides a set of criteria for the evaluation of the strengths and weaknesses of a problem statement as it appears in a research report. The critiquer assesses the clarity of the problem statement as well as the related subproblems, the specificity of the population, and the implications for testability. The interrelatedness between the problem statement, the literature review, the theoretical framework, and the hypotheses should be apparent. The appropriateness of the research design suggested by the problem statement is also evaluated. Finally, the purpose of the study (that is, *why* the researcher is doing the study) should be differentiated from the problem statement or the research question to be answered.

A clearly and concisely stated research problem provides a firm foundation to depart from when conducting or critically appraising a research study. The time-consuming process of developing a problem statement may often seem overwhelming or frustrating. However, the product, as evaluated by the research consumer, is most often worth the struggle.

References

Baillie, V., Norbeck, J.S., and Barnes, L.A. (1988). Stress, social support and psychological distress of family caregivers of the elderly, *Nursing Research,* **37**:217-222.

Brown, S.A. (1988). Effects of educational interventions in diabetes care: a meta-analysis of findings, *Nursing Research,* **37**:223-229.

Dodd, M.J. (1984). Measuring informational intervention for chemotherapy knowledge and self-care behavior, *Research in Nursing and Health,* 7:43-50.

Downs, F.S., and Newman, M.A. (1977). *A sourcebook of nursing research,* 2nd ed., Philadelphia, F.A. Davis Co.

Farr, L.A., Campbell-Grossman, J.M., and Mack, J.M. (1988). Circadian disruption and surgical recovery, *Nursing Research,* **37**:170-175.

Kerlinger, F.N. (1986). *Foundations of behavioral research,* 3rd ed., New York, Holt, Rinehart & Winston, Inc.

Meier, P. (1988). Bottle and breast-feeding effects on transcutaneous oxygen pressure and temperature in preterm infants, *Nursing Research,* **31**:36-41.

Mullooly, V.M., Levin, R.F., and Feldman, H.R. (1988). Music for postoperative pain and anxiety, *The Journal of the New York State Nurses Association,* 19:4-7.

Munro, B.H., Creamer, A.M., Haggerty, M.R., and Cooper, F.S. (1988). Effect of relaxation therapy on post–myocardial infarction patients' rehabilitation, *Nursing Research,* **37**:231-235.

Shannahan, M.D., and Cottrell, B.H. (1985). Effect of the birth chair on duration of second stage labor, fetal outcome, and maternal blood loss, *Nursing Research,* **34**:89-92.

Strumpf, N.E., and Evans, L.K. (1988). Physical restraint of the hospitalized elderly: perceptions of patients and nurses, *Nursing Research,* **37**:132-137.

5

The Literature Review

Margaret Grey

LEARNING OBJECTIVES

After reading this chapter the student should be able to do the following:

◇ Define the purposes of the literature review.

◇ List the most utilized sources of nursing and related literature.

◇ Critically evaluate literature reviews in selected research studies.

KEY TERMS

concept	primary source
conceptual literature	review of the literature
construct	secondary source
data-based literature	variable

To critically evaluate literature reviews in published research papers, it is important for the student to understand how a review is conducted so that he or she can judge whether an adequate review is presented.

Every research project should be an outcome of all previous thinking and research in the chosen area. Just how does this logical flow of ideas occur? It occurs through the conscious part of the research process that is known as the **review of the literature.** Now, you are probably thinking, "I know all about that because I've had to review published literature on a certain topic for term papers." Although literature reviews for term papers are similar in that they must summarize what is known about an area, the literature review conducted for the purpose of supporting a research project is different in two important ways. First, the literature review places the current study in the context of previous research. As such, it includes both **conceptual literature** and **data-based literature.** *Conceptual literature* is published material dealing with the theory that underlies the research. *Data-based literature* is composed of all the published research studies dealing with the problem of interest. Second, this type of review requires a critical examination of the related literture. The review must identify the weaknesses, strengths, conflicts, and gaps in the literature covering the topic area. Thus it is not simply a narration of "so-and-so said." Rather, the literature review relates what others said, how and why they said it, and how much confidence the author has in the findings. The goal of this chapter is to present the purposes and scope of the literature review, as well as the criteria for evaluating a literature review in a research report.

OVERVIEW

The literature review can be defined as an extensive, exhaustive, systematic, and critical examination of publications relevant to the research project (Seaman and Verhonick, 1982). As such, the literature review begins with locating as many relevant materials as possible and ends with writing a critical summary of the available knowledge.

By reviewing the literature the researcher hopes to accomplish two main goals: (1) identifying and becoming familiar with all of the relevant published material and (2) composing this foundation so that it puts this study into the context of all of the previous research. These overall goals of the literature review are accomplished through the following five specific purposes of the review (Fox, 1982):

1. To develop the theoretical framework for the study. This aspect of the literature review is discussed in detail in the next chapter. Primarily based on the conceptual literature, the development of the theoretical framework for the study is especially important for the development of nursing and nursing research, because it allows for the findings of research studies to contribute to the development of nursing theory. For this outcome to be possible, researchers must demonstrate familiarity with all points of view in the field, not just with those that support their personal notions. It is particularly important that researchers distinguish between summaries of the work of others and their own views.

2. To understand the status of research in the problem area. This is the most familiar purpose of the literature review. Here the researcher reviews the data-based literature and the reports of studies conducted in the area of interest. This step clarifies the gaps in our current understanding of a problem and helps to identify how this proposed research will fit into the study of the larger problem area. To understand the depth of this step the researcher should realize that the following five basic questions must be answered:

- *When* was this problem studied?
- *What* has been studied about this problem?
- *Where* has this problem been investigated?
- *Who* has been studied?
- *What* is known about this problem?

The answers to these five questions give the researcher an overall picture of the work that has been done in the topic area to date. Students who are new to the research process often ask how far back the literature review should go. This is not an easy question to answer. The basic decision depends on how much literature is new in an area and how much is older. If the researcher finds that there is nothing in the recent literature, then she must go as far back as necessary to give a complete picture of what is known about the problem area, and the literature review might span 20 to 30 years. If, on the other hand, the topic is a new area of inquiry, the review may span only a few years. The only way the researcher knows the answer to this question is to continue to go back in the literature until no new information is found.

3. To provide clues to methodology and instrumentation. The third purpose of the literature review answers the following important question:

- *How* has this problem been studied in the past?

This aspect of the literature review shows the researcher what has and has not been tried in regard to approaches and methods and what types of data-gathering instruments exist.

4. To estimate the potential for success of the proposed study. Having reviewed the work of others in the problem area, the researcher needs to assess at this stage whether or not the proposed study has potential for answering the research question. This assessment is based on the success others have had in studying the problem and the usefulness of their findings. As discussed in Chapter 3, the researcher has an ethical and legal obligation not to proceed with a study that has no potential for success. Therefore the nurse must be willing to abandon or change the proposed research at this point so that subjects are not enrolled in a useless study.

5. To serve as a sounding board. Finally, the literature review helps the researcher to know when the problem has been specified enough. The researcher knows that a problem is well specified when certain papers are clearly related to the problem and others are not directly related. Until the researcher can make this distinction, the review is not complete and the problem has not been specified enough. In other words, the literature discriminates which variables are important to the present investigation and which variables can be ignored for the contemplated study.

A recent paper by Mercer, Nichols, and Doyle (1988) is an excellent illustration of the use of conceptual and data-based literature to support a study. These authors studied the life histories of mothers and nonmothers to identify differences in developmental trajectories over the life cycle. In their introduction they present an overview of the theoretical concepts underlying the study by defining and reviewing the concepts of transitions, developmental change, and developmental processes. They expand on these conceptual definitions in the "Relevant Literature" section of their paper by providing a summary of the previous research on women's developmental transitions. The literature also provides support for the researchers' choice of measurement techniques. The use of the literature review for Purposes 4 and 5 above are less obvious, but the reader can assume that the authors also accomplished these purposes, because the study was successful and the problem for study was well specified.

These purposes of the literature review and how they fit with the research process will become clearer as we study how a literature review is conducted. The process of conducting such a review is delineated so that you can assess the adequacy of a published review. You will need to see these steps reflected in the studies that you critique. In addition, the steps may be useful to you when writing term papers, care plans, and clinical reports.

HOW THE LITERATURE REVIEW IS CONDUCTED

As with any written work, the author of a research paper needs to define the scope of the problem to be addressed. For researchers, this step is the identification of the relevant **concepts, constructs,** and **variables** to be included in the review. This step goes hand-in-hand with the specification of the research problem discussed in the previous chapter. For instance, a researcher may be interested in the general problem of stress. One could undertake a review of the massive literature on stress from a number of angles, such as the physiology of the stress response, the effect of a particular stressful event such as hospitalization, or the effect of social support on people undergoing stressful experiences. If the problem is quite broad to begin with, the researcher may use the literature review to narrow the scope of the problem to one that is manageable. In so doing the researcher begins to define the important concepts and variables that need to be addressed.

If, on the other hand, the researcher comes to the literature review stage with a well-formulated problem that states all of the relevant variables and defines them, the literature review is already outlined.

Either way, the researcher needs to identify the related literature. Usually this is done by starting with the broad topic being studied and reading summary papers or reviews written by experts in the field. In this initial step the researcher becomes familiar with the previous research in the area and the views of others working in the area. Summary papers may be found in books or journals. Thus the logical place to begin a literature search is in the card catalog of the library, looking under the topic area in question. For example, a researcher interested in some aspect of stress would look under "Stress" in the card catalog. If the topic is a well-studied one such as stress, many listings may be found and the process of refining the problem begins. Suppose the researcher has decided to study the problem of social support and stress; all of the books dealing with stress physiology would not be relevant and thus would not need to be reviewed. If books existed on social support and stress, the researcher would begin the review by reading them carefully to get an understanding of the major views on this problem.

By now you may be getting a mental picture of a researcher sitting in the library surrounded by books written on the chosen topic and are wondering how the researcher can keep it all straight. The age-old method of keeping bibliography cards is priceless in this regard. Bibliography cards can be quite detailed or they may merely provide notes to jog the memory about the piece reviewed. All cards should contain the following information: bibliographic information, including authors' names, title of the book or article, publication information, and a summary of the major points made in the work. Keeping bibliography cards allows the researcher to know what literature has already been consulted, whether it was useful or not, and the appropriate sources to be cited when writing the research report.

Books provide only one source of literature. Since books are usually summaries of previous theory and research in an area, they provide a foundation for building the conceptual framework of the research. However, books take longer to publish than journal articles and so their information is sometimes not up to date. In addition, books do not usually provide in-depth reports of individual research projects and thus cannot provide the data-based literature needed to build an understanding of the status of research in a specific problem area.

The search for published articles dealing with a specific problem begins by using either literature indexes or computerized data bases. Both serve the purpose of identifying articles dealing with the topic of interest. Several such indexes exist and help in the search. The most commonly used indexes in nursing research are listed in the box on p. 82. An index is a list of articles, by topics. Computerized data bases are also lists of published articles cross-referenced by author and subject, but these are available on-line rather than in hard copies in the library (see Chapter 18). As more bibliographic indexes are computerized and made available and as more individuals have access to microcomputers, more literature searches will begin with computerized data bases. Such literature searching can be more expedient than a traditional search through multiple hardbound indexes. When used well, microcomputer-based bibliographic searching can provide a high-quality, customized list of citations. This list can be the foundation of the literature review (Smith, 1988).

Indexes Commonly Used in Nursing Research

Nursing Indexes

1. *The International Nursing Index*

This index references articles from more than 200 nursing journals and nursing articles from more than 2000 nonnursing journals. References are listed alphabetically by author and subject and cover articles beginning with 1966.

2. *The Nursing Studies Index*

This annotated guide to reported studies, research methods, and historical and biographical materials covers English periodicals, books, and pamphlets. This index includes nursing literature for the period 1900 to 1959.

3. *The Nursing Research Index*

This index appears annually in the last issue of *Nursing Research* and contains alphabetical listings of research studies published in the last year by author and subject.

4. *Computerized Index of Nursing and Allied Health Literature (CINAHL)*

This computerized data base provides subject/author access to all English-language nursing journals and to journals from the medical and behavioral sciences.

Nonnursing Indexes

1. *Cumulative Index Medicus*

This index includes more than 2000 biomedical journals published worldwide as well as several nursing journals. Entries are listed alphabetically by author and subject.

2. *The Social Science Citation Index*

This index covers all areas of the social sciences and includes more than 1000 social science journals, from history and economics to sociology. Many topics included are relevant to areas of nursing research.

3. *The Science Citation Index*

This index covers the technological and scientific references that may be useful in physiologic research in nursing.

4. *The Educational Resources Information Center (ERIC)*

ERIC publishes a monthly index called *The Current Index to Journals in Education* that references articles by subject and author from more than 500 journals. Authors dealing with nursing education or client education might find this index useful.

5. *Psychological Abstracts*

This index publishes abstracts of more than 120 books and 800 journals yearly in the fields of psychology and behavioral science.

Whether generated by hand or by computer, the researcher eventually acquires a list of relevant articles. The task then is to locate and critically review these papers so that the researcher becomes totally familiar with all points of view in the problem area. The list may include both primary sources and secondary sources. **Primary sources,** for example, are first-hand accounts, research reports written by the researcher, or client records. **Secondary sources** are at least once removed from the primary author. Common secondary sources include summaries of research studies, textbooks, and biographies. Whereas secondary sources are useful in guiding the researcher to all of the relevant work in the chosen area, literature reviews should be built chiefly on primary sources, because secondary sources may be contaminated by the bias of the individual writing the summary. Since the purpose of the literature review is to place the study in the context of previous work, it should be as unbiased as possible.

Having read and summarized the conceptual and data-based literature available on a certain problem area, the researcher writes the review, clarifying for the reader what has been studied about the problem in the past, how it has been studied, and who has been studied. In addition, the review should make clear what is known about the problem or what is assumed to be known, what is not known, and how this particular piece of research will help to answer what is not known. The written literature review should take the reader from the general problem area to the specific hypotheses or research questions studied in the piece of research presented. The reader should be provided with an understanding of the researchers' thoughts from defining the problem to presenting the study findings.

ORGANIZATION OF THE LITERATURE REVIEW

Both beginning researchers and readers of research articles are often troubled by questions about the depth and breadth of the literature review. How broad the review needs to be depends on a number of factors. One factor is the length of the report. Journal editors usually require the literature review to be brief so the report can concentrate on the findings of the particular study. The nature of the problem itself may dictate how many peripherally related studies need to be addressed. A problem that has been heavily studied may require the researcher to be familiar with many articles, each directly relevant to the problem. On the other hand, a new problem that has not been extensively studied may require the researcher to become familiar with articles that are only peripherally related to the problem so that a meaningful framework can be developed. The question of depth is also determined by the relevance of the article to the stated problem. In general the more closely the article is related to the problem, the more detail needs to be presented. Studies that are indirectly related are often summarized quite briefly.

As with any written work, the organization of the literature review is of paramount importance. The review is written so that the development of the major concepts for study is made explicitly clear to the reader. Thus the literature review should include an introduction, a summary of the related literature, and a summary of the current knowledge of the problem. Usually the researcher begins with the broader topic area and progressively limits the problem to the one being studied with more detailed summaries of previous work in the area. The review should organize and summarize the literature so that it is clear to the reader how the researcher chose to study this particular aspect of a problem. Often the review of the literature is organized by variables of importance to the study. Thus the researcher may introduce the independent variable and summarize the literature relevant to it, then outline the dependent variables of interest and what is known about their relationship to the independent variable, and finally discuss any antecedent or intervening variables of importance. The summary of the literature would then indicate what the proposed relationships among these variables would be expected to be on the basis of the previous work in the field.

Researchers may present the literature as a written history that reflects the progress of knowledge in a problem area over time. In such reports the authors begin with the earliest research in the field and summarize for the reader how the research has progressed to the present study. This approach is often used when a group of researchers has carried out a program of research over several years.

Another approach to presenting the literature review is illustrated in the paper by Kunnel, O'Brien, Hazard Munro, and Medoff-Cooper (1988) (Appendix C). This commonly used method for organizing the review of relevant literature focuses on each relevant concept in turn. In this paper, for example, the authors discuss the literature related to the importance of newborn body temperature, site of measurement, and measuring time. They conclude with a discussion of the conflicts in the literature and the need for further data. Note that the review does not merely summarize the previous work; rather, the review is critical of the previous work, which allows the researchers to draw conclusions about the state of knowledge.

Some journals require the literature review to be incorporated into the discussion section. In such cases a brief introduction supports the extent and nature of the problem studied. The bulk of the research literature is presented in the discussion section, where the author can compare present results with previous findings. This approach allows the author to be more concise and places the emphasis in the paper on the results of the present study and their interpretation.

In any case, the reader should be able to pick out contradictions and inconsistencies in the previous research findings that led to the present study. It should also be clear to the reader that the researcher has not merely reported the results of previous studies but has applied their findings to the current work. This application of findings to the present study allows the researcher to be critical of previous work. By critical, we do not mean "picky," but we mean capable of determining the worth of the studies.

Although it is important that the literature review reflect the author's views on the topic as they relate to the literature available in the problem area, it is equally important that the review be objective. In other words, reports of studies that contradict the author's hypothesis should not be omitted; rather, such studies should be analyzed for the potential reasons for these discrepancies. Often these discrepancies form the basis of further research in an area.

Critiquing Criteria

1. What type of report is this? If it is abridged, the literature review is likely to be brief.
2. Does the review of the literature follow immediately after the introduction and the statement of the problem?
3. Are all relevant concepts and variables included in the review?
4. Does the review follow a logical sequence leading to the summary of the current knowledge of the problem?
5. Is there a summary of the literature reviewed, the gaps in current knowledge about the problem, and how this study intends to fill in those gaps?
6. Are both conceptual literature and data-based literature included?
7. Are the sources for the literature review mostly primary or mostly secondary sources?
8. Can you follow the logic of the author in building the literature review?
9. Is there evidence that the review is unbiased?

CRITIQUING THE LITERATURE REVIEW

Evaluating a literature review is a difficult task. To a certain extent it is difficult to evaluate a review if the reader is not familiar with the topic studied. However, there are several areas to consider when reading literature reviews in published research reports. Criteria for evaluating the literature review are summarized in the box above.

The first area to consider is the type of report. We have said that journals frequently require literature reviews to be brief and to the point. Thus the reviews found in journal articles are likely to be condensed. It is useful to page through the rest of the journal where the current article is found. Is this review similar to others? If so, the brevity of the review may reflect the requirements of the journal. If the report is a dissertation or thesis, the reader should expect that the literature review will be complete and cover all relevant areas.

Next, the reader should determine if the literature review follows immediately after the introduction. Since the purpose of the literature review is to place the current work in the context of previous work, the review should follow the statement of the problem. In addition, this placement allows the reader to follow precisely the thinking of the researcher in the development of the specific hypotheses within the problem area.

Since the literature review's purpose is to inform the reader to what extent the researcher has placed the current investigation in the context of previous work, this thinking should be reflected in what is read. A good review builds a case for the need

Table 5-1 **Excerpt from a Weak Literature Review and How to Improve It**

Weak	Better
Goebel et al. (1984) studied the effectiveness of a postpartum educational program on infant car seat usage. Excerpts from their review are as follows:	Blouse et al.* demonstrated in a survey that parents feel that using safety belts for children is too much work.
"Some parents say it is too much work to use safety belts for children. . . .	"Since previous work by Truck* has shown that a child's weight is multiplied 10 to 20 times during the impact of an automobile accident, it is clear that even the strongest parent will not be able to restrain an infant sitting in the parent's lap.
"Even the strongest parents cannot safely restrain an infant sitting in the parent's lap. . . .	
"In addition to the safety of the child, the parents' psychological comfort is another incentive for the use of car seats."	"Other studies have suggested that the use of child restraints will increase the parents' psychological comfort."

*These references are fictitious.

for this study to be conducted in light of what has previously been accomplished and how this study will extend current knowledge of the problem area. It should be very clear what the researcher is accepting as true for this study on the basis of previous work in the area. It should be equally clear what areas the researcher considers to be in need of further research. The specific study in question should then be designed around these gaps in current knowledge. In addition, if the study relates explicitly to a particular theory, that relationship should be stated.

Another purpose of the review is to demonstrate to the reader that the researcher is familiar with *all* points of view in the topic area. The complete review covers all conceptual and data-based literature that is directly relevant to the specific problem under study. If, because of space restrictions, the review needs to be summarized, the reader should expect that this is reflected in the report. As much as possible, the sources referred to should be primary sources, rather than secondary sources. Table 5-1 illustrates how a written literature review should reflect the studies cited and how the importance of the study should be based on previous data and not the opinion of the researcher.

Finally, the literature review should be judged by how well it shows the need for this study to have been conducted. It should be quite obvious to the reader exactly what the gaps in knowledge are and how this study intends to contribute to filling in the gaps. This criterion requires that the review be written in a logical sequence, flowing from the general problem to the specific problem, and finally providing justification for the hypotheses generated.

Critiquing a literature review is difficult, but the reader should be able to see how the researcher built the study based on the previous work in the topic area. If there are areas that are not addressed or if the review seems biased to the researcher's point of view, the review may be considered to be deficient. Since it is important that all research build on previous work, this step of the research process is critical to the overall worth of the study.

Example of critique of a literature review

The paper by Brooten, Kumar, Brown, Butts, Finkler, Bakewell-Sachs, Gibbons, and Delivoria-Papadopoulos (1986) (Appendix A) provides an excellent example of the use of the literature and one common method of presenting the literature review. The first paragraph of the paper clearly presents the problem under study—that infants of low birth weight are at high risk for multiple problems, including prolonged hospitalization and rehospitalization. Previous research on the extent of the problem is used to support the need for the research.

Although it is brief, the literature review discusses each of the relevant concepts under study: home care, hospitalization, failure to thrive, foster placement, and cost. The review is clear in its progression from problem of low birth weight to testing an approach to dealing with these infants in a cost-effective manner. The literature cited is primarily data based and from primary sources. There is no evidence of bias.

SUMMARY

The purpose of this chapter was to introduce the student to the process of the literature review so that the student can critically evaluate published research.

The literature review was defined as an extensive, exhaustive, systematic, and critical examination of publications relevant to the research project. Such literature reviews utilize both conceptual and databased literature in the problem area. Reviews may utilize both primary and secondary sources but should arise mostly from primary sources.

The literature review helps the researcher to identify and become familiar with all relevant published material in the problem area and to write this foundation so that the review places the study in the context of all previous research in the area. The literature review also serves the following five specific purposes: to develop the conceptual framework for the study, to understand the status of research in the problem area, to provide clues to methodology and instrumentation, to estimate the potential for success of the proposed study, and to serve as a sounding board.

The chapter also presented information on how a literature search is conducted and written. This information on commonly used indexes relevant to nursing research was presented so that the student can begin to judge whether all the necessary steps are reflected in the written report.

Finally, suggestions for critically reading the review of the literature are given. In addition, examples of statements from one review and recommendations for change are given.

References

Brooten, D., Kumar, S., Brown, L.P., Butts, P., Finkler, S.A., Bakewell-Sachs, S., Gibbons, A., and Delivoria-Papadopoulos, M. (1986). A randomized clinical trial of early hospital discharge and home follow-up of very-low-birth-weight infants, *New England Journal of Medicine,* **315:**934-939.

Fox, D. (1982). *Fundamentals of research in nursing,* Norwalk, Conn., Appleton-Century-Crofts.

Goebel, J.B., Copps, T.J., and Sulayman, R.F. (1984). Infant car seat usage: effectiveness of a postpartum educational program, *Journal of Obstetric and Gynecological Nursing,* **13:**33-36.

Kunnel, M.T., O'Brien, C., Hazard Munro, B., and Medoff-Cooper, B. (1988). Comparisons of rectal, femoral, axillary, and skin-to-mattress temperatures in stable neonates, *Nursing Research,* **37:**162-164, 189.

Mercer, R.T., Nichols, E.G., and Doyle, G.C. (1988). Transitions over the life cycle: a comparison of mothers and nonmothers, *Nursing Research,* **37:**144-151.

Seaman, C.C.H., and Verhonick, P.J. (1982). *Research methods for undergraduate students in nursing,* Norwalk, Conn., Appleton-Century-Crofts.

Smith, L.W. (1988). Micro-computer-based bibliographic searching, *Nursing Research,* **37:** 125-127.

6

The Theoretical Framework

Harriet R. Feldman

LEARNING OBJECTIVES

After reading this chapter the student should be able to do the following:

- Identify the purpose and nature of a theoretical framework.
- Describe the process involved in developing a theoretical framework.
- Contrast the borrowed versus new theory approaches in the development of nursing science.
- Formulate conceptual and operational definitions.
- Describe how a theoretical framework guides research.
- Identify how hypotheses are generated.
- Define nursing theory.
- Identify the phenomena of concern to nursing.
- Describe the points of critical appraisal used to evaluate the appropriateness, cohesiveness, and consistency of a theoretical framework.

A theoretical framework is analogous to the frame of a house. Just as the foundation supports a house, a theoretical framework provides a foundation and rationale for predictions about the relationship between variables of a research study. This chapter addresses the nature and purpose of a theoretical framework in a research study and shows how to develop and critique a theoretical framework. The following definitions serve as a guide to the ensuing discussion of these topics.

DEFINITION OF A THEORY

Theory has been defined in a number of ways. For example, Chinn and Jacobs (1987, p. 2) say theory is a "systematic abstraction of reality that serves some purpose." They describe each part of the definition as follows: *Systematic* implies a specific organizational pattern, *abstraction* means that theory is a representation of reality, and *purposes* include description, explanation, and prediction of phenomena and control of some reality. Kerlinger's definition of theory is perhaps the one most widely used. It takes a basic view of science; that is, the development of general explanations about natural phenomena via theories. To be more precise, Kerlinger (1986) states that "a theory is a set of interrelated constructs (concepts), definitions, and propositions that present a systematic view of phenomena by specifying relations among variables, with the purpose of explaining and predicting the phenomena" (p. 9). Included in this definition, as in the one developed by Chinn and Jacobs (1987), are abstraction, expressed in the term **construct,** a systematic process, and a statement of purpose.

DEFINITION OF A THEORETICAL FRAMEWORK

A *theoretical framework* provides a context for examining a problem; that is, the theoretical *rationale* for developing hypotheses, just as a direction indicator on a compass (N-S-E-W) provides a context for using a road map. It is also a frame of reference that is a base for observations, definitions of variables, research designs, interpretations, and generalizations, much the same way that the frame that rests on a foundation defines the overall design of a house. Finally, a theoretical framework serves as a guide to systematically identifying a logical, precisely defined relationship between variables. Suppose a nurse researcher were interested in studying interven-

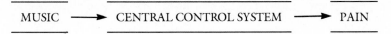

Fig. 6-1   Inventory of relationship between music and pain.

tions for reducing postoperative pain in patients with cholecystectomies and found out through a search of the literature that pain perception can be altered by distraction. The nurse might study the use of a distractor (for example, music) for these patients. Thus she would be studying the relationship between music and postoperative pain in these patients. The theoretical framework of this study of the relationship between two variables, music and postoperative pain, is the gate control theory of pain (Melzack and Wall, 1965), which says that pain can be affected by altering such pain-inhibiting mechanisms as a central control system in the cerebral cortex. Distraction can alter this inhibiting mechanism by overriding the competitive sensation of pain. Fig. 6-1 illustrates this theoretical relationship.

When an investigator reports research, he or she is obliged to clearly state the theoretical basis for hypothesis formulation (which is the researcher's prediction about the outcome of the study), study findings, and outcome interpretations. As in the analogy previously presented, each piece of lumber that comprises the frame of the house must be connected to another piece, as in the relationship between two or more variables. The frame must rest squarely on a solid foundation, just as the relationship between two variables rests firmly on a theoretical framework. The "fit" must be precise or the house will fall; similarly, the theoretical fit must be precise or the prediction made about the relationship between the variables will in all likelihood not be supported through testing of the **hypothesis.**

HOW TO USE A THEORETICAL FRAMEWORK AS A GUIDE IN A RESEARCH STUDY

The theoretical framework of a research study places the problem in a theoretical context, bringing meaning to the problem and study findings. It summarizes the existing knowledge in the field of inquiry and identifies the linkages among the **concepts,** thereby establishing a basis for predicting specific outcomes or generating hypotheses (Fig. 6-2). These linkages or **propositions** spell out how defined concepts are interrelated, and they lay a foundation for the development of methods that test the validity and strength of identified relationships or hypotheses. The examples that follow will clarify how theory guides the research process.

Suppose you were interested in alternatives to medication for the treatment of postoperative pain. An examination of the literature might lead you to relaxation training as an intervention. The following series of questions might occur to you:

⋄ On what basis has a linkage between pain and relaxation been established?
⋄ What is the nature of the linkage?
⋄ How can this linkage or relationship be tested?
⋄ What methods can be used for the purpose of testing?

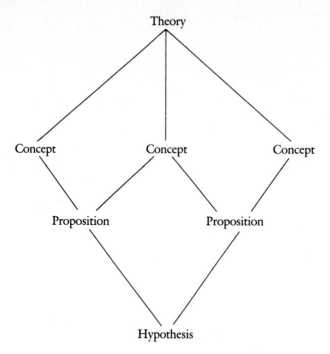

Fig. 6-2   Process of hypothesis generation.

To answer these questions you must begin by exploring a theoretical framework that is suitable for pursuing the research problem. Either a nursing or nonnursing theory can provide a frame to guide the way toward developing hypotheses.

Wells (1982) examined the relationship between relaxation and postoperative pain. In establishing a theoretical explanation for linking these variables, she alluded to the gate control theory of pain, citing two components of the pain experience, physiological and psychological, and the interaction of these components. Citing Melzack and Wall (1965, p. 236), she stated, "The physiological component involves adequate stimulus initiating neural transmission to higher centers in the brain. Localization and integration with motivational and affective input occurs in the cortical and sub-cortical structures. Descending control from the higher centers alters the transmission of additional impulses from the periphery." She further stated that the "psychological component involves the interaction of many factors: focus of attention; coping style; cultural background; previous experience with pain; anxiety; and perceived control" (p. 236). Specific aspects of the postoperative pain experience for adult patients with cholecystectomies, such as abdominal muscle tension and neural input from structures affected by the incision, were identified. In describing the relaxation response she referred to both physiological and psychological effects of this technique. She explicitly concluded that "a relaxation technique applied to postoperative pain may reduce the physiological input due to secondary reflex muscle

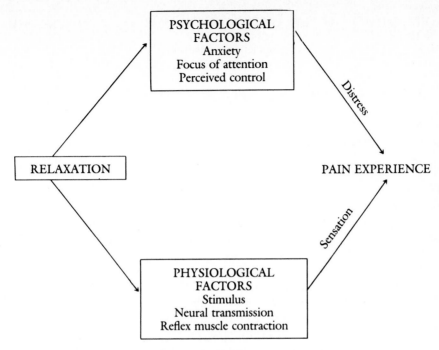

Fig. 6-3   Inventory of relationship between relaxation and pain.

contraction as well as alter the psychological variables of focus of attention, anxiety, and perceived control" (p. 236).

Fig. 6-3 illustrates the linkage between the proposed independant variable (relaxation), and dependant variable (pain), showing that by influencing certain psychological and physiological components of the pain experience, that experience could be altered. Taking this rationale a step further the following hypotheses can be generated:

1. Clients who practice a relaxation technique will experience reduced postoperative muscle tension in involved muscle groups as compared with clients who do not practice a relaxation technique.

2. Clients who practice a relaxation technique will experience reduced intensity of postoperative pain as compared with clients who do not practice a relaxation technique.

3. Clients who practice a relaxation technique will experience reduced postoperative pain distress as compared with clients who do not practice a relaxation technique.

4. Clients who practice a relaxation technique will report reduced postoperative anxiety.

The first hypothesis evolved from the theoretical linkage between relaxation and physiological factors associated with pain. The second and third hypotheses evolved from the theoretical physiological and psychological factors, respectively, associated

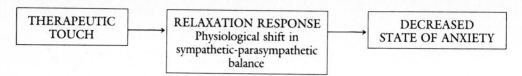

Fig. 6-4   Inventory of relationship between therapeutic touch and anxiety.

with pain. The fourth hypothesis evolved from the theoretical linkage between relaxation and psychological factors associated with pain.

Once hypotheses are generated they are tested. This involves selecting the individual subjects to participate in the study, using instruments that will validly and reliably measure the variables, developing a method of systematically collecting the information needed to test hypothesized relationships, and selecting statistical measures that will determine the extent and meaning or significance of the relationships. Furthermore the outcomes of the study must be viewed in terms of their support or nonsupport of the chosen theoretical rationale.

As you can see the theoretical framework plays an important role in guiding the entire process of the research study. If the framework is logically sound and substantiated by previous research studies, there is a strong possibility that the predictions or hypotheses evolving from that framework will be supported; however, if the hypotheses are not based firmly on a theoretical rationale, there can be no confidence in the findings. Research consumers must be able to identify the theoretical framework that was used and evaluate whether or not it is consistent with the concepts, definitions, and hypotheses stated by the investigator.

How the theoretical rationale provides a basis for hypothesis development in a research study may not always be made explicit in the research report. For example, Heidt (1981, p. 32), in her study of therapeutic touch and anxiety, pointed out "the potential of this intervention (therapeutic touch) for eliciting in the subject a state of physiological relaxation." She further discussed repatterning energy fields and the use of self therapeutically as two facets of therapeutic touch. Nowhere in the discussion of the theoretical background of the study did she state how therapeutic touch relates to anxiety reduction or how relaxation might form a connecting link between these two variables. Fig. 6-4 illustrates how this relationship might have been conceived. Study hypotheses were not explicitly substantiated in the investigator's presentation of the theoretical rationale, leaving theoretical interpretations to the reader.

In some cases the theoretical rationale is inappropriately used. For example, a theory designed to explain a particular behavior in infants may not be appropriate for the study of those behaviors in adults. Similarly, a theory developed from Rogers' (1970) interactive conceptual model is not appropriate for the study of cause-and-effect relationships. The inappropriate use of theory, aside from being logically unsound, can lead to erroneous conclusions about the problem being studied.

In other cases the theoretical rationale may be weak. For example, perhaps the theory was not sufficiently tested, the assumptions (see Chapter 2) were incompatible, the concepts were ill defined, or the terms were inconsistent with the theory.

PURPOSE OF HAVING A THEORETICAL FRAMEWORK IN A RESEARCH STUDY

You may be wondering why you need a theoretical framework in a research study. You may ask, "Why can't I just match any two variables that make sense to me and look at their relationship?" As an analogy, consider the first time you traveled by car to an unfamiliar place. How did you get to your destination? Did you use a map? Did you follow someone's directions? Did you stick to the prescribed route, or did you try a shortcut? Did you turn left instead of right because it seemed logical, or did you use known information to make that decision? The map served as a guide to your destination, and when conducting research a theoretical rationale serves as a guide or map to systematically identifying a logical, precisely defined relationship between variables. Other purposes of a theoretical rationale include providing clear descriptions of variables, suggesting ways or methods to conduct the study, and guiding the interpretation, evaluation, and integration of study findings.

HOW TO DEVELOP A THEORETICAL FRAMEWORK

Although in the role of research consumer you will not be expected to develop a theoretical framework, an understanding of the process will assist you in critiquing this aspect of a research study. Therefore the basis for and intricacies of developing a theoretical framework will be discussed; numerous examples are provided.

Selection of concepts

A *concept* is an image or symbolic representation of an abstract idea. It is formed by generalizing from particular characteristics. For example, health is a concept formed by generalizing from particular behaviors, such as being mobile, being free of infection, and communicating appropriately. Other concepts include pain, intelligence, weight, grieving, self-concept, and achievement. Concepts facilitate the delineation of ideas so that systematic inquiry can proceed. Some concepts are directly observable (such as a chair or rain) and others are indirectly observable (for example, anxiety or intelligence). A theoretical framework specifies the relationship between concepts in a study.

Since concepts are the basis for refining ideas and developing theory, it is important to select those concepts that clearly reflect the subject matter being pursued. In evaluating a piece of research, you must consider whether or not the concepts or variables as defined are examined both in general and specifically in the context of the problem under investigation (see Chapter 4). Furthermore consider if they are being measured with the appropriate instruments (see Chapter 14).

Identifying the interrelationships among concepts

In the process of examining the concepts or variables that guide the research effort, relationships emerge. For example, from a review of the literature in a particular area such as stress, information about related variables can be found (e.g., onset of illness, certain physiological responses, and learning ability). Relationships can also be identified through systematic observation and experience. A relationship may be invariable, tentative, or inconclusive. One type of invariable relationship is a scientific law; for example, Newton's three laws of motion. In this case no known contradiction has been observed. A tentative or inconclusive relationship is a hypothesis, which expresses a relationship between two or more variables and does not convey truth or falsity. Both laws and hypotheses are types of propositions (see Chapter 2).

The literature review is the part of the research report that generally specifies the theoretical rationale and should explicitly identify propositions in relation to the individual variables described. The hypotheses should express relationships between variables in an unambiguous, precise manner, and they should be based on the propositions that evolved from the theoretical framework (see Chapters 5 and 7).

Formulating definitions

As stated earlier, concepts are representations of abstract ideas. To develop a theoretical framework that can generate and test hypotheses, concepts must be clearly defined. If you think back to the earlier illustration about traveling to an unfamiliar place, how do you think you would have arrived if the directions simply read, "First you take one road, then turn at another, and proceed to three more roads?" Without a clear conception of which road to take, what direction to turn, and how far to proceed, you would probably get lost. The same process applies to any concept. For example, how would you define pain or anxiety or intelligence? In addition to knowing the names of the roads to travel, other specifics are clearly needed, such as what type of vehicle you will use, what town you will travel through, how you will know when you have arrived, and how far you will travel. These parameters delineate the procedure to follow by identifying what *operations* must occur to make the trip. When defining concepts for the purpose of systematic examination, you must include both conceptual and operational information.

Conceptual definitions

Concepts, no matter what their level of abstraction, must be defined as unambiguously as possible so that they can be easily communicated to others. Even the word *can* is open to varied interpretations; for example, "a container," "being able to," or a "commode." A *conceptual definition* conveys the general meaning of the concept, as does a dictionary definition. It reflects the theory used in the study of that concept. The following are examples of **conceptual definitions:**

> *Recovery:* the process of healing that takes place after an injury
> *Concept:* an image or symbolic representation of an abstract idea
> *Postoperative pain:* discomfort an individual experiences after a surgical procedure
> *Mothering:* " . . . an interaction between a human adult and a child that conveys a positive affect and is reciprocal in nature. The interaction involves reciprocal contact, touching, and vocalization" (Chinn and Jacobs, 1987, p. 103)
> *State anxiety:* "a transitional emotional state aroused in a situation that presents a perceived threat to self-integrity" (Mullooly, Levin, and Feldman, 1988, p. 5)

Since these are general definitions, they do not include an indication of how the concepts will be measured.

Operational definitions

Operationalization adds another dimension to the conceptual definition by delineating the procedures or operations required to measure the concept. It supplies the information needed to collect data on the problem being studied. Some concepts are easily defined in operational terms; for example, pulse can be measured numerically after finding the radial pulse and counting the number of beats or pulsations for a minute. Other concepts are more difficult to operationally define, such as anxiety, leaving it up to the investigator to locate and select an instrument that best measures the concept as defined. The following are examples of **operational definitions:**

> *Sensation pain rating:* the periodic self-report of the intensity of the sensation component of the pain experienced, by subjects using the Pilowsky and Kaufman (1965) visual analog scale
>
> *Extended skin-to-skin contact:* "at least half of the infant's naked body touching the mother's naked trunk for 15 minutes or more during the first hour following delivery" (Curry, 1982, p. 74)
>
> *Body attitude:* "individuals' general attitudes about the outward form and appearance of their bodies" (Drake, Verhulst, Fawcett, and Barger, 1988, p. 89), as measured by the Body Attitude Scale
>
> *Social support:* "a characteristic of the social situation that buffers the effect of stress on the health of the individual" (Northouse, 1988, p. 91), as measured by the Social Support Questionnaire

Each of these examples has a conceptual definition and at least one index of measurement that makes it operational. To summarize, an operational definition provides specificity and direction for the concept to guide the development of the research study. Once the concept is operationalized (made measurable), it is termed a *variable*, and at that point it begins to play a significant role in formulating the theoretical rationale. In the role of research consumer you are responsible for evaluating whether or not variables are clearly defined, both conceptually and operationally. If the meaning of the variable is vague or if the measurement used does not reflect the same meaning as the variable, comparisons of the research with the other investigations will not be valid and the research will be impossible to replicate.

Some research reports present conceptual definitions, followed in another section (e.g., methodology or instrumentation) by a description of measurement. Other reports present operational definitions; still others may present no definitions, leaving interpretations about the meaning of the variables to the reader. Of course, in the latter instance it is easy to get lost en route.

FORMULATING THE THEORETICAL RATIONALE

Through the literature review an investigator becomes aware of or confirms suspected theoretical connections between variables. For example, in reviewing the literature on stress Baillie, Norbeck, and Barnes (1988, p. 217) found that "of the variables that potentially mediate stress, social support has been studied most frequently." The literature review also uncovered the stress-buffering model of social support, which theoretically supported the hypothesis that "social support will have a buffering effect on the relationship between perceived caregiver stress and psychological distress" (p. 218). Another example concerns temperature-taking sites in neonates. Kunnel, O'Brien, Hazard Munro, and Medoff-Cooper (1988) probably decided to study different sites for temperature taking in neonates because of their clinical experience with the standard practice of temperature taking at the rectal site. Through their literature review they found that "the risk of rectal perforation associated with rectal temperature taking is increased in the neonate" (p. 162) because of a change in the colon's angle at a depth of 3 cm, and that "previous studies have failed to provide empirical data necessary to establish the most clinically satisfactory alternative site and the optimal time for measurement of the temperature" (p. 162). In the first example Baillie et al. used a deductive approach to studying the relationship between stress, social support, and psychological distress. They began with the concepts *stress* and *social support;* identified a model that links social support, as a stress buffer, with psychological distress; and derived a hypothesis about the relationship between the variables social support, stress, and psychological distress. In the second example Kunnel et al. used an inductive approach. A number of clinical observations served as the initial impetus for drawing conclusions (i.e., generating hypotheses about the determination of optimal temperature-taking sites in neonates).

In evaluating the formulation of the theoretical rationale you should be certain that the internal structures, such as concepts and their definitions, have clarity and continuity and that the approach to understanding phenomena, whether inductive or deductive, is logical. For example, you should evaluate the breadth and depth of the literature review, the presence or absence of unambiguous definitions of concepts and variables, and the advancement of a logical and explicit theoretical rationale firmly based on these structures.

BORROWED VERSUS NEW THEORY

When you develop a theoretical framework for nursing research studies, you acquire knowledge by two approaches. Either it is developed primarily in disciplines other than nursing and borrowed for the purpose of answering nursing questions, or it is derived by identifying and asking questions about phenomena that are unique to nursing. There are pros and cons to each approach, and these views will be briefly described.

To date, most nursing research has been based on theories borrowed from other disciplines. Phillips (1977, p. 4) sees this as a problem and states, "the process of borrowing theories and models from other disciplines has hampered nurses in learning how to ask questions which are of specific concern to nursing or in conceptualizing how the borrowed knowledge is to be used to generate theory to expand nursing science." Further concerns expressed by Feldman (1980, p. 87) are whether or not "such theories have been substantially supported in other disciplines" and whether or not they are "generalizable to nursing." The advantages of using a borrowed theory are that many of the theories of other disciplines are well developed and have been supported by substantial hypothesis testing, and that nursing science will be advanced if the overall research effort demonstrates the synthesis of borrowed knowledge to reflect a nursing focus.

Theories of learning and self-esteem can be used to illustrate how to "borrow" theories from other disciplines for the purpose of asking nursing questions. For example, theories of learning in adults take a self-directed approach. A nursing question that uses this theory is, "Do diabetic clients who use self-directed learning techniques perform foot care more frequently and more correctly than diabetic clients who do not use self-directed learning techniques?" As another example, self-esteem theory involves the evolution of a sense of identity so that the individual develops a self-evaluation; that is, in terms of approval/disapproval, adequate/inadequate, acceptable/unacceptable, and capable/incapable parameters. This self-evaluation is intended to influence interactions with others and with the environment. A nursing question that uses this theory is "What is the relationship between self-esteem and engagement in social interactions in the retired, older population?"

A case can be made for developing new theories that are unique to nursing. Having a knowledge base specifically created to reflect a nursing focus helps nursing define its uniqueness, hence its difference from other disciplines. Nursing theory development is in its infancy and is far from being refined and tested enough to be able to rely on its validity. The following are examples of theories derived from nursing models. Nursing research is currently being conducted to test their validity.

Orem's (1980) model of self-care has generated theories of self-care, self-care deficits, and nursing systems. King's (1981) model of personal, interpersonal, and social systems has generated a theory of goal attainment. Rogers' (1970) life process, interactive person-environment model has generated a theory of "integrality." These theories contribute to the development of nursing as a unique scientific discipline. Other examples were presented in Chapter 2. In contrast, you may wonder if all of nursing's knowledge base should be unique. You may ask if it is useful even to have such a base. Answers to these questions are controversial, and you are referred to the readings of Johnson (1968), Phillips (1977), Feldman (1980), and Fawcett (1983) for various perspectives.

To summarize, the development of borrowed and new theories is evidence of the growth of nursing science. The contributions based on borrowed theories are most appropriate when data are related specifically to nursing; new theories based on nursing models are steadily increasing. As a consumer of nursing research it is important for you to evaluate the theoretical rationale of research studies in terms of relevance to nursing. You should ask if the investigator states the relevance of the problem to nursing, if the borrowed theories and the reported studies from other disciplines are related to nursing data, and if the findings are related to nursing; that is, nursing practice, nursing education, and/or nursing administration.

THE CONTRIBUTION OF NURSING MODELS TO RESEARCH

In the previous discussion of *borrowed versus new theory*, it was pointed out that theories unique to nursing help nursing define how it is different from other disciplines. Nursing theories reflect particular views of the person, health, and other concepts that contribute to the development of a body of knowledge specific to nursing's concerns. But what is *nursing* theory? What are nursing's phenomena of concern? Where do nursing theories originate if they are not borrowed from other disciplines?

Fawcett (1978, p. 25) defines *nursing theory* as "a set of propositions consisting of defined and interrelated units which presents a systematic view of the person, the environment, health, and nursing by specifying relations among relevant variables." The phenomena of concern to nursing are the person, the environment, health, and nursing. Therefore theories that deal with these phenomena are termed *nursing theories*. These phenomena, as stated, are not conceptualized or operationalized. Clearly, terms must be defined before relationships among them can be specified. The next logical question is "How are these phenomena defined?" The *person* for example can be viewed as active or waiting to be acted upon, inherently good or inherently bad, as an energy field (Rogers, 1970), or as an integrated whole (Orem, 1971). The answer to the question of defining phenomena lies in the *conceptual models* that form the bases for constructing nursing theories.

"A conceptual model is a highly abstract umbrella of related multidimensional concepts . . . [It] provides a perspective for a science, telling the scientist what to look at" (Fawcett, 1978, pp. 18-19). A conceptual model is developed inductively, by use of unsystematic observations, intuition, and other unstructured approaches. Theoretical models, on the other hand, postulate relationships based on available theories, empirical research findings, and other structured approaches.

Several well-known conceptual models in nursing have served as a basis for theory development. Among them are Rogers' (1970) life process interactive person-environment model; King's (1980) model of personal, interpersonal, and social systems; Orem's (1980) model of self-care; and Roy's (1984) adaptation model. Each of these models addresses the four phenomena of concern to nursing but from different perspectives. For example, Rogers' conceptual model views the person and the environment as energy fields coextensive with the universe; that is, person-environment interactions are mutual and simultaneous. King's conceptual model, however, views the person and the environment as separate and views interactions as cause-and-effect processes.

You may wonder how these conceptual models actually guide the research effort. The following description should clarify this process. Rogers' (1970) conceptual framework guided Goldberg and Fitzpatrick (1980) in their use of movement therapy with aged clients. Based on the concept of the person as "a holistic being whose interaction with the environment changes the state of being" (p. 339), Goldberg and Fitzpatrick described movement therapy as a positive integrating force or an integrated and holistic intervention. This intervention was proposed to be associated with positive changes in self-esteem, morale, agitation, attitude toward the individual's own aging, and lonely dissatisfaction. Study hypotheses, methods used to measure the variables such as self-esteem and morale, and the procedure for collecting data about the variables were based on Rogers' interactive framework. Among other findings, Goldberg and Fitzpatrick reported for the group who received movement therapy a significant improvement in total morale and attitude toward clients' own aging. It was concluded that movement therapy is a holistic, effective nursing intervention that adds support to the validity of Rogers' conceptual framework.

With this background on what nursing models are, what the phenomena of concern to nursing are, and how nursing theories develop, we can summarize the contribution of a nursing model to research. Chapter 2 focused on the scientific approach to the research process, including the philosophy of science, the sources of human knowledge, and the characteristics of the scientific approach. The development of nursing knowledge was said to depend on both philosophy and science. Additionally, the individual researcher's own philosophy of human behavior and other related phenomena was said to guide the intent of the research effort. Similarly, a nursing conceptual model serves as the philosophical view of specific phenomena of concern to nursing, from which nursing theories originate. As such, it is instrumental in guiding the nursing research effort.

CRITIQUING THE THEORETICAL FRAMEWORK

The criteria for critiquing a theoretical framework are found in the box on p. 104. The theoretical framework provides the context that clarifies and specifies problems, develops and tests hypotheses, evaluates research findings, and makes generalizations. As research consumers it is important for nurses to know how to critically appraise both the conceptual and theoretical bases for research. The following discussion is intended to assist you in this process.

Initially, you will probably focus on the concepts being studied. Concepts should clearly reflect the area of investigation. Using the general concept of stress when anxiety is more appropriate to the research focus creates difficulties in defining variables and delineating hypotheses.

Next, you must evaluate the completeness and appropriateness of the operational definitions of each concept. Once they are defined, you must consider whether or not the variables are examined in general and specifically in the context of the problem under investigation. The literature review is the source for this kind of discussion.

Finally, it is important to appraise the instruments used to measure the variables in terms of appropriateness. Does the instrument measure the variables as defined and is the instrument consistent with the theoretical framework? How do the instruments hold up when compared with other instruments? Are all of the subparts consistently measuring the same characteristics? Do the instruments maintain their stability when repeatedly used over time?

A second aspect of appraising the theoretical rationale relates to the interrelationships among concepts, or *hypotheses*. Briefly stated, hypotheses should express relationships between variables precisely and unambiguously. They should be based on the propositions that come from the theoretical framework and should directly answer

Critiquing Criteria

1. Is there evidence of a conceptual framework?
2. Is the theoretical framework clearly identified?
3. Is the conceptual framework consistent with what is being studied?
4. Are the concepts clearly and operationally defined?
5. Does the operationalization adequately reflect each conceptual definition?
6. Was sufficient literature reviewed to support the proposed relationships?
7. Is the theoretical basis for hypothesis formulation clearly articulated? Is it logical?
8. Are the relationships among propositions clearly stated?
9. Is the conceptual framework consistent throughout; that is, is the basic philosophical view of the phenomena of concern maintained throughout the study?
10. If the theory is borrowed from a discipline other than nursing, are the data related specifically to nursing?
11. Are the study findings related to the theoretical rationale?

the research problem identified early in the report. A more detailed discussion of critiquing hypotheses appears in Chapter 7.

When you evaluate the theoretical framework itself, it is important to examine both the depth and breadth of the literature review. Has the investigator included sufficient information "so that the reader could be assured that the investigator had considered a broad spectrum of possibilities for investigating the problem" (Downs and Newman, 1977, p. 4)? Is there consistency throughout in terms of the philosophical view of phenomena? Are previous studies sufficiently described so that their validity can be determined? Is there a firm basis for linking the variables and determining the direction of hypotheses? Can the theory be empirically tested? Does the research contribute to the understanding of the phenomena of interest? Are the findings discussed in relation to the theoretical framework? In summary, you must evaluate whether or not the theoretical framework or the map led you to your findings of destination in a logical and systematic way.

SUMMARY

This chapter provides information about the nature and purpose of a theoretical framework. It addresses the relationship between theory and research, emphasizing the importance of theory as a guide to systematically identify and study the logical, precise relationships between variables.

A concept is an image or symbolic representation of an abstract idea. Concepts help us refine the ideas that form the basis for developing theory. To facilitate the process of refinement, concepts must be clearly defined. Additionally, operationalization of the definitions serves to delineate the procedures or operations required to measure the concept.

Theory is defined as "a set of interrelated constructs, definitions, and propositions that present a systematic view of phenomena by specifying relations among variables, with the purpose of explaining and predicting the phenomena" (Kerlinger, 1986, p. 9). A theoretical rationale provides a road map or context for examining problems and developing and testing hypotheses. It brings meaning to the problem and study findings by summarizing existing knowledge in the field of inquiry and identifying linkages among concepts.

In developing a theoretical framework for nursing, knowledge may be acquired from other disciplines or directly from nursing. In either case, that knowledge is used to specifically answer nursing questions. Nursing conceptual models provide a context for constructing theories that deal with phenomena of concern to nursing; that is, the person, the environment, health, and nursing. They help nursing define how it is different from other disciplines.

Of significance to the research consumer is the evaluation or critique of the theoretical rationale of a research study. It is important to consider not only the clarity and logic of the theoretical rationale itself but whether or not the operational definitions, measurement instruments, and methods of carrying out collection of data about the variables, hypotheses, and findings are consistent with the theory.

References

Baillie, V., Norbeck, J., and Barnes, L. (1988). Stress, social support, and psychological distress of family caregivers of the elderly, *Nursing Research,* **37**:217-222.

Chinn, P., and Jacobs, M. (1987). *Theory and nursing: a systematic approach,* 2nd ed., St. Louis, The C.V. Mosby Co.

Cleland, V. (1967). The use of existing theories, *Nursing Research,* **16**:118-121.

Curry, M.A. (1982). Maternal attachment behavior and the mother's self-concept: the effect of early skin-to-skin contact, *Nursing Research,* **31**:73-78.

Downs, F., and Newman, M. (1977). *A sourcebook of nursing research,* 2nd ed., Philadelphia, F.A. Davis Co.

Drake, M., Verhulst, D., Fawcett, J., and Barger, D. (1988). Spouses' body image changes during and after pregnancy: a replication in Canada, *Image,* **20**:88-92.

Fawcett, J. (1978). The "what" of theory develop-

ment. In *Theory development: what, why, how?* New York, National League for Nursing.

Fawcett, J. (1983). Hallmarks of success in nursing theory development. In P. Chinn: *Advances in nursing theory development,* Rockville, Md., Aspen Systems Corp., pp. 3-17.

Feldman, H. (1980). Nursing research in the 1980s: issues and implications, *Advances in Nursing Science,* **3**:85-92.

Goldberg, W., and Fitzpatrick, J. (1980). Movement therapy with the aged, *Nursing Research,* **29**:339-346.

Heidt, P. (1981). Effects of therapeutic touch on anxiety level of hospitalized patients, *Nursing Research,* **30**:32-37.

Johnson, D. (1968). Theory in nursing: borrowed and unique, *Nursing Research,* **17**:206-209.

Kerlinger, F. (1986). *Foundations of behavioral research,* 2nd ed., New York, Holt, Rinehart & Winston, Inc.

King, I. (1981). *A theory for nursing: systems, concepts, process,* New York, John Wiley & Sons, Inc.

Kunnel, M., O'Brien, C., Hazard Munro, B., and Medoff-Cooper, B. (1988). Comparisons of rectal, femoral, axillary, and skin-to-mattress temperatures in stable neonates, *Nursing Research,* **37**:162-164.

Melzack, R., and Wall, P. (1965). Pain mechanisms: a new theory, *Science,* **150**:971-979.

Mullooly, V., Levin, R., and Feldman, H. (1988). Music for postoperative pain and anxiety, *Journal of the New York State Nurses Association,* **19**:4-7.

Newman, M. (1972). Nursing's theoretical revolution, *Nursing Outlook,* **20**:449-453.

Newman, M. (1977). Movement tempo and the experience of time. In F. Downs and M. Newman, eds.: *A sourcebook of nursing research,* 2nd ed., Philadelphia, F.A. Davis Co.

Northouse, L. (1988). Social support in patients' and husbands' adjustment to breast cancer, *Nursing Research,* **37**:91-95.

Orem, D. (1971). *Nursing: concepts of practice,* New York, McGraw-Hill Book Co.

Orem, D. (1980). *Nursing: concepts of practice,* 2nd ed., New York, McGraw-Hill Book Co.

Phillips, J. (1977). Nursing systems and nursing models, *Image,* **9**:4-7.

Pilowsky, I., and Kaufman, A. (1965). An experimental study of a typical phantom pain, *British Journal of Psychiatry,* **3**:1185-1187.

Rogers, M. (1970). *An introduction to the theoretical basis of nursing,* Philadelphia, F.A. Davis Co.

Roy, Sr., C. (1984). *Introduction to nursing: an adaptation model,* 2nd ed., Englewood Cliffs, N.J., Prentice-Hall, Inc.

Wells, N. (1982). The effect of relaxation on postoperative muscle tension and pain, *Nursing Research,* **31**:236-238.

Additional Readings

Benoliel, J. (1977). The interaction between theory and research, *Nursing Outlook,* **25**:108-113.

Ellis, R. (1968). Characteristics of significant theories, *Nursing Research,* **17**:217-222.

Fawcett, J. (1989). *Analysis and evaluation of conceptual models of nursing,* 2nd ed., Philadelphia, F.A. Davis Co.

Jacox, A. (1974). Theory construction in nursing: an overview, *Nursing Research,* **23**:4-13.

Leddy, S., and Pepper, M. (1985). *Conceptual bases of professional nursing,* Philadelphia, J.B. Lippincott Co.

National League for Nursing. (1978). *Theory development: what, why, how?* New York.

Newman, M. (1979). *Theory development in nursing,* Philadelphia, F.A. Davis Co.

Quint, J. (1967). The case for theories generated from empirical data, *Nursing Research,* **16**:109-114.

Walker, L. (1971). Toward a clearer understanding of nursing theory, *Nursing Research,* **20**:428-435.

7

The Hypothesis

Judith Haber

LEARNING OBJECTIVES

After reading this chapter the student should be able to do the following:

◇ Identify the characteristics of a hypothesis.

◇ Discuss the relationship of the hypothesis to the other research process components.

◇ Describe the advantages and disadvantages of directional and nondirectional hypotheses.

◇ Compare and contrast the use of statistical versus research hypotheses.

◇ Discuss the appropriate use of research questions in a research study.

◇ Formulate a hypothesis.

◇ Identify the criteria used for critiquing a hypothesis.

◇ Apply the critiquing criteria to the evaluation of a hypothesis in a research report.

KEY TERMS

conceptual definition   operational definition
dependent variable   research hypothesis
directional hypothesis   statistical hypothesis
hypothesis   testability
independent variable   theory
nondirectional hypothesis

A hypothesis attempts to answer the question posed by the research problem. It is a vehicle for testing the validity of the theoretical framework's assumptions. Actually, a hypothesis is a bridge between **theory** and the real world. In the scientific realm researchers derive hypotheses from theories and subject the hypotheses to empirical testing. As such, a hypothesis is an integral component of the scientific method (see Chapter 2). The theory's validity is not directly examined. Instead, it is through the hypothesis that the merit of a theory can be evaluated. The hypothesis of a research study is analogous to a compass that indicates in which direction the research study will proceed.

This chapter will present the purpose and characteristics of the hypothesis, its interrelationship with the research process, and the criteria for critiquing hypotheses.

DEFINITION

Hypotheses flow from the problem statement, literature review, and theoretical framework. Fig. 7-1 illustrates this flow. A *hypothesis* is an assumptive statement about the relationship between two or more variables. A hypothesis converts the question posed by the research problem into a declarative statement that predicts an expected outcome.

Each hypothesis represents a unit or subset of the research problem. For example, a research problem might pose the question "Is there a relationship between maternal-infant sleep rhythms, maternal social support systems, and postpartum blues?" This problem can be broken down into the following two subproblems:

1. Is there a relationship between maternal-infant sleep rhythms and postpartum blues?
2. Is there a relationship between maternal social support systems and postpartum blues?

A hypothesis can then be generated for each unit of the research problem, the subproblems. The hypotheses of the research problem already mentioned might be stated in the following way:

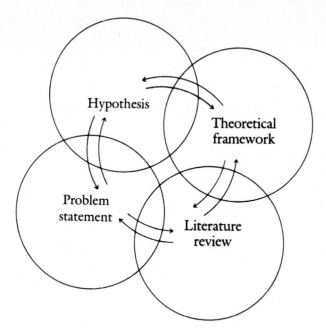

Fig. 7-1 Interrelationship between problem statement, literature review, theoretical framework, and hypothesis.

Hypothesis 1: Synchrony in maternal-infant sleep rhythms will be negatively related to postpartum blues.

Hypothesis 2: Perception of positive maternal social support systems will be negatively related to postpartum blues.

The critiquer of a research report will want to evaluate whether the hypotheses of the study represent subsets of the main research problem as illustrated by the examples just given.

Hypotheses are formulated before the study is actually conducted, because they will provide direction for the collection, analyses, and interpretation of data. Hypotheses have three purposes. Their first purpose is to provide a bridge between theory and reality, and in this sense they unify the two domains. Their second purpose is to be powerful tools for the advancement of knowledge, since they enable the researcher to objectively enter new areas of discovery. Their third purpose is to provide direction for any research endeavor by tentatively identifying the anticipated outcome.

CHARACTERISTICS

Nurses who are conducting research or nurses critiquing published research studies must have a working knowledge about what constitutes a "good" hypothesis. Such knowledge will enable them to have a standard for evaluating their own work or the work of others. The following discussion about the characteristics of hypotheses will present criteria to be used when formulating or evaluating a hypothesis.

The relationship statement

The first characteristic of a hypothesis is that it is a declarative statement that identifies the predicted relationship between two or more variables. This implies that there is a systematic relationship between an **independent variable** and a **dependent variable.** The direction of the predicted relationship is also specified in this statement. Phrases such as *greater than; less than; positively, negatively,* or *curvilinearly related* (∪- or ∩-shaped); and *difference in* connote the directionality that is proposed in the hypothesis. It is not unusual for a beginning researcher to generate a hypothesis that omits one of the two required variables or that fails to make a prediction about the direction of the relationship. For example, the prediction "Children who have asthma will respond favorably to postural drainage treatments" is not a scientifically acceptable hypothesis. There is only one stated variable, postural drainage treatments. This statement could be revised to make it an acceptable hypothesis containing two variables and a relational statement. The hypothesis would then be stated in the following manner: "Asthmatic children who receive postural drainage treatments (independent variable) will have less bronchial congestion (dependent variable) than have children with no postural drainage." In this hypothesis the two variables are explicitly identified, and the relational aspect of the prediction is contained in the phrase *less than.*

The nature of the relationship, either causal or associative, is also implied by the hypothesis. A causal relationship is one where the researcher is able to predict that the independent variable (X) causes a change in the dependent variable (Y). It is rare in research that one is in a firm enough position to take a definitive stand about a cause-and-effect relationship. For example, a researcher might hypothesize that relaxation training would have a significant effect on the physical and psychological health status of patients who have suffered myocardial infarction. However, it would be difficult for a researcher to predict a strong cause-and-effect relationship because of the multiple intervening variables, such as age, medication, and life-style changes, that might also influence the subject's health status. Variables are more commonly related in noncausal ways; that is, the variables are systematically related but in an associative way. This means that there is a systematic movement in the associated values of the two phenomena. For example, there is strong evidence that cigarette smoking is related to lung cancer. It is tempting to state that there is a causal relationship between cigarette smoking and lung cancer. However, do not overlook the fact that not all cigarette smokers will have lung cancer and not all of those who have lung cancer are cigarette smokers. Consequently, it would be scientifically unsound to take a position advocating the presence of a causal relationship between these two variables. Rather, one can only say that there is an associative relationship between the variables of cigarette smoking and lung cancer, a relationship where there is a strong systematic association between the two phenomena.

Testability

The second characteristic of a hypothesis is its **testability.** This means that the variables of the study must lend themselves to observation, measurement, and analysis. The hypothesis is either supported or not supported after the data have been collected and analyzed. The predicted outcome proposed by the hypothesis will or will not be congruent with the actual outcome when the hypothesis is tested. Hypotheses advance scientific knowledge by confirming or refuting theories.

Hypotheses may fail to meet the criteria of testability because the researcher has not made a prediction about the anticipated outcome, the variables are not observable or measurable, or the hypothesis is couched in terms that are value laden. Table 7-1 illustrates each of these points and provides a remedy for each problem.

Theory base

A sound hypothesis is consistent with an existing body of theory and research findings. Regardless of whether a hypothesis is arrived at inductively or deductively (see Chapter 2), it must be based on a sound scientific rationale. The reader of a research report should be able to identify the flow of ideas from the problem statement to the literature review, to the theoretical framework, and through the hypotheses (see Chapters 5 and 6). Table 7-2 illustrates this process in relation to the problem statement "What is the effect of perceived caregiver stress and social

Table 7-1 **Hypotheses That Fail to Meet the Criteria of Testability**

Problematic hypothesis	Problematic issue	Revised hypothesis
Anxiety is related to learning.	No predictive statement about the relationship is made; therefore the relationship is not verifiable.	Anxiety is curvilinearly (∩-shaped) related to problem-solving behavior.
Clients who receive preoperative instruction have less postoperative stress than have clients who do not.	The "postoperative stress" variable must be specifically defined so that it is observable or measurable, or the relationship is not testable.	Clients who attend preoperative education classes have less postoperative emotional stress than have clients who do not.
Small-group teaching will be better than individualized teaching for dietary compliance in diabetic clients.	"Better than" is a value-laden word that is not objective. Moral and ethical questions containing words such as "should," "ought," "better than," and "bad for" are not scientifically testable.	Dietary compliance will be greater in diabetic clients receiving diet instruction in small groups than in diabetic clients receiving individualized diet instruction.

Table 7-2 Flow of Data Between Problem Statement, Literature Review, Theoretical Framework, and Hypothesis

Problem statement	Literature review	Theoretical framework	Hypotheses

What is the effect of perceived caregiver stress and social support on the psychological distress of family caregivers of the elderly?	1. Studies related to emotional, physical, social and financial difficulties associated with caregiving.
	2. Studies related to antecedent variables related to caregiver strain, burden, or diminished well-being.
	  a. Demographic characteristics of caregivers and of elders.
	  b. Characteristics of the caregiving situation.
	  c. Variables that mediate the effect of caregiver stress such as social support.
		1. Family caregivers of the elderly experience significant amounts of stress in relation to the burden of caregiving.
		2. The amount of stress varies and is proposed to be a perceptual phenomenon.
		3. Social support is proposed to be a variable that mediates (buffers) stress.
		4. Social support is positively related to coping effectiveness and reduced burden.
		5. Satisfaction with social support is correlated with mental health.
			1. Perceived stress of caregiving will be positively related to psychological distress.
			2. Satisfaction with social support will be negatively related to psychological distress.
			3. Social support will have a buffering effect on the relationship between perceived caregiver stress and psychological distress.

support on the psychological distress of family caregivers of the elderly?" (Baillie, Norbeck, and Barnes, 1988). In this example it is clear that there is an explicitly developed, relevant body of scientific data that provides the theoretical grounding for the study. The hypotheses, as stated in Table 7-2, are logically derived from the theoretical framework. However, the research consumer should be cautioned about assuming that the theory-hypothesis link will always be present. In an analysis of nursing practice research from 1977 to 1986, Moody, Wilson, Smyth, Tittle, and Vancott (1988) indicate that only slightly more than half (51%) of the 720 articles analyzed had some type of theoretical perspective.

Wording the hypothesis

As you read the scientific literature and become more familiar with it, you will observe that there are a variety of ways to word a hypothesis. Regardless of the specific format used to state the hypothesis, the statement should be worded in clear, simple, and concise terms. If this criterion is met, the reader will understand the following:

1. The variables of the hypothesis
2. The population being studied
3. The predicted outcome of the hypothesis

This information may be further clarified by the definition section of a study (see Chapters 6 and 15).

Directional versus nondirectional hypotheses

Hypotheses can be formulated directionally or nondirectionally. A **directional hypothesis** is one that specifies the expected direction of the relationship between the independent and dependent variables. The reader of a directional hypothesis may observe that the existence of a relationship is proposed as well as the nature or direction of that relationship. The following is an example of a directional hypothesis: women with high-risk pregnancies who experience antenatal hospitalization and their partners will report less optimal family functioning than women with low-risk pregnancies and their partners (Mercer, Ferketich, DeJoseph, May, and Sollid, 1988). Examples of directional hypotheses can also be found in Table 7-3 in examples 2 to 5, 7, and 8.

In contrast, whereas a **nondirectional hypothesis** indicates the existence of a relationship between the variables, it does not specify the anticipated direction of the relationship. The following is an example of a nondirectional hypothesis: "There is a relationship between perception of self-competence and breast-feeding behavior." Other examples of nondirectional hypotheses are illustrated in Table 7-3, examples 1 and 6.

Nurses who are learning to critique research studies should be aware that both the directional and nondirectional forms of hypotheses statements are acceptable. However, they should also be aware that there are definite pros and cons pertaining to each one.

Proponents of the nondirectional hypothesis state that this format is more objective and impartial than the directional hypothesis. It is argued that the directional hypothesis is potentially biased, because the researcher, in stating an anticipated outcome, has demonstrated a commitment to a particular position.

On the other side of the coin, proponents of the directional hypothesis argue that researchers naturally have hunches, guesses, or expectations concerning the outcome of their research. It was the hunch, the curiosity, or the guess that initially led them to speculate about the problem. The literature review and the conceptual framework provided the theoretical foundation for deriving the hypothesis. Consequently it might be said that a deductive hypothesis derived from a theory will almost always be directional (see Chapter 6). The theory will provide a critical rationale for proposing that relationships between variables will have particular outcomes. When there is no theory or related research to draw on for rationale, or when findings in previous research studies are ambivalent, the nondirectional hypothesis may be appropriate.

Table 7-3 Examples of How Hypotheses Are Worded

Hypothesis	Variables*	Type of hypothesis	Type of design suggested
1. There will be a relationship between self-concept and suicidal behavior	IV: Self-concept DV: Suicidal behavior	Nondirectional Research	Nonexperimental
2. Synchrony of maternal and newborn sleep rhythms will be negatively related to postpartum blues	IV: Synchrony of maternal and newborn sleep rhythms DV: Postpartum blues	Directional Research	Nonexperimental
3. Structured preoperative education is more effective than structured postoperative education in reducing the client's perception of pain	IV: Preoperative education IV: Postoperative education DV: Perception of pain	Directional Research	Experimental
4. The incidence and degree of severity of subject discomfort will be less after administration of medications by the Z-track intramuscular injection technique than after administration of medications by the standard intramuscular injection technique	IV: Z-track intramuscular injection technique IV: Standard intramuscular injection technique DV: Subject discomfort	Directional Research	Experimental

*IV, Independent variable; DV, dependent variable.

In summary, the evaluator of a hypothesis should know that there are several advantages to directional hypotheses, making them appropriate for use in most studies. The advantages are the following:

1. Directional hypotheses indicate to the reader that a theory base has been used to derive the hypotheses and that the phenomena under investigation have been critically thought about and interrelated. The reader should realize that nondirectional hypotheses may also be deduced from a theory base. However, because of the exploratory nature of many studies utilizing nondirectional hypotheses, the theory base may be less well developed.

Table 7-3 Examples of How Hypotheses Are Worded — cont'd

Hypothesis	Variables*		Type of hypothesis	Type of design suggested
5. Progressive relaxation will be more effective in reducing indices of physiological arousal than hypnotic relaxation or self-relaxation in patients undergoing cardiac rehabilitation	IV:	Progressive relaxation	Directional Research	Experimental
	IV:	Hypnotic relaxation		
	IV:	Self-relaxation		
	DV:	Physiological arousal indices		
6. There will be a relationship between years of nursing experience and attitude toward patients with acquired immune deficiency syndrome	IV:	Age of the nurse	Nondirectional Research	Nonexperimental
	DV:	Attitude toward rape		
7. There will be a positive relationship between trust and self-disclosure in marital relationships	IV:	Trust	Directional Research	Nonexperimental
	DV:	Self-disclosure		
8. There will be a greater decrease in posttest state anxiety scores in subjects treated with noncontact therapeutic touch than in subjects treated with contact therapeutic touch	IV:	Noncontact therapeutic touch	Directional Research	Experimental
	IV:	Contact therapeutic touch		
	DV:	State anxiety		

2. They provide the reader with a specific theoretical frame of reference within which the study is being conducted.
3. They suggest to the reader that the researcher is not sitting on a theoretical fence, and as a result, the analyses of data can be accomplished in a statistically more sensitive way.

The important thing for the critiquer to keep in mind regarding directionality of the hypotheses is whether or not there is a sound rationale for the choice the researcher has proposed regarding directionality.

Statistical versus research hypotheses

Readers of research reports may observe that a hypothesis is further categorized as either a research or a statistical hypothesis. A **research hypothesis,** also known as a scientific hypothesis, consists of a statement about the expected relationship between the variables. A research hypothesis indicates what the outcome of the study is expected to be. A research hypothesis can be either directional or nondirectional. If the researcher obtains statistically significant findings for a research hypothesis, the hypothesis is supported. For example, in their study on stress and social support in family caregivers of the elderly, Baillie, Norbeck, and Barnes (1988) hypothesized that "satisfaction with social support will be negatively related to psychological distress." The authors report statistically significant findings for this hypothesis, and as such, the hypothesis is supported; that is, the predicted outcome was supported by the study findings. The examples in Table 7-3 represent research hypotheses.

A **statistical hypothesis,** also known as a null hypothesis, states that there is no relationship between the independent and dependent variables. The examples in Table 7-4 illustrate statistical hypotheses. If in the data analysis a statistically significant relationship emerges between the variables at a specified level of significance, the null hypothesis is rejected. Rejection of the statistical hypothesis is equivalent to acceptance of the research hypothesis. For example, in a study that compared levels of anxiety and depression in mothers of term and preterm infants (Brooten, Gennaro, Brown, Butts, Gibbons, Bakewell-Sachs, and Kuman, 1988), a null or statistical hypothesis would state that mothers of term and preterm infants do not differ in levels of anxiety and depression. The researchers found that mothers of preterm infants were *significantly* more depressed and anxious than mothers of term infants. Since the difference between the two groups was greater than that expected by chance, the null hypothesis was rejected (see Chapter 16).

Some researchers refer to the null hypothesis as a statistical contrivance that obscures a straightforward prediction of the outcome. Others state that it is more exact and conservative statistically, and that failure to reject the null hypothesis implies that there is insufficient evidence to support the idea of a real difference. Readers of research reports will note that, in general, research hypotheses are more commonly stated than statistical hypotheses. It is more desirable to state the researcher's expectation. The reader then has a more precise idea of the proposed outcome. In any study that involves statistical analysis, the underlying null hypothesis is usually assumed without being explicitly stated.

THE RELATIONSHIP BETWEEN THE HYPOTHESIS AND THE RESEARCH DESIGN

Regardless of whether the researcher uses a statistical or a research hypothesis, there is a suggested relationship between the hypothesis and the research design of the study. The type of design, experimental or nonexperimental (see Chapters 8 to 10), will influence the wording of the hypothesis. For example, when an experimental design is utilized, the research consumer would expect to see hypotheses that reflect relationship statements:

Table 7-4 **Examples of Statistical Hypotheses**

Hypothesis	Variables*	Type of hypothesis	Type of design suggested
Oxygen inhalation by nasal canula of up to 6 L/min does not affect oral temperature measurement taken with an electronic thermometer	*IV:* Oxygen inhalation by nasal cannula *DV:* Oral temperature	Statistical	Experimental
The incidence of prenancy in adolescent girls attending birth control education classes will not differ from that of girls who do not attend birth control education classes	*IV:* Birth control education classes *DV:* Adolescent pregnancy	Statistical	Experimental

⬦ X_1 is more effective than X_2 on Y
⬦ The effect of X_1 on Y is greater than that of X_2 on Y
⬦ The incidence of Y will not differ in subjects receiving X_1 and X_2 treatments
⬦ The incidence of Y will be greater in subjects after X_1 than after X_2

Such hypotheses indicate that an experimental treatment will be used and that two groups of subjects, experimental and control groups, are being used to test whether or not the difference predicted by the hypothesis actually exists.

In contrast, hypotheses related to nonexperimental designs reflect associative relationship statements:

⬦ X will be negatively related to Y
⬦ There will be a positive relationship between X and Y.

Additional examples of this concept are illustrated in Table 7-2.

RESEARCH QUESTIONS

Research studies do not always contain hypotheses. As you become more familiar with the scientific literature, you will notice that exploratory studies usually do not have hypotheses. This is particularly common where there is a dearth of literature or related research studies in a particular area that is of interest to the researcher. The researcher, interested in finding out more about a particular phenomenon, may engage in a fact-finding or relationship-finding mission guided only by research questions. The outcome of the exploratory study may be that data about the phenomenon are amassed and the researcher is then able to formulate hypotheses for a future study.

Research questions tend to be more general than the research problems discussed in Chapter 4. However, the more specific they are, the more they provide direction for the study. The following are some examples of research questions:

1. What are the factors that produce success on state board exams for associate degree nursing students?
2. What are the hospital unit organizational factors that contribute to quality nursing care?
3. How does the use of nursing diagnosis improve client care?
4. What are the community resources that homebound elderly clients need to remain in the community?

In other studies, research questions are formulated in addition to hypotheses to answer questions related to ancillary data. Such questions do not directly pertain to the proposed outcomes of the hypotheses. Rather, they may provide additional and sometimes serendipitous findings that are enriching to the study and valuable in providing direction for further study. Sometimes they are the kernels of new or future hypotheses.

The evaluator of a research study needs to determine whether or not it was appropriate to formulate a research question rather than a hypothesis, given the nature and context of the study.

CRITIQUING THE HYPOTHESIS

Hypotheses represent the core of an empirical research study. As such it is important not only that nurses understand how to formulate hypotheses but that they also know how to critically appraise them. Consequently we will now turn our attention to the evaluation of hypotheses in research reports.

When reviewing a research report, several criteria for critiquing the hypotheses should be used as a standard for evaluating the strengths and weaknesses of the hypotheses.

1. When reading a research study the research consumer may find the hypotheses clearly delineated in a separate hypothesis section of the research article, after the literature review and/or theoretical framework section(s). In many cases the hypotheses are not explicitly stated and are only implied in the results section of the article. As such, they must be inferred by the critiquer from the purpose statement and the type of analysis used. The reader must be cognizant of this variation and not think that because hypotheses do not appear at the beginning of the article, they do not exist in the particular study. Even when hypotheses are stated at the beginning of an article, they are reexamined in the results section as the findings are presented and discussed. However, the critiquer should expect hypotheses to be appropriately reflected depending on the purpose of the study and format of the article.

2. The hypothesis should directly answer the research problem that was posed at the beginning of the report. Its placement in the research report logically follows the problem statement, the literature review, and the theoretical framework, because the hypothesis should reflect the culmination and expression of this conceptual process.

It should be consistent with both the literature review and the theoretical framework. The flow of this process, as depicted in Table 7-2, should be explicit and apparent to the reader. If this criterion is met, the reader feels reasonably assured that the basis for the hypothesis is theoretically sound.

3. As the reader examines the actual hypothesis, several aspects of the statement should be critically appraised. First, the hypothesis should consist of a declarative statement that objectively and succinctly expresses the relationship between an independent and a dependent variable. In wording a complex versus a simple hypothesis, there may be more than one independent and dependent variable.

Second, the reader can expect that often there will be more than one hypothesis, particularly if there is more than one independent and dependent variable. If you recall, an earlier section of the chapter indicated that each hypothesis should be specific to one relationship. Consequently, if there are multiple variables in the problem or if the problem statement is broken down into subproblems, the reader may anticipate that there should be several hypotheses.

Third, the variables of the hypothesis should be understandable to the reader. Often in the interest of formulating a succinct hypothesis statement, the complete meaning of the variables is not apparent. The critiquer must realize that sometimes a researcher is caught between the "devil and the deep blue sea" on that issue. It may be a choice between having a complete but verbose hypothesis paragraph, or a less complete but concise hypothesis. The solution to this dilemma is for the researcher to have a definition section in the research report. The inclusion of **conceptual** and **operational definitions** (see Chapter 6) provides the complete explication of the variables. The critiquer is then able to examine the hypothesis side by side with the definitions and determine the exact nature of the variables under consideration. An excellent example of this process appears in a research article by Trainor (1982). The researcher hypothesized that

> *Visitors would demonstrate a significantly greater level of acceptance of their own ostomy than nonvisitors.*

This is an appropriately worded hypothesis. However, it is not completely clear what the variable "visitor" implies. It is only when one examines the definitions of "visitor" and "nonvisitor" that the exact nature of the variables becomes clear to the reader:

> *Visitor:* a person with an ostomy who is a member of a local United Ostomy Association chapter and who has visited other ostomates
>
> *Nonvisitor:* a person with an ostomy who is a member of a local United Ostomy Association chapter but who has neither trained as a visitor nor visited other ostomates

The context of the variables is now revealed to the evaluator.

Fourth, although a hypothesis can legitimately be nondirectional, it is preferable to indicate the direction of the relationship between the variables in the hypothesis. The reader will find that when there is a dearth of data available for the literature review—that is, the researcher has chosen to study a relatively undefined area of interest—the nondirectional hypothesis may be appropriate. There simply may not be enough information available to make a sound judgment about the direction of the proposed relationship. All that could be proposed is that there will be a relationship between two variables. Essentially, the critiquer wants to determine the appropriateness of the researcher's choice regarding directionality of the hypothesis.

4. The notion of **testability** is central to the soundness of a hypothesis. One criterion related to testability is that the hypothesis should be stated in such a way that it can be clearly supported or not supported. Whereas the previous statement is very important to keep in mind, the reader should also understand that ultimately neither theories nor hypotheses are ever proved beyond the shadow of a doubt through hypothesis testing. Researchers who claim that their data have "proved" the validity of their hypothesis should be regarded with grave reservation. The reader should realize that, at best, findings that support a hypothesis are considered tentative. If repeated replication of a study yields the same results, greater confidence can be placed in the conclusions advanced by the researchers. An important thing to remember about testability is that although hypotheses are more likely to be accepted with increasing evidence, they are never ultimately proven.

Another point about testability for the consumer to consider is that the hypothesis should be objectively stated and devoid of any value-laden words. Value-laden hypotheses are not empirically testable. Quantifiable words such as *greater than, less than, decrease, increase,* and *positively, negatively,* and *curvilinearly related* convey the idea of objectivity and testability. The reader should be immediately suspicious of hypotheses that are not stated objectively.

5. The evaluator of a research study should be cognizant of the fact that the way that the proposed relationship of the hypothesis is phrased suggests the type of research design that will be appropriate for the study. For example, if a hypothesis proposes that treatment X_1 will have a greater effect on Y than treatment X_2, an experimental or quasiexperimental design is suggested (see Chapter 9). If a hypothesis proposes that there will be a positive relationship between variables X and Y, a nonexperimental design is suggested (see Chapter 10). A review of Table 7-3 will provide you with additional examples of hypotheses and the type of research design that is suggested by each hypothesis. The reader of a research report should evaluate whether or not the selected research design is congruent with the hypothesis. This factor has important implications for the remainder of the study in terms of the appropriateness of sample selection, data collection, data analysis, interpretation of findings, and ultimately the conclusions advanced by the researcher.

6. If the research report contains research questions rather than hypotheses, the reader will want to evaluate whether or not this is appropriate to the study. The criterion for making this decision, as presented earlier in this chapter, is whether or not the study is of an exploratory nature. If it is, then it is appropriate to have research questions rather than hypotheses. Ancillary research questions should be evaluated as to whether or not they answer additional questions secondary to the hypotheses.

Critiquing Criteria

1. Does the hypothesis directly answer the research question?
2. Is the hypothesis concisely stated in a declarative form?
3. Are the independent and dependent variables identified in the statement of the hypothesis?
4. Are the variables measurable or potentially measurable?
5. Is each of the hypotheses specific to one relationship so that each hypothesis can be either supported or not supported?
6. Is the hypothesis stated in such a way that it is testable?
7. Is the hypothesis stated objectively, without value-laden words?
8. Is the direction of the relationship in each hypothesis clearly stated?
9. Is each hypothesis consistent with the literature review?
10. Is the theoretical rationale for the hypothesis explicit?
11. Are the research questions stated in relation to the auxiliary data except in the case of an exploratory study?

Sometimes the substance of an additional research question is more appropriately posed as another hypothesis in that it relates in a major way to the original research problem.

Conclusion

After you have explored the scientific literature and evaluated enough hypotheses, you will have an appreciation for how carefully a hypothesis must be worded. The hypothesis represents the core of the scientific method. The remainder of a study revolves around testing the hypothesis. To determine the merit of a hypothesis that has been formulated or reviewed in the literature, the reader must have and use criteria to objectively evaluate it. Criteria for critiquing the hypothesis are given in the box above.

SUMMARY

A hypothesis attempts to answer the question posed by the research problem. When testing the validity of the theoretical framework's assumptions, the hypothesis bridges the theoretical and real worlds.

A hypothesis is a declarative statement about the relationship between two or more variables that predicts an expected outcome. Characteristics of a hypothesis include a relationship statement, implications regarding testability, and consistency with a defined theory base. Hypotheses can be formulated in a directional or a nondirectional manner. Hypotheses can be further categorized as either research or statistical hypotheses.

Research questions may be utilized instead of hypotheses in exploratory research studies. Research questions may also be formulated in addition to hypotheses to answer questions related to ancillary data.

The critiquing process provides a set of criteria for the evaluation of the strengths and weaknesses of a hypothesis as it is presented in a research report. The reader evaluates the wording of the hypothesis in terms of the clarity of the relational statement, the implications for testability, and its congruence with a theory base. The appropriateness of the hypothesis in relation to the type of research design suggested by the design is also examined. The appropriate use of research questions is also evaluated.

The hypothesis represents the core of a research study. The remainder of the study revolves around the testing of the hypothesis. The hypothesis must be as accurate as possible, because it is analogous to a compass indicating the direction for the research endeavor to proceed.

References

Baillie, V., Norbeck, J.S., and Barnes, L.A. (1988). Stress, social support, and psychological distress of family caregivers of the elderly, *Nursing Research,* **37**:217-222.

Brooten, D., Gennaro, S., Brown, L.P., Butts, P., Gibbons, A.L., Bakewell-Sachs, S., and Kuman, S.P. (1988). Anxiety, depression and hostility in mothers of preterm infants, *Nursing Research,* **37**:213-216.

Campbell, D.T., and Stanley, J.C. (1963). *Experimental and quasi-experimental designs for research,* Chicago, Rand-McNally College Publishing Co.

Downs, F.S., and Newman, M.A. (1977). *A source book of nursing research,* Philadelphia, F.A. Davis Co.

Keen, M.F. (1986). Comparison of intramuscular injection techniques to reduce site discomfort and lesions, *Nursing Research,* **35**:207-210.

Kerlinger, F.N. (1986). *Foundations of behavioral research,* New York, Holt, Rinehart & Winston.

Mercer, R.T., Ferketich, S.L., DeJoseph, J., May, K.A., and Sollid, D. (1988). Effect of stress on family functioning during pregnancy, *Nursing Research,* **37**:268-275.

Moody, L.E., Wilson, M.E., Smyth, K., Tittle, M., and Vancott, M.L. (1988). Analysis of a decade of nursing practice research: 1977-1986, *Nursing Research,* **37**:374-379.

Munro, B.H., Creamer, A.M., Haggerty, M.R., and Cooper, F.S. (1988). Effect of relaxation therapy on post–myocardial infarction patient's rehabilitation, *Nursing Research,* **37**:231-235.

Newman, M.A. (1979). *Theory development in nursing,* Philadelphia, F.A. Davis Co.

Trainor, M.A. (1982). Acceptance of ostomy and the visitor role in a self-help group for ostomy patients, *Nursing Research,* **31**:102-106.

Van Dalen, D.B. (1979). *Understanding educational research,* New York, McGraw-Hill Book Co.

8

Introduction to Design

Geri LoBiondo-Wood

LEARNING OBJECTIVES

After reading this chapter the student should be able to do the following:

⋄ Define research design.

⋄ Identify the purpose of the research design.

⋄ Describe the concepts that affect the research design.

⋄ Define control as it affects the research design.

⋄ Compare and contrast the elements that affect control.

⋄ Begin to evaluate what degree of control should be exercised in the design.

⋄ Define internal validity.

⋄ Identify the threats to internal validity.

⋄ Define external validity.

⋄ Identify the conditions that affect external validity.

⋄ Evaluate the design using the critiquing questions.

KEY TERMS

constancy	instrumentation
control	internal validity
control group	maturation
experimental group	mortality
external validity	randomization
extraneous variable	reactivity
history	selection bias
homogeneity	testing

The word *design* implies the organization of elements into a masterful work of art. In the world of art and fashion, design conjures up images of processes and techniques that are used to express a total concept. When an individual creates, process and form are employed. The form, process, and degree of adherence to structure depend on the aims of the creator. The same can be said of the research process. The research process and the development of research design need not be a sterile procedure but one where the researcher develops a masterful work within the limits of a problem and the related theoretical basis. The framework that the researcher creates is the design. When reading a study the research consumer should be able to recognize that the problem statement, purpose, literature review, theoretical framework, and hypothesis all interrelate with, complement, and assist in the operationalization of the design (Fig. 8-1).

Nursing is concerned with a variety of structures that require varying degrees of process and form, such as the administration of holistic and quality client care, staff organization, student education, and continuing education. When client care is administered, the nursing process based on assessment, planning, intervention, and evaluation is utilized. Before these four steps can be accomplished, a certain level of knowledge is required. This knowledge is derived from theory, practice, and experience. Validation of these areas is derived from research. To understand and utilize research it is necessary to have knowledge of the process and an equally important in-depth knowledge of the content of the subject area being studied. Previous chapters have stressed the importance of theory and subject matter knowledge. How a researcher structures, implements, or designs an investigation affects the results of a research project.

For the consumer to understand the implications of research and to utilize research, the central issues in the design of a research project should be understood. This chapter will provide an overview of the meaning, purpose, and importance of research design, whereas Chapters 9 to 12 will present specific types of designs.

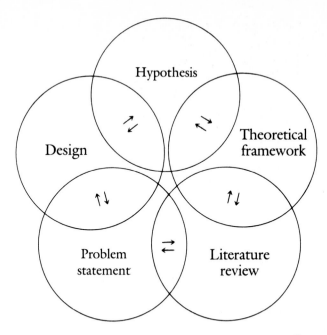

Fig. 8-1 Interrelationship between design, problem statement, literature review, theoretical framework, and hypothesis.

PURPOSE OF RESEARCH DESIGN

The purpose of the research design is to provide the scheme for answering specific research questions. The design then becomes the vehicle for the hypothesis. The principles of scientific inquiry are utilized to answer research questions. Therefore the design involves a plan, structure, and strategy. These three concepts of design guide a researcher in writing the hypothesis, during the operationalization or the carrying out of the project, and in the analysis and evaluation of the data. The overall purpose of the research design is twofold: to aid in the solution of research questions and to maintain control. All research attempts to answer questions. The design is coupled with the methods and procedures, and together they are the mechanisms for finding solutions to research questions. **Control** is defined as the measures that the researcher utilizes to hold the conditions of the investigation uniform. In this way the researcher avoids possible impingement of bias on the dependent variable that may affect the outcome.

A research example that demonstrates how the design can aid in the solution of a research question and maintain control is the study by Brooten, Kumar, Brown, Butts, Finkler, Bakewell-Sachs, Gibbons, and Delivoria-Papadopoulas (1986) (Appendix A). The purpose of the study was to examine if it is safe and economical to discharge infants of very low birth weight (< 1500 g) early if they meet certain conditions. To maintain control the investigators randomly assigned infants to one of two groups. To participate in the study the infants in the control group had to be clinically well and feeding well and had to have had no routine home follow-up care. To further maintain control the infants in the early discharge group were discharged before they weighed 2200 g. They had to be clinically well, fed by nipple every 4 hours, able to be maintained in an open crib in room air, and have no evidence of serious apnea or bradycardia. The mother or primary caretaker had to demonstrate satisfactory caretaking skills, and the home environment needed to be adequate. By establishing these specific criteria of safety and subject eligibility and by maintaining control, the researchers were able to say what type of infant would most benefit from the early discharge program. A variety of considerations, including the type of design chosen, affect the accomplishment of this end. These considerations include objectivity in the conceptualization of the problem, accuracy, economy, control of the experiment, **internal validity,** and **external validity.** There are statistical principles behind the many forms of control, but a clear conceptual understanding is of greater importance for the research consumer.

OBJECTIVITY IN THE CONCEPTUALIZATION

Objectivity in the conceptualization of the problem is derived from a review of the literature and development of a theoretical framework (Fig. 8-1). Using the literature the researcher assesses the depth and breadth of available knowledge concerning the problem. The literature review and theoretical framework should demonstrate to the reader that the researcher reviewed the literature with a critical and objective eye (see Chapters 2 and 5), since this affects the type of design chosen. For example, a question regarding the relationship of the length of a breast-feeding teaching program may suggest either a correlational or an experimental design (see Chapters 9 and 10), whereas a question regarding the growth in size of a woman's body during pregnancy and maternal perception of the unborn child may suggest a survey or case study (see Chapters 11 and 12). Therefore it should be obvious how the researcher's literature review reflects the following:
- When the problem was studied
- What aspects of the problem was studied
- Where it was investigated
- By whom it was investigated

The review that incorporates these aspects allows the consumer to judge the objectivity of the problem area and therefore whether the design chosen matches the problem.

ACCURACY

Accuracy is also accomplished through the theoretical framework, review of the literature, and as a result of the researcher's preparation (see Chapters 5 and 6). Accuracy means that all aspects of a study systematically and logically follow from the identified problem statement. The beginning researcher is wise to answer a question involving few variables that will not require the use of sophisticated designs. The simplicity of a research project does not render it useless or of a lesser value for practice. Although the project is simple, the researcher should not forego accuracy. The consumer should feel that the investigator used the appropriate type of design to answer the research question with a minimum of contamination. The issues of contamination or control will be discussed later in this chapter. Also, many clinical problems have not yet been researched. Therefore a preliminary or pilot study would be a wise approach. The key is the accuracy, validity, and objectivity used by the researcher in attempting to answer the question. Accordingly, the researcher should read various levels of studies and assess how and if the criteria for each step of the research process were followed. Research consumers will find that many nursing journals publish not only sophisticated clinical research projects but smaller clinical studies that can be applied to practice.

An example of a preliminary study that investigated a clinical problem was conducted by Keefe (1988). Concerned that postpartum rooming-in, which has gained increasing popularity in the United States, could have a positive as well as a negative impact, she conducted a two-group comparison study. The study was designed to test whether there were differences in sleep patterns for a group of mother-infant dyads who roomed-in at night as compared with a group who were separated at night. This study then looked at an important clinical problem—the potential for maternal sleep deprivation—that could potentially affect maternal recovery. The researcher acknowledges the limitations of the study and the need for future research. Although this study does not give clinicians all the data to decide whether or not the practice of rooming-in has positive results, it does provide a beginning study of the question and suggests avenues of future inquiry for nursing practice and research.

ECONOMY

When critiquing the research design the evaluator also needs to be aware of the pragmatic consideration of economy. Sometimes the reality of this does not truly sink in until one does research. It is important to consider economy when reviewing a study, including availability of the subjects, timing of the research, time required for the subjects to participate, cost in terms of such items as reproduction, and analysis of the data (Table 8-1). These pragmatic considerations are not presented as a step in the research process as are the theoretical framework or methods, but they do affect every step of the process. As such, the reader of a study should consider these when assessing the investigation. The student researcher may or may not have monies or accessible services. When critiquing an investigation, note the credentials of the author and if the investigation was part of a student project or part of a fully funded granted project. If the project was a student project, the standards of critiquing are applied more liberally than for a prepared, experienced researcher or clinician. Finally, the pragmatic issues raised affect the scope and breadth of an investigation and therefore its generalizability.

Table 8-1 **Pragmatic Considerations in Determining Feasibility of a Research Problem**

Factor	Pragmatic consideration
Time	The research problem must be one that can be studied within a realistic period of time. All researchers have deadlines for completion of a project. It is essential that the scope of the problem be circumscribed enough to provide ample time for the completion of the entire project. Research studies generally take longer than anticipated to complete.
Subject availability	The researcher needs to determine whether or not a sufficient number of eligible subjects will be available and willing to participate in the study. If one has a captive audience, like students in a classroom, it may be relatively easy to enlist their cooperation. When a study involves the subjects' independent time and effort, they may be unwilling to participate when there is no apparent reward for doing so. Other potential subjects may have fears about harm or confidentiality and may be suspicious of the research process in general. Subjects with unusual characteristics are often difficult to locate. In general, people are fairly cooperative about participating, but a researcher must consider needing a larger subject pool than will actually participate. At times, when reading a research report the researcher may note how the procedures were liberalized or the number of subjects was altered. This was probably a result of some unforeseen pragmatic consideration.
Facility and equipment availability	All research projects require some kind of equipment. The equipment may be questionnaires, telephones, stationery, stamps, technical equipment, or other apparatus. Most research projects require the availability of some kind of facility. The facility may be a hospital site for data collection or laboratory space, or a computer center for data analyses.
Money	Research projects require some expenditure of money. Before embarking on a study the researcher probably itemized the expenses and projected the total cost of the project. This provides a clear picture of the budgetary needs for items like books, stationery, postage, printing, technical equipment, telephone and computer charges, and salaries. These expenses can range from about $50 for a small-scale student project to hundreds of thousands of dollars for a large-scale federally funded project.
Researcher experience	The selection of the research problem should be based on the nurse's realm of experience and interest. It is much easier to develop a research study related to a topic that is either theoretically or experientially familiar. Selecting a problem that is of interest to the researcher is essential for maintaining enthusiasm when the project has its inevitable ups and downs.
Ethics	Research problems that place unethical demands on subjects may not be feasible for study. Researchers must take ethical considerations seriously. The consideration of ethics may affect the choice between an experimental or nonexperimental design.

INTRODUCTION TO DESIGN **133**

CONTROL

A researcher attempts to use a design to maximize the degree of control over the tested variables. *Control* involves holding the conditions of the study constant and establishing specific sampling criteria as described by Brooten et al. (1986). An efficient design can maximize results, decrease errors, and control preexisting or impaired conditions that may affect outcome. To maximize efforts the researcher should maximize control. To accomplish these tasks the research design and methods should demonstrate the researcher's efforts at control. For example, in a study by Farr, Keene, Samson, and Michael (1984), the researchers attempted to determine if a relationship existed between the degree of circadian alteration and the subject reentrainment to typical circadian profiles.

Their hypotheses were the following:

I. Normal circadian rhythms are altered in response to surgical trauma.

II. Normal circadian rhythms uncouple in response to surgical trauma.

III. Alterations in normal circadian rhythms are an additional stress to that of surgical trauma, and therefore should affect reentrainment or return to normal rhythmic state.

To test these hypotheses and apply control the investigators included in their study individuals who were active in the daytime; in relatively good health; free of renal problems, hypertension, and endocrine disorders; and taking no medications known to interfere with catecholamine secretion, adrenal cortical secretions, or electrolyte excretion. Subjects were also excluded if postoperative complications developed. This study illustrates how investigators in one study planned their design to apply controls. Control is important in all designs. When various research designs are critiqued, the issue of control is always raised but with varying levels of flexibility. The issues to be discussed here will become clearer as you review the various types of designs discussed in later chapters (see Chapters 9 to 12). Control is accomplished by ruling out *extraneous variables* that compete with the independent variables as an explanation for the relationship or outcome of the study. The **extraneous variable** is one that interferes with the operations of the phenomena being studied, such as age and sex. Means of controlling extraneous variables include the following:

◇ Use of a homogeneous sample
◇ Use of consistent data collection procedures
◇ Manipulation of the independent variable
◇ Randomization

The following example will be used to illustrate and define these concepts:

> An investigator might be interested in how a new stop-smoking program (independent variable) affects smoking behavior (dependent variable). The independent variable is assumed to affect the outcome or dependent variable. But the investigator needs to be relatively sure that the decrease in smoking is truly related to the stop-smoking program rather than to some other variable, such as motivation. The design of the research study alone does not inherently provide control. But an appropriately designed study with the necessary controls built in can increase the researcher's ability to answer this research question.

Homogeneous sampling

In the stop-smoking study, extraneous variables may affect the dependent variable. The characteristics of a study's subjects are common extraneous variables. Age, sex, and even newer smoking laws may affect the outcome in the stop-smoking example. These variables may therefore affect the outcome, even though they are extraneous or outside of the study's design. As a control for these and other similar problems, the researcher's subjects should demonstrate **homogeneity** or similarity with respect to the extraneous variables relevant to the particular study (see Chapter 15). These extraneous variables are not fixed but need to be reviewed and decided on, based on the specific problem and its theoretical base. By using a sample of homogeneous subjects, the researcher has used a straightforward step of control.

For example, Koniak-Griffin and Ludington-Hoe (1988) designed a study to assess the longitudinal effects of a home-based program of different methods of stimulation provided during the infant's first 3 months, on 4 months' and 8 months' developmental status and temperament of normal infants. To assure themselves of a homogenous sample of normal infants, the researchers purposefully selected from mother-infant pairs who had uncomplicated, full-term pregnancies that ended in the delivery of a healthy infant. This control step limits the *generalizability* or the application of the outcomes to other populations when analyzing and discussing the outcomes (see Chapter 19). Results can then be generalized only to a similar population of individuals. You may say that this is limiting. This is not necessarily so because no treatment or program may be applicable to all populations, and the consumer or user of research findings needs to take the differences in populations into consideration. It is better to have a "clean" study that can be used to make generalizations about a specific population than a "messy" one that can be used to generalize little or nothing.

If the researcher feels that one of the extraneous variables is important, then it may be included in the design. In the smoking example, if individuals are working in an area where smoking is not allowed and this is considered to be important, then the researcher could built it into the design and set up a control for it. This can be done by comparing two different work areas, one where smoking is allowed and one where it is not. The important concept to keep in mind is that before the data are collected the researcher should have identified, planned for, or controlled the important extraneous variables.

Constancy in data collection

Another basic, yet critical, component of control is **constancy** in data collection conditions or procedures. *Constancy* refers to the notion that the data collection procedures should reflect to the consumer a cookbook-like recipe of how the researcher controlled the conditions of the study. This means that environmental conditions, timing of data collection, data collection instruments, and data collection procedures used to gain the data are the same for each subject (see Chapter 13). An example of a well-controlled laboratory experiment was done by Lim-Levy (1982). Lim-Levy's study was performed to determine the effect of oxygen inhalation by nasal cannula on oral temperatures. To control conditions one electronic thermometer was used; subjects were requested verbally and in writing to refrain from vigorous activity, eating, drinking, and smoking for 1 hour before the procedure; mouth breathers were excluded; subjects were requested to sit quietly for at least 15 minutes before the experiment; and a comfortable sitting area was provided for the subjects. This type of control aided the researcher's ability to draw conclusions, discuss, and cite the need for further research in this area. For the consumer it demonstrates a clear, consistent, and specific means of data collection. Another method of ensuring constancy of data collection methods is training the data collectors similarly.

Not all of the problems nurses wish to research are amenable to laboratory study. Studies set in clinical settings also need constancy of data collection procedures to demonstrate to the consumer the efforts taken to address the concept of control.

Manipulation of independent variable

A third and very effective means of control is manipulation of the independent variable. This refers to administration of a program, treatment, or intervention to only one group within the study but not to the other subjects in the study. The first group is known as the **experimental group,** and the other group is known as the **control group.** In a *control group* the phenomena under study are held at a constant or comparison level. For example, suppose a researcher wants to study the level of infection rates between a new type of surgical dressing and an old type. The older method represents the control group and the new method the experimental group. Experimental designs use manipulation. Nonexperimental designs do not manipulate the independent variable. This does not decrease the usefulness of a nonexperimental design, but the use of a control group in an experimental design is related to the level of the problem and, again, its theoretical framework. But if the problem is amenable to a design that incorporates manipulation of the independent variable, it can increase the theoretical and statistical power of the researcher to draw generalizable results; that is, if all of the other considerations of control are equally addressed (see Chapters 9 and 10). Again the reader should be cautioned that the lack of manipulation of the independent variable does not mean a weaker study. The level of the problem, the amount of theoretical work, and the research that has preceded a project all affect the researcher's choice of a design.

Randomization

Researchers may also choose other forms of control such as randomization. **Randomization** is employed when the required number of subjects from the population are obtained in such a manner that each subject in a population has an equal chance of being selected. Randomization eliminates bias, aids in the attainment of a representative sample, and can be employed in various designs (see Chapters 9 and 15). Curry (1982) used one method of randomization when assigning primiparous women to receive or not to receive extended skin-to-skin contact with their newborns in the immediate postpartum period to assess if there were differences in various maternal attachment behaviors and self-concept.

Randomization can also be done with paper and pencil type instruments. By randomly ordering items on the instruments the investigator can assess if there is a difference in response that can be related to the order of the items. This may be especially important in longitudinal studies where bias from giving the same instrument to the same subjects on a number of occasions can be a problem (see Chapters 10 and 15).

CONTROL AND FLEXIBILITY

The same level of control cannot be exercised in all types of designs. The various types of designs that will be introduced to you in Chapters 9 to 12 will fully illuminate the issues that are being introduced to you within this chapter. At times, when a researcher wants to explore a new area where little or no literature on the concept exists, the researcher will probably use an exploratory design. In this type of study the researcher is interested in describing or categorizing a phenomenon in a group of individuals. Rubin's (1967a and 1967b) early work on the development of maternal tasks during pregnancy is an example of exploratory research. In this research she attempted to categorize conceptually the various maternal tasks of pregnancy. Rubin interviewed women throughout their pregnancies and from these extensive interviews developed a framework of the maternal tasks of pregnancy. In critiquing this type of study the issue of control should be applied in a highly flexible manner because of the preliminary nature of the work.

If it is determined from a review of a study that the researcher intended to conduct a correlational study, or a study that looks at the relationship between or among the variables, then the issue of control takes on more importance (see Chapter 10). Control needs to be strictly exercised as far as it is possible. At this intermediate level of design it should be clear to the reviewer that the researcher considered the extraneous variables that may have accounted for the outcomes.

All aspects of control are strictly applied to studies that utilize an experimental design (see Chapter 9). The reviewer should be able to locate in the research report how the researcher met the following criteria: the conditions of the research were constant throughout the study, assignment of subjects was random, and an experimental group and control group were utilized. The Lim-Levy study (1982) is an example where all the aspects of control were addressed. Because of the control exercised by Lim-Levy the reviewer can see that the highest level of control was applied and that extraneous variables were thereby considered.

INTERNAL AND EXTERNAL VALIDITY

When reading research one needs to feel that the results of a study are valid, based on precision, and faithful to what the researcher wanted to measure. For a study to form the basis of further research, practice, and theory development, it must be believable and dependable. There are two important criteria for evaluating the credibility and dependability of the results: internal validity and external validity.

Internal validity

Internal validity asks if the independent variable really made the difference. This requires the researcher to rule out other factors or threats as rival explanations of the relationship between the variables. Thus internal validity refers to the causal relationship. Internal validity problems revolve around the issues of control. Six major threats to internal validity are defined by Campbell and Stanley (1966). These should be considered by the researcher in planning the design and by the consumer before implementing results in practice. If these threats are not considered, they could negate the results of the research. How these threats may affect specific designs will be addressed in Chapters 9 to 12. The following are threats to internal validity:

1. *History.* In addition to the independent variables, another specific event that may have an effect on the dependent variable may occur either inside or outside the experimental setting; this is referred to as **history.** For example, in a study of the effects of a breast-feeding teaching program on the length of time of breast-feeding, an event such as government-sponsored advertisements on the importance of breast-feeding featured on television and newspapers may be a threat of history.

    Another example may be that of an investigator testing the effects of a breast self-examination teaching program on the incidence of monthly breast self-examination. Concurrently the President's wife is diagnosed as having breast cancer. The event of this diagnosis in a public figure engenders a great deal of media and press attention. In the course of the media attention medical experts are interviewed widely and the importance of breast self-examination is supported. If the researcher finds that breast self-examination behavior is improved, the researcher may not be able to conclude that the change in behavior is due to the teaching program, but it may be due to the diagnosis given the President's wife and the resultant media coverage.

2. *Maturation.* **Maturation** refers to the developmental, biological, or psychological processes that operate within an individual as a function of time and are external to the events of the investigation. For example, suppose one wishes to evaluate the effect of a specific teaching method on baccalaureate students' achievements on a skills test. The investigator would record the students' abilities before and after the teaching method. Between the pretest and posttest the students have grown older and wiser. This growth or change is unrelated to the investigation and may explain differences between the two testing periods rather than the experimental treatment.

    An example of a study in which the investigator took precautions to avoid the threat of maturation is a study conducted by Vessey (1988). Vessey wanted to investigate the relationship between two methods of teaching on children's knowledge of their internal bodies. Posttests of student learning were conducted 1 week after the teaching sessions were completed. This relatively short interval is a strength of the study and allows the investigator to conclude that the results were due to the design of the study and not maturation in a population of children who are learning new skills rapidly.

3. *Testing.* **Testing** is defined as the effect of taking a pretest on the score of a posttest. The effect of taking a pretest may sensitize an individual and improve the score of the posttest. Individuals generally score higher when they take a test a second time regardless of the treatment. The differences between posttest and pretest scores may not be a result of the independent variable but rather of the experience gained through testing.

An example in which testing might have accounted for the results was in a study conducted by Lowe and Roberts (1988). The study was designed to assess the congruence between in-labor report and postpartum recall of labor pain. The researchers measured labor pain on several occasions during labor and the postpartum period. They found that postpartal women tended to devalue early labor pain and inflate transitional labor pain when compared to their in-labor report. The researchers noted in discussing the results that the bias of repeated measures of pain during labor may have primed the postpartum responses, and that the practice of reporting pain repeatedly on the same instrument during labor and memory may have influenced the results.

4. *Instrumentation.* **Instrumentation** threats are changes in the measurement of the variables or observational techniques that may account for changes in the obtained measurement. Lim-Levy's use (1982) of the same equipment and procedures for each data collection session is an example of how a researcher took steps to avoid the threat of instrumentation.

Kunnel, O'Brien, Hazard Munro, and Medoff-Cooper (1988) used four identical mercury-in-glass thermometers that were tested for accuracy by immersing them in a temperature-controlled circulating water bath and then checking the readings against the readings on the National Bureau of Standards thermometer; this is an example of how researchers took steps to avoid the threat of instrumentation.

Another example that fits into this area is related to techniques of observation. If an investigator has several raters collecting observational data, all must be trained in a similar manner. If they are not similarly trained, a lack of consistency may occur in their ratings and therefore a major threat to internal validity will occur.

5. *Mortality.* **Mortality** is the loss of study subjects from the first data collection point (pretest) to the second data collection point (posttest). If the subjects who remain in the study are not similar to those who dropped out, the results could be affected. In a study of how a media campaign affects the incidence of breast-feeding, if most dropouts were non-breast-feeding women, the perception given could be that exposure to the media campaign increased the number of breast-feeding women, whereas it was the effect of experimental mortality that led to the observed results.

An example of a study in which the results may be due to death of subjects is that conducted by Murphy (1988). The study was a longitudinal one to examine the relationships between stress, potential mediators of stress, and health outcomes. Data were collected over a 3-year period. A number of the subjects did not participate at the second data collection. Murphy (1988), citing her earlier research (1986) and that of Green, Grace, Lindy, Titchener, and Lindy (1983), believed that possibly some of the bereaved who continued in the study were worse off than those who dropped out. She further concluded that it is unknown whether individuals who are more distressed participate in follow-up studies more frequently than those who perceive their emotional distress to be lower.

6. *Selection bias.* If the precautions are not used to gain a representative sample, a bias of subjects could result from the way the subjects were chosen. Selection effects are a problem in studies where the individuals themselves decide whether or not to participate in a study. Suppose an investigator wishes to assess if a new breast-feeding program contributes to the incidence and length of time of breast-feeding. If the new program is offered to all, chances are that women who are more motivated to learn about breast-feeding will take part in the program. Assessment of the effectiveness of the program is problematic, because the investigator cannot be sure if the new program increased the number of women who breast-fed their newborns or if only highly motivated individuals joined the program. The way to avoid **selection bias** in this case is to randomly assign the women to either the new teaching method group or a control group that receives a different type of instruction.

External validity

External validity deals with possible problems of generalizability of the investigation's findings to additional populations and to other environmental conditions. External validity questions under what conditions and with what types of subjects the same results can be expected to occur. The goal of the researcher is to select a design that maximizes both internal and external validity. This is not always possible; if this is the case then the researcher needs to establish a minimum requirement of meeting the criteria of external validity.

The factors that may affect external validity are related to selection of subjects, study conditions, and type of observations. These factors are termed *effects of selection, reactive effects,* and *effects of testing.* The reader will notice the similarity in names of the factors of selection and testing and those of threats to internal validity. When considering them as internal threats the consumer assesses them as they relate to the independent and dependent variables *within* the study, and when assessing them as external threats the consumer considers them in terms of the generalizability or utility *outside the study* to other populations and settings. Problems of internal validity are generally easier to control. Generalizability issues are more difficult to deal with, because it means that the researcher is assuming that other populations are similar or like the one being tested. A discussion of each of the external validity factors follows:

1. *Effect of selection.* Selection refers to the generalizability of the results to other populations. An example of the effects of selection occurs when the researcher is not able to attain the ideal sample population. At times, numbers of available subjects may be low or not accessible to the researcher; the researcher may then need to choose a nonprobability method of sampling over a probability method (see Chapter 15). Therefore the type of sampling method utilized and how subjects are assigned to research conditions affect the generalizability to other groups or the external validity.

   An example of the effect of selection is depicted with the following example. Aaronson (1989) studied perceived and received social support during pregnancy and its effects on health behavior practices during pregnancy. The sample consisted of 529 pregnant women who responded to questionnaires and a phone interview. In the discussion of the findings she cautions the reader to avoid extensive generalizations. The investigator states:

   > One note of caution, however, is necessary. The findings and conclusions of this study are based on a relatively homogenous, middle class sample. Consequently, the findings cannot be generalizations to more ethnically diverse groups or to those of lower socioeconomic status. (p. 7)

   Her remarks caution the reader to avoid extensive generalizations and let the reader know that there are limitations of the findings.

2. *Reactive effects.* **Reactivity** is defined as the subjects' responses to being studied. Subjects may respond to the investigator not because of the study procedures but merely as an independent response to being studied. This is also known as the *Hawthorne effect,* named after Western Electric Corporation's Hawthorne plant where a study of working conditions was conducted. The researchers developed several different working conditions (i.e., turning up the lights, playing music, and changing work hours). They found that no matter what was done the workers' productivity increased. They concluded that production increased as a result of the workers knowing that they were being studied rather than because of the experimental conditions.

3. *Effect of testing.* Administration of a pretest in an experimental situation affects the generalizability of the findings to other populations. Just as pretesting affects the posttest results within a study, pretesting affects the posttest results and generalizability outside the study. For example, suppose a researcher wants to conduct a study with the aim of changing attitudes toward acquired immune deficiency syndrome (AIDS). To accomplish this an education program on the risk factors for AIDS is incorporated. To test if the education program changes attitudes toward AIDS, tests are given before and after the teaching intervention. The pretest on attitudes allows the subjects to examine their attitudes regarding AIDS. The subjects' responses on follow-up testing

may be different than those of individuals who were given the education program and who did not see the pretest. Therefore, when a study is conducted and a pretest is given, it may prime the subjects and affect their ability to generalize to other situations.

There are other threats to external validity that are dependent on the type of design and methods of sampling utilized by the researcher, but these are beyond the scope of this textbook. Detailed coverage of the issues related to internal and external validity is offered by Campbell and Stanley (1966).

CRITIQUING THE RESEARCH DESIGN

Criteria for critiquing the research design are given in the box on p. 142.

Critiquing the design of a study requires one to first have knowledge of the overall implications that the choice of a particular design may have for the study as a whole. The concept of the research design is an all-inclusive one that parallels the concept of the theoretical framework. The research design is similar to the theoretical framework in that it deals with a piece of the research study that affects the whole. For one to knowledgeably critique the design in light of the entire study, it is important to understand the factors that influence the choice and the implications of the design. In this chapter the meaning, purpose, and important factors of design choice as well as the vocabulary that accompanies these factors have been introduced.

Several criteria for evaluating the design can be drawn from the preceding chapter. One should remember that these criteria are applied differently with various designs. Different application does not mean that the consumer will find a haphazard approach to design. It means that each design has particular criteria that allow the evaluator to classify the design as to type, such as experimental or nonexperimental. These criteria need to be met and addressed in conducting an experiment. The particulars of specific designs will be addressed in Chapters 9 through 12. The following discussion pertains primarily to the overall evaluation of a research design.

The research design should reflect that an objective review of the literature and the establishment of a theoretical framework guided the choice of the design. There is no explicit statement researching this in a research study. A consumer can evaluate this by critiquing the theoretical framework (see Chapter 6) and literature review (see Chapter 5). Is the problem new and not researched extensively? Has a great deal been done on the problem, or is it a new or different way of looking at an old problem? Depending on the level of the problem, certain choices are made by the investigators. Manderino and Bzdek (1984) conducted a study to examine the efficacy of videotaped information and modeling as pain-reducing techniques for women during labor and delivery. They utilized various theory and research studies to design their study as objectively and accurately as possible. Before the study began the investigators identified methodological problems in the research that they cited and built various design controls into their study (Manderino and Bzdek, 1984, p. 10).

Critiquing Criteria

1. Is the type of design employed appropriate to the structured question?
2. Does the researcher utilize the various concepts of control that are consistent with the type of design chosen?
3. Does the design utilized seem to reflect the issues of economy?
4. Does the design utilized seem to flow from the proposed problem statement, theoretical framework, literature review, and hypothesis?
5. What are the controls for the threats to internal validity?
6. What are the controls for the threats to external validity?

The consumer should be alert for the means used by investigators to maintain control, such as homogeneity in the sample, consistent data collection procedures, how or if the independent variable was manipulated, and whether randomization was utilized. As the reader will see in Chapter 9, all of these criteria must be met for an experimental design. As the reader begins to understand the types of designs and levels of research, namely, quasiexperimental and nonexperimental designs such as survey and interrelationship designs, the reader will find that these concepts are applied in varying degrees, or, as in the case of a survey study, the independent variable is not manipulated at all (see Chapter 10). The level of control and its applications presented in Chapters 9 to 12 will provide the remaining knowledge to fully critique the aspects of the design in a study.

Once it has been established whether the necessary control or uniformity of conditions has been maintained, the evaluator needs to determine if the study is believable or valid. The evaluator should ask if the findings are the result of the variables tested and internally valid or if there could be another explanation. To assess this aspect the threats to internal validity should be reviewed. If the investigator's study was systematic, well grounded in theory, and followed the criteria for each of the processes, then the reader will probably conclude that the study is internally valid.

In addition, the critical reader needs to know if a study has external validity or generalizability to other populations or environmental conditions. External validity can be claimed only after internal validity has been established. If the credibility of a study (internal validity) has not been established, then a study could not be generalized (external validity) to other populations. Determination of external validity goes hand in hand with the sampling frame (see Chapter 15). If the study is not representative of any one group or phenomena of interest, then external validity may be limited or not present at all. The evaluator will find that establishment of internal and external validity needs not only knowledge of the threats to internal and external validity but also a knowledge of the phenomena being studied. A knowledge of the phenomena being studied allows critical judgments to be made regarding the linkage of theories and variables for testing. The critical reader should find that the design follows from the theoretical framework, literature review, problem statement, and hypotheses. The evaluator should feel, based on clinical knowledge as well as the knowledge of the research process, that the investigators in a study are not comparing apples to oranges.

SUMMARY

The purpose of the design is to provide the format of a masterful and creative piece of research. As you will find in the following chapters, there are many types of designs. No matter which type of design the researcher uses, the purpose always remains the same. The consumer of research should be able to locate within the study a sense of the question that the researcher wished to answer. The question should be proposed with a plan or scheme for the accomplishment of the investigation. Depending on the question, the consumer should be able to recognize the steps taken by the investigator to ensure control.

The choice of the specific design depends on the nature of the problem. To specify the nature of the problem requires that the design reflects the investigator's attempts to maintain objectivity, accuracy, pragmatic considerations, and, most importantly, control. Control not only affects the outcome of a study, but also its future utility. The design should also reflect how the investigator attempted to control threats to both internal and external validity. Internal validity needs to be established before external validity can. Both are considered within the sampling structure.

No matter which design the researcher chooses, it should be evident to the reader that the choice was based on a thorough examination of the problem within a theoretical framework. The design, problem statement, literature review, theoretical framework, and hypothesis should all interrelate to demonstrate a woven pattern (see Fig. 8-1). It should also be kept in mind that the choice of the design is affected by pragmatic issues and, at times, two different designs may be equally valid for the same problem. The main issues of control have been only minimally addressed here and will be covered in depth as they pertain to specific designs.

References

Aaronson, L.S. (1989). Perceived and received support: effects on health behavior during pregnancy, *Nursing Research,* **38**:4-9.

Brooten, D., Kumar, S., Brown, L.P., Butts, P., Finkler, S.A., Bakewell-Sachs, S., Gibbons, A., and Delivoria-Papadopoulos, M. (1986). A randomized clinical trial of early hospital discharge and home follow-up of very-low-birth-weight infants, *The New England Journal of Medicine,* **315**:934-939.

Campbell, D., and Stanley, J. (1966). *Experimental and quasi-experimental designs for research,* Chicago, Rand McNally.

Curry, M.A. (1982). Maternal-attachment behavior and the mother's self-concept, *Nursing Research,* **31**:73.

Farr, L., Keene, A., Samson, D., and Michael, A. (1984). Alterations in circadian excretion of urinary variables and physiological indicators of stress following surgery, *Nursing Research,* **33**:140-146.

Green, B.L., Grace, M.C., Lindy, J.D., Titchener, J.L., and Lindy, J.G. (1983). Levels of functional impairment following a civilian disaster: The Beverly Hills Supper Club fire. *Journal of Consulting and Clinical Psychology,* **51**:573-580.

Keefe, M.R. (1988). The impact of infant rooming-in on maternal sleep at night, *JOGNN,* **17**:122-126.

Koniak-Griffin, D. and Ludington-Hoe, S.M. (1988). Developmental and temperament outcomes of sensory stimulation in healthy infants, *Nursing Research,* **37**:70-76.

Kunnel, M.T., O'Brien, C., Hazard Munro, B., and Medoff-Cooper, B. (1988). Comparisons of rectal, femoral, axillary, and skin-to-mattress temperatures in stable neonates, *Nursing Research,* **37**:162-164.

Lim-Levy, F. (1982). The effect of oxygen inhalation on oral temperature, *Nursing Research,* **31**:150-153.

Lowe, N.K., and Roberts, J.E. (1988). The convergence between in-labor report and postpartum recall of parturition pain, *Research in Nursing and Health,* **11**:11-22.

Manderino, M.A., and Bzdek, V.M. (1984). Effects of modeling and information on reactions to pain: a childbirth-preparation analogue, *Nursing Research,* **33**:9-14.

Murphy, S.A. (1986). Stress, coping and mental health outcomes following a natural disaster: bereaved family members and friends compared, *Death Studies,* **10**:411-429.

Murphy, S.A. (1988). Mental distress and recovery in a high-risk bereavement sample three years after untimely death, *Nursing Research,* **37**: 30-35.

Rubin, R. (1967a). Attainment of the maternal role, part I: processes, *Nursing Research,* **16**:237-245.

Rubin, R. (1967b). Attainment of the maternal role, part II: models and referents, *Nursing Research,* **16**:342-346.

Vessey, J.A. (1988). Comparison of two teaching methods on children's knowledge of their internal bodies, *Nursing Research,* **37**:262-267.

Additional Readings

Cook, T.D., and Campbell, D.T. (1979). *Quasi-experimentation: design analysis issues for field settings,* Boston, Houghton-Mifflin Co.

Judd, C.M., and Kenny, D.A. (1981). *Estimating the effects of social interventions,* Cambridge, Cambridge University Press.

Kerlinger, F.N. (1986). *Foundations of behavioral research,* 3rd ed., New York, Holt, Rinehart & Winston, Inc.

Schantz, D., and Linderman, C.A. (1982). The research design, *The Journal of Nursing Administration,* **82**:35-38.

9

Experimental and Quasiexperimental Designs

Margaret Grey

LEARNING OBJECTIVES

After reading this chapter the student should be able to do the following:

◇ List the criteria necessary for inferring cause-and-effect relationships.

◇ Distinguish the differences between several experimental and quasiexperimental designs.

◇ Define internal validity problems associated with several experimental and quasiexperimental designs.

◇ Critically evaluate the findings of selected studies that test cause-and-effect relationships.

KEY TERMS

antecedent variable	intervening variable
control	manipulation
dependent variable	quasiexperimental design
experimental design	randomization
independent variable	

The purpose of this chapter is to acquaint you with the issues involved in interpreting studies that utilize **experimental design** and **quasiexperimental design.** One of the fundamental purposes of scientific research in any profession is to determine cause-and-effect relationships. In nursing, for example, we are concerned with developing effective approaches to maintaining and restoring wellness. Testing such nursing interventions to determine how well they actually work is accomplished by using experimental and quasiexperimental designs. These designs differ from nonexperimental designs in one important way: the researcher actively brings about the desired effect and does not passively observe behaviors or actions. In other words, the researcher is interested in making something happen, not merely observing the routine.

Experimental designs are particularly suitable for testing cause-and-effect relationships because they help to eliminate potential alternative explanations for the findings. To infer causality requires that the following three criteria be met: the causal variable and effect variable must be associated with each other, the cause must precede the effect, and the relationship must not be explainable by another variable. When the reader critiques studies that utilize experimental and quasiexperimental designs, the primary focus will be on the validity of the conclusion that the experimental treatment, or the **independent variable,** caused the desired effect on the outcome, or **dependent variable.** The validity of the conclusion depends on just how well the researcher has controlled the other variables that may explain the relationship studied. Thus the focus of this chapter will be to explain how the various types of experimental and quasiexperimental designs control extraneous variables.

It should be made clear, however, that most research in nursing is not experimental. This is because nursing, unlike the physical sciences, is just beginning to identify the content and theory that are the exclusive province of nursing science. In addition, an experimental design requires that all of the relevant variables have been defined so that they can be manipulated and studied. In most problem areas in nursing this requirement has not been met. Therefore nonexperimental designs utilized in identifying variables and determining their relationship to each other often need to be done before experimental studies are performed.

THE TRUE EXPERIMENTAL DESIGN

An *experiment* is a scientific investigation that makes observations and collects data according to explicit criteria. True experiments have three identifying properties— randomization, control, and manipulation. These properties allow for other explanations of the phenomenon to be ruled out and thereby provide the strength of the design for testing cause-and-effect relationships.

Randomization

Randomization involves the assignment of subjects to either the experimental or control group on a purely random basis. That is, each subject has an equal and known probability of being assigned to either group. Random assignment to groups allows for the elimination of any systematic bias in the groups with respect to attributes that may affect the dependent variable being studied. The procedure for random assignment assumes that any important intervening variables will be equally distributed between the groups and, as discussed in Chapter 8, minimizes variance. Note that random assignment to groups is different from random sampling discussed in Chapter 15.

Control

By **control** we mean the introduction of one or more constants into the experimental situation. Control is acquired by manipulating the causal or independent variable, by randomly assigning subjects to a group, by very carefully preparing experimental protocols, and by using comparison groups. In experimental research the comparison group is the control group, or the group that receives the usual treatment, rather than the innovative experimental one.

Manipulation

We have said that experimental designs are characterized by the researcher "doing something" to at least some of the involved subjects. This "something," or the independent variable, is *manipulated* by giving it to some participants in the study and not to others or by giving different amounts of it to different groups. The independent variable might be a treatment, a teaching plan, or a medication. It is the effect of this **manipulation** that is measured to determine the result of the experimental treatment.

◇   ◇   ◇

The concepts of control, randomization, and manipulation and their application to experimental design are sometimes confusing for students. To see how these properties allow researchers to have confidence in the causal inferences that they make by allowing them to rule out other potential explanations, we will examine the use of these properties in one report. Brooten, Kumar, Brown, Butts, Finkler, Bakewell-Sachs, Gibbons, and Delivoria-Papadopoulos (1986) used a clinical experiment to study the safety, efficacy, and cost savings of early hospital discharge of very-low-birth-weight infants. Infants with birth weights of 1500 or less were *randomly assigned* to one of two groups after parental consent was given. This means that each infant had an equal chance of being assigned to the control or experimental group. The use of random assignment to group helps to ensure that the two study groups are comparable on preexisting factors that might affect the outcomes of interest, such as socioeconomic status and infant's gestational age. Note that the researcher checks statistically to see if the procedure of random assignment did in fact produce groups that are similar.

The two study groups were a routine care group and an early discharge group with home follow-up by a nurse specialist. The degree of *control* exerted over the experimental conditions is illustrated by the detailed description in the report of the home follow-up services provided by the nurse specialists. This ensures that each member of the experimental group receives similar treatment. The *control group* provides a comparison against which the experimental group can be judged.

In this study, time of discharge (early versus usual) is *manipulated*. Infants in the experimental group were discharged early with nurse specialist follow-up, whereas the control group received routine care and follow-up.

The use of the true experimental design allowed the investigators to rule out many of the potential threats to the internal validity of the findings such as selection, history, and maturation (see Chapter 8). By exerting clear and careful control over the experimental situation, the researchers were able to make the assertion that early discharge was safe and cost-effective.

The strength of the true experimental design lies in its ability to help the researcher and the reader to control the effects of any extraneous variables that might constitute threats to internal validity. Such extraneous variables may be either antecedent or intervening. The **antecedent variable** occurs before the study but may affect the dependent variable and confuse the results. Factors such as age, sex, socioeconomic status, and health status might be important antecedent variables in nursing research, because they may affect dependent variables such as recovery time and ability to integrate health care behaviors. Antecedent variables that might affect the dependent variables in the Brooten et al. (1986) study might include infant gestational age, complicating illnesses, parental socioeconomic status, and prenatal care. Randomization helps to ensure that groups will be similar on these variables so that differences in the dependent variable may be attributed to the experimental treatment. It should be noted, however, that the researcher should check and report how the groups actually compared on such variables. The **intervening variable** occurs during the course of the study and is not part of the study, but it affects the dependent variable. An example of an intervening variable that might affect the outcomes in the early discharge study (Brooten et al., 1986) would be a change in the hospital's discharge policy. Certainly, if the hospital changed its policy toward earlier discharges, the study would be affected.

Types of experimental designs

There are several different experimental designs (Campbell and Stanley, 1966). Each is based on the classic design called the *true experiment* diagramed in Fig. 9-1. In this and the following illustrations, a simple notation will be used to describe the design.

R   01   ×   02

R   01   02

Fig. 9-1   The true experiment.

R stands for random assignment of subjects to group, X is the experimental treatment, and O stands for the observations or measurements made of the dependent variable. All true experimental designs have subjects randomly assigned to groups, have an experimental treatment introduced to some of the subjects, and have the effects of the treatment observed. Designs vary primarily in the number of observations that are made.

As shown, subjects are randomly assigned to the two groups, experimental and control, so that antecedent variables are controlled. Then pretest measures or observations are made so that the researcher has a baseline for determining the effect of the independent variable. The researcher then introduces the experimental variable to one of the groups and measures the dependent variable again to see if it has changed. The control group gets no experimental treatment but is also measured later for comparison with the experimental group. The degree of difference between the two groups at the end of the study indicates the confidence that the researcher has that a causal link exists between the independent and dependent variables. Because random assignment and the control inherent in this design minimize the effects of many threats to internal validity, it is a strong design for testing cause-and-effect relationships. However, the design is not perfect. Some threats cannot be controlled in true experimental studies (see Chapter 8). Mortality effects are often a problem in such studies, because people tend to drop out of studies that require their participation over a period of time. If there is a difference in the number of people who drop out of the experimental group from that of the control group, a mortality effect might explain the findings. When reading such a work, examine the sample and the results carefully to see if deaths occurred. Testing is also a problem in these studies, because the researcher is usually giving the same measurement twice, and subjects tend to score better the second time just by learning the test. Researchers can get around this problem in one of two ways. They might use different forms of the same test for the two measurements, or they might use a more complex experimental design called the Solomon four-group design.

The *Solomon four-group design,* shown in Fig. 9-2, has two groups that are identical to those utilized in the classic experimental design, plus two additional groups, an experimental after-group and a control after-group. As the diagram shows, all four groups have randomly assigned subjects as with experimental studies, but the addition of these last two groups helps to rule out testing threats to internal validity that the before and after groups may experience. Suppose a researcher is interested in the effects of some counseling on chronically ill clients' self-esteem, but just taking a measure of self-esteem may influence how the subjects report themselves. For example, the items might make the subjects think more about how they view themselves so that the next time they fill out the questionnaire, their self-esteem might appear to have improved. In reality, however, their self-esteem may be the same as it was before; it

$$
\begin{array}{llll}
R & 01 & \times & 02 \\
R & 01 & & 02 \\
R & & \times & 02 \\
R & & & 02
\end{array}
$$

Fig. 9-2   The Solomon four-group design.

just looks different because they took the test before. The use of this design with the two groups that do not receive the pretest allows for evaluating the effect of the pretest on the posttest in the first two groups. Although this design helps to evaluate the effects of testing, the threat of death remains a problem as with the classic experimental design.

Another frequently utilized experimental design is the *after-only design* shown in Fig. 9-3. This design is composed of two randomly selected groups, and neither group is pretested or measured. Again, the independent variable is introduced to the experimental group and not the control group. The process of randomly assigning the subjects to groups is assumed to be sufficient to ensure a lack of bias so that the researcher can still determine if the treatment created significant differences between the two groups. This design is particularly useful when testing effects are expected to be a major problem and the number of available subjects is too limited to use a Solomon four-group design. A complex example of the use of the after-only experimental design is provided by Olds, Henderson, Tatelbaum, and Chamberlin (1988) who studied a comprehensive program of home visiting for prenatal and postpartum women. Since all the dependent variables could not be measured at entry into the study, such as the child's development and the mother's return to work, the authors chose an after-only design. They randomly assigned families to one of four treatment groups, which included either home visits or comparison services (free transportation for prenatal and well-child care and/or sensory and developmental screening for the child). The authors were able to demonstrate that the nurse-visited families did better on a variety of outcomes than did the other three groups.

Field and laboratory experiments

Experiments can also be classified by setting. Field experiments and laboratory experiments share the properties of control, randomization, and manipulation, and they utilize the same design characteristics, but they are conducted in various environments. Laboratory experiments take place in an artificial setting that is created specifically for the purpose of research. In the laboratory the researcher has almost total control over the features of the environment, such as temperature, humidity, noise level, and subject conditions. On the other hand, field experiments are exactly what the name implies—experiments that take place in some real, existing social setting such as a hospital or clinic where the phenomenon of interest usually occurs. Since most experiments in the nursing literature are field experiments and control is such an important element in the conduction of experiments, it should be obvious that studies conducted in the field are subject to treatment contamination by factors specific to the setting that the researcher cannot control. However, studies conducted in the

$$R \quad \times \quad O$$
$$R \qquad O$$

Fig. 9-3 The after-only experimental design.

laboratory are by nature "artificial," because the setting is created for the purpose of research. Thus laboratory experiments, although stronger in relationship to internal validity questions than field work, suffer more from problems with external validity. For example, a subject's behavior in the laboratory may be quite different from the person's behavior in the real world, a dichotomy that presents problems in generalizing findings from the laboratory to the real world. When research reports are read, then, it is important to consider the setting of the experiment and what impact it might have on the findings of the study. Consider the study of temperatures in neonates by Kunnel, O'Brien, Hazard Munro, and Medoff-Cooper (1988), reprinted in Appendix C. The authors compared four sites of temperature taking. The study could have been accomplished in a laboratory with animals as models, which would have allowed complete control over the external environment of the study, a variable that might be important in measuring temperature. However, there is no guarantee that the animals would be the same as neonates so the study would lose some external validity.

ADVANTAGES AND DISADVANTAGES OF THE EXPERIMENTAL DESIGN

As we have said, experimental designs are the most appropriate for testing cause-and-effect relationships. This is because of the design's ability to control the experimental situation. Therefore it offers better corroboration that *if* the independent variable is manipulated in a certain way, *then* certain consequences can be expected to ensue. Such studies are important because one priority in the development of nursing and nursing research is the development of prescriptive theory (see Chapter 1). Brooten et al. (1986) were able to conclude from their study that the infants of low birthweight who were discharged early and received follow-up from the nurse specialist had outcomes that were as good as or better than those of infants who received routine care. This study and others like it allow nurses to anticipate in a scientific manner the probable effects of their nursing actions.

Still, experimental designs are not the ones most commonly utilized. There are several reasons that most nursing research studies are not experimental. First, experimentation assumes that all of the relevant variables involved in a phenomenon have been identified. For many areas of nursing research this simply is not the case, and descriptive studies need to be completed before experimental interventions can be applied. Second, there are some significant disadvantages to these designs.

One problem with an experimental design is that many variables important in predicting outcomes of nursing care are not amenable to experimental manipulation. It is well known that health status varies with age and socioeconomic status. No matter how careful a researcher is, no one can assign subjects randomly by age or a certain level of income. In addition, some variables may be technically manipulable, but their nature may preclude actually doing so. For example, the ethics of a researcher who tried to randomly assign groups for a study of the effects of cigarette smoking and asked the experimental group to smoke two packs of cigarettes a day would be seriously questioned. It is also potentially true that such a study would not work, since nonsmokers randomly assigned to the smoking group would be unlikely to comply with the research task.

Another problem with experimental designs is that they may be difficult or impractical to perform in field settings. It may be quite difficult to randomly assign clients on a hospital floor to different groups when they might talk to each other about the different treatments. Experimental procedures may also be disruptive to the usual routine of the setting. If several different nurses are involved in administering the experimental program, it may be impossible to ensure that the program is administered in the same way to each subject.

Finally, just being studied may influence the results of the study. This is called the *Hawthorne effect.* Named for the study at the Hawthorne plant of the General Electric Company where it was first noted, this effect means that just because subjects know they are participating in a study, they may answer questions or perform differently. In the Hawthorne experiment the researchers were trying to determine the effect of environmental factors on workers' productivity. Many different changes were made in the environment, and their effects on productivity were measured. No matter what the researchers did—improved the lighting or dimmed it, piped in music loudly or softly, or made no change—once the study began, productivity increased with each change. The increase in productivity was not a result of the environmental changes but rather was caused by the attention being paid to the workers! (See Chapter 8.)

Because of these problems in carrying out true experiments, researchers frequently turn to another type of research design to evaluate cause-and-effect relationships. Such designs, because they look like experiments but lack some of the control of the true experimental design, are called quasiexperiments.

QUASIEXPERIMENTAL DESIGNS

In a quasiexperimental design full experimental control is not possible. *Quasiexperiments* are research designs where the researcher initiates an experimental treatment but where some characteristic of a true experiment is lacking. Control may not be possible because of the nature of the independent variable or the nature of the available subjects. Usually what is lacking in a quasiexperimental design is the element of randomization. In other cases the control group may be missing. However, like experiments, quasiexperiments involve the introduction of an experimental treatment.

Compared with the true experimental design, quasiexperiments are quite similar in their utilization. Both types of designs are used when the researcher is interested in testing cause-and-effect relationships. However, the basic problem with the quasiexperimental approach is a weakened confidence in making causal assertions. Because of the lack of some controls in the research situation, quasiexperimental designs are

$$01 \quad \times \quad 02$$
$$01 \qquad 02$$

Fig. 9-4   The nonequivalent control group design.

subject to contamination by many, if not all, of the threats to internal validity discussed in Chapter 8.

There are many different quasiexperimental designs. We will discuss only the ones most commonly utilized in nursing research. Again we will use the notations introduced earlier in the chapter.

Refer back to the true experimental design shown in Fig. 9-1 and compare it to the *nonequivalent control group design* shown in Fig. 9-4. You should note that this design looks exactly like the true experiment except that subjects are not randomly assigned to groups. Suppose a researcher is interested in the effects of a new diabetes education program on the physical and psychosocial outcome of newly diagnosed clients. If conditions were right, the researcher might be able to randomly assign subjects to either the group receiving the new program or the group receiving the usual program, but for any number of reasons, that design might not be possible. For example, nurses on the floor where clients are admitted might be so excited about the new program that they cannot help but include the new information for all clients. So the researcher has two choices, to abandon the experiment or to conduct a quasiexperiment. To conduct a quasiexperiment the researcher might find a similar unit that has not been introduced to the new program and study the newly diagnosed diabetic clients who are admitted to that floor as a comparison group. The study would then involve this type of design.

The nonequivalent control group design is very commonly used in nursing research studies conducted in field settings. The basic problem with the design is the weakened confidence the researcher can have in assuming that the experimental and comparison groups are similar at the beginning of the study. Threats to internal validity such as selection, maturation, testing, and mortality are possible with this design. However, the design is relatively strong, because the gathering of the data at the time of the pretest allows the researcher to compare the equivalence of the two groups on important antecedent variables before the independent variable is introduced. In our example the motivation of the clients to learn about their diabetes might be important in determining the effect of the new teaching program. The researcher could include in the measures taken at the outset of the study some measure of motivation to learn. Then differences between the two groups on this variable can be tested, and if significant differences exist, they can be controlled statistically in the analysis. Nonetheless the strength of the causal assertions that can be made on the basis of such designs depends on the ability of the researcher to identify and measure or control possible threats to internal validity.

Now suppose that the researcher did not think to measure the subjects before the introduction of the new treatment, but afterward decided that it would be useful to have data demonstrating the effect of the program. Perhaps, for example, a third party

$$\times \quad O$$
$$O$$

Fig. 9-5   The after-only nonequivalent control group design.

asks for such data to determine whether the extra cost of the new teaching program should be paid. The study that could then be conducted would look like that drawn in Fig. 9-5.

This design, the *after-only nonequivalent control group design,* is similar to the after-only experimental design, but randomization is not utilized to assign subjects to group. This design makes the assumption that the two groups are equivalent and comparable before the introduction of the independent variable. Thus the soundness of the design and the confidence that we can put in the findings depend on the soundness of this assumption of preintervention comparability. Often it is very difficult to support the assertion that the two nonrandomly assigned groups are comparable at the outset of the study, because there is no way of assessing its validity. In the example of the teaching program for newly diagnosed diabetic clients, measuring the subjects' motivation after the teaching program would not tell us whether their motivations differed before they received the program, and it is possible that the teaching program would motivate individuals to learn more about their health problem. Therefore the researcher's conclusion that the teaching program improved physical status and psychosocial outcome would be subject to the alternative conclusion that the results were an effect of preexisting motivations (selection effect) in combination with greater learning in those so motivated (selection-maturation interaction). Nonetheless this design is frequently utilized in nursing research, because there often are limited opportunities for data collection and because it is particularly useful when testing effects may be problematic. Consider again the example of the after-only experimental design. Suppose Olds et al. (1988), who studied the effects of home visits on infant outcomes in at-risk families, had not randomly assigned subjects to groups. The study would then be an example of an after-only nonequivalent control group design. If they had chosen to conduct the study using this design, and if they had found the same results, they would have been less confident of the results, since selection effects may have been significant.

A *preexperimental design* that is commonly employed in clinical nursing studies is the *one-group pretest-posttest design.* This design is similar to the nonequivalent control group design except for the absence of the control group. It can be diagramed as in Fig. 9-6. Hill, Levine, and Whelton (1988) used the one-group pretest-posttest design to determine the impact of the 1984 Joint National Consensus Report on High Blood Pressure on the practice of a sample of Maryland physicians. The authors were not able to control the physicians or the report, but they were able to determine actions before and 1 year after dissemination of the report.

The one-group pretest-posttest design is employed when the researcher does not have access to an equivalent group and cannot use random assignment. The design then loses two important characteristics of experimentation—randomization and

01 $\times$ 02

Fig. 9-6 The one-group pretest-posttest design.

control over extraneous variables. Although this design is better than not studying the effect of nursing care, it suffers from many problems in interpretation of the results. In the diabetes example, how would the reader know if the improvement in the clients' physical status and psychosocial adjustment were not the result of the types of clients that happened to be admitted over the study period (selection)? Perhaps some event occurred on the study unit during the time of the project that would cause the researcher to conclude that the program had no impact (history). Any number of alternative conclusions could be drawn from these and similar data.

One approach that is utilized by researchers when only one group is available is to study that group over a longer period of time. This quasiexperimental design is called a *time series design* and is pictured in Fig. 9-7. Time series designs are useful for determining trends. Samet, Wiggins, Key, and Becker (1988) wanted to determine the effect of ethnicity on mortality rate related to lung disease. They used data from the National Health and Examination Surveys of 1958 to 1982 to determine mortality rates for Hispanic whites, other whites, and native Americans. These national surveys are performed periodically by the National Center for Health Statistics, and they help to determine the health status of the American people. The data collected are available for analysis by individuals who are interested in looking at different questions than the Center analyses. In this case, mortality statistics were analyzed to determine if ethnicity played a role in deaths from lung disease. This is considered a quasiexperiment because the researchers are interested in the causes of death in relation to lung disease. However, since they could not assign ethnicity, they examined trends in the different groups over time and were able to determine that Hispanic and native Americans had higher mortality rates than white Americans.

To rule out some alternative explanations for the findings of a one-group pretest-posttest design, researchers can measure the phenomenon of interest over a longer period of time and introduce the experimental treatment sometime during the course of the data collection period. Even with the absence of a control group, the broader range of data collection points help to rule out such threats to validity as history effects. Obviously our problem related to the earlier example of teaching diabetic clients will not lend itself to this design, because we do not have access to the clients before the diagnosis.

An example of how a time series design would strengthen causal conclusions is provided by Perry (1981). Perry studied the effect of a rehabilitation program on a group of clients with chronic lung disease, but she had only the one group to study. Thus it is difficult to be confident that the changes she found and attributed to the rehabilitation program might not have happened without the program. On the other hand, the use of the time series design would have allowed Perry to follow the clients for a longer period of time and to be more confident that the program worked. The time series weakens the alternative explanation that the program worked because of

$$01 \quad 02 \quad 03 \quad 04 \quad \times \quad 05 \quad 06 \quad 07 \quad 08$$

Fig. 9-7 The time series design.

something else that happened during the study period. However, the testing threat to validity looms large in these designs, since measures are repeated so many times.

Advantages and disadvantages of quasiexperimental designs

Given the problems inherent in interpreting the results of studies utilizing quasiexperimental designs, you may be wondering why anyone would use them. Quasiexperimental designs are used very frequently because they are practical, feasible, and generalizable. These designs are more adaptable to the real-world practice setting than the controlled experimental designs. In addition, for some hypotheses these designs may be the only way to evaluate the effect of the independent variable of interest.

The weaknesses of the quasiexperimental approach involve mainly the inability to make clear cause-and-effect statements. However, if the researcher can rule out any plausible alternative explanations for the findings, such studies can lead to furthering knowledge about causal relationships. Researchers have several options for ferreting out these alternative explanations. They may control them a priori by design or control them statistically, or in some cases, common sense or knowledge of the problem and the population can suggest that a particular explanation is not plausible. Nonetheless it is very important to replicate such studies to support the causal assertions developed through the use of quasiexperimental designs.

The literature on cigarette smoking is an excellent example of how findings from many studies, experimental and quasiexperimental, can be linked to establish a causal relationship. A large number of well-controlled experiments with laboratory animals randomly assigned to smoking and nonsmoking conditions have documented that lung disease will develop in smoking animals. Whereas such evidence is suggestive of a link between smoking and lung disease in humans, it is not directly transferable because animals and humans are different. But we cannot randomly assign humans to smoking and nonsmoking groups for ethical and other reasons. So researchers interested in this problem have to use quasiexperimental data to test their hypotheses about smoking and lung disease. Several different quasiexperimental designs have been used to study this problem and all had similar results — that there is a causal relationship between cigarette smoking and lung disease. Despite this massive evidence the tobacco associations continue to insist that because the studies are not experimental, another explanation for the relationship may exist. One possible explanation that infrequently comes up is that the tendency to smoke is linked to the tendency for lung disease to develop, and so the smoking itself is merely an unimportant intervening variable!

QUALITY ASSURANCE AND EXPERIMENTATION

As the science of nursing expands and the cost of health care rises, nurses and others have become increasingly concerned with the ability to document the costs and the benefits of nursing care. This is a very complex process, but at its heart is the ability to measure the results of nursing care. Such studies are usually associated with quality assurance. Studies of quality assurance do exactly what the name implies; in such studies we are concerned with the determination of the quality of nursing and health care and with assuring the public that they are receiving quality care.

Quality assurance in nursing is in its infancy. We are just beginning to apply techniques of experimentation to the study of delivering nursing care. Many early quality assurance studies documented whether or not nursing care had met predetermined standards. These were important studies, but they do not allow us to compare different ways of providing care. The use of experimental and quasiexperimental designs in quality assurance studies will allow for the determination not only of whether care is adequate but which method of care is best under certain conditions. The study by Brooten et al. (1986) was so important, not only to nursing but to health care in general, because the authors were able to demonstrate not only that the intervention was as safe and efficacious as routine care but that there was a significant cost savings.

CRITIQUING EXPERIMENTAL AND QUASIEXPERIMENTAL DESIGNS

We have said that various designs for research studies differ in the amount of control the researcher has over the antecedent and intervening variables that may impact the results of the study. True experimental designs offer the most possibility for control, and preexperimental designs offer the least. Quasiexperimental designs lie somewhere between. Research designs must balance the needs for internal validity and external validity to produce useful results. In addition, judicious use of design requires that the chosen design be appropriate to the problem, free of bias, and capable of answering the research question.

Questions that the reader should pose when reading studies that test cause-and-effect relationships are listed in the box on p. 160. All of these questions should help the reader to judge whether it can be confidently believed that a causal relationship exists.

For studies where either experimental or quasiexperimental designs are utilized, first try to determine the type of design that was used. Often a statement describing the design of the study appears in the abstract and in the methods sections of the paper. If such a statement is not present, the reader should examine the paper for evidence of the following three characteristics: control, randomization, and manipulation. If all are discussed, the design is probably experimental. On the other hand, if the study involves the administration of an experimental treatment but does not involve the random assignment of subjects to groups, the design is quasiexperimental.

Then try to identify which of the various designs within these two types of designs was used. Determining the answer to these questions gives you a head start, because each design has its inherent threats to validity, and this step makes it a bit easier to critically evaluate the study. The next question to ask is whether the researcher required a solution to a cause-and-effect problem. If so, the study is suited to these

Critiquing Criteria

1. What design is used in the study?
2. Is the design experimental or quasiexperimental?
3. Is the problem one of a cause-and-effect relationship?
4. Is the method used appropriate to the problem?
5. Is the design suited to the setting of the study?

Experimental Designs

1. What experimental design is used in the study?
2. Is it clear how randomization, control, and manipulation were applied?
3. Are there any reasons to believe that there are alternative explanations for the findings?
4. Are all threats to validity, including mortality, addressed in the report?
5. Whether the experiment was conducted in the laboratory or a clinical setting, are the findings generalizable to the larger population of interest?

Quasiexperimental Designs

1. What quasiexperimental design is used in the study?
2. What are the most common threats to the validity of the findings of this design?
3. Have all plausible alternative explanations been addressed?
4. Are the author's explanations of threats to validity acceptable?
5. What does the author say about the limitations of the study?
6. Are there other limitations related to the design that are not mentioned?

designs. Finally, think about the conduct of the study in the setting. Is it realistic to think that the study could be conducted in a clinical setting without some contamination?

The most important question to ask yourself as your read experimental studies is "What else could have happened to explain the findings?" Thus it is important that the author provide adequate accounts of how the procedures for randomization, control, and manipulation were carried out. The paper should include a description of the procedures for random assignment to such a degree that the reader could determine just how likely it was for any one subject to be assigned to a particular group. The description of the independent variable should also be detailed. The inclusion of this information helps the reader to decide if it is possible that the treatment given to some subjects in the experimental group might be different from what was given to others in the same group. In addition, threats to validity such as testing and the occurrence of deaths should be addressed. Otherwise there is the potential for the findings of the study to be in error and less believable to the reader.

This question of potential alternative explanations or threats to internal validity for the findings is even more important when critically evaluating a quasiexperimental study, because quasiexperimental designs cannot possibly control many plausible alternative explanations. A well-written report of a quasiexperimental study will systematically review potential threats to the validity of the findings. Then the reader's work is to decide if the author's explanations make sense.

As with all research, studies using these designs need to be generalizable to a larger population of people than those actually studied. Thus it is important to decide whether the experimental protocol eliminated some potential subjects and whether this affected not only internal validity but also external validity.

SUMMARY

This chapter has reviewed two types of design commonly used in nursing research to test hypotheses about cause-and-effect relationships. Experimental and quasiexperimental designs are useful for the development of nursing, because they test the effects of nursing actions and lead to the development of prescriptive theory.

True experiments are characterized by the ability of the researcher to control extraneous variation, to manipulate the independent variable, and to randomly assign subjects to research groups. Experiments conducted either in clinical settings or in the laboratory provide the best evidence in support of a causal relationship because the following three criteria can be met:

1. The independent and dependent variables are related to each other.
2. The independent variable chronologically precedes the dependent variable.
3. The relationship cannot be explained by the presence of a third variable.

However, there are many times when experimental designs are impractical or unethical; therefore researchers will frequently turn to quasiexperimental designs to test cause-and-effect relationships. Quasiexperiments may lack either the randomization or comparison group characteristics of true experiments or both of these factors. Their usefulness in studying causal relationships depends on the ability of the researcher to rule out plausible threats to the validity of the findings, such as history, selection, maturation, and testing effects.

Finally, questions for the student to ask regarding the finding of experimental and quasiexperimental designs were presented. The overall purpose of critiquing such studies is to assess the validity of the findings and to determine if these findings are worth incorporating into the nurse's personal practice.

References

Brooten, D., Kumar, S., Brown, L.P., Butts, P., Finkler, S., Bakewell-Sachs, S., Gibbons, A., and Delivoria-Papadopoulos, M. (1986). A randomized clinical trial of early hospital discharge and home follow-up of very-low-birth-weight infants, *New England Journal of Medicine,* **315:**934-939.

Campbell, D., and Stanley, J. (1966). *Experimental and quasiexperimental designs for research,* Chicago, Rand McNally.

Gennaro, S. (1988). Postpartal anxiety and depression in mothers of term and preterm infants, *Nursing Research,* **37**:82-85.

Hill, M.N., Levine, D.M., and Whelton, P.K. (1988). Awareness, use, and impact of the 1984 Joint National Committee Consensus Report on High Blood Pressure, *American Journal of Public Health,* **78**:1190-1194.

Kruszewski, A.Z., Long, S.H., and Johnson, J.E. (1979). Effect of positioning on discomfort from intramuscular injections in the dorsogluteal site, *Nursing Research,* **28**:103-105.

Kunnel, M.T., O'Brien, C., Hazard Munro, B., and Medoff-Cooper, B. (1988). Comparisons of rectal, femoral, axillary, and skin-to-mattress temperatures in stable neonates, *Nursing Research,* **37**:162-164, 189.

Olds, D.L., Henderson, C.R., Tatelbaum, R., and Chamberlin, R. (1988). Improving the life-course development of socially disadvantaged mothers: a randomized trial of nurse home visitation, *American Journal of Public Health,* **78**:1436-1445.

Perry, J.A. (1981). Effectiveness of teaching in the rehabilitation of patients with chronic bronchitis and emphysema, *Nursing Research,* **30**:219-222.

Samet, J.M., Wiggins, C.L., Key, C.R., and Becker, T.M. (1988). Mortality from lung cancer and chronic obstructive pulmonary disease in New Mexico, 1958-82, *American Journal of Public Health,* **78**:1182-1186.

Selltiz, C., Wrightsman, L.S., and Cook, S.W. (1976). *Research methods in social relations,* New York, Holt, Rinehart, & Winston, Inc.

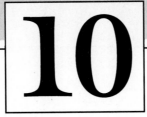

Nonexperimental Designs

Geri LoBiondo-Wood
Judith Haber

LEARNING OBJECTIVES

After reading this chapter the student should be able to do the following:

◇ Describe the overall purpose of nonexperimental designs.

◇ Describe the characteristics of survey and interrelationship designs.

◇ Define the differences between survey and interrelationship designs.

◇ List the advantages and disadvantages of surveys and each type of interrelationship design.

◇ Discuss relational inferences versus causal inferences as they relate to nonexperimental designs.

◇ Identify the criteria used to critique nonexperimental research designs.

◇ Apply the critiquing criteria to the evaluation of nonexperimental research designs as they appear in research reports.

KEY TERMS

correlational study   nonexperimental research
cross-sectional study   prediction study
developmental study   prospective study
ex post facto study   retrospective data
interrelationship study   retrospective study
longitudinal study   survey study

Nonexperimental research designs are used in studies where the researcher wishes to construct a picture of a phenomenon or make account of events as they naturally occur. In experimental research the independent variable is manipulated; in nonexperimental research it is not. In nonexperimental research the independent variables have already occurred, so to speak, and the investigator cannot directly control them by manipulation (Pedhazur, 1982). Thus in an experimental design the researcher actively manipulates one or more variables, but in a nonexperimental design the researcher explores relationships.

The reader of research reports will find that most of the studies that are conducted and reported utilize a nonexperimental design. Many phenomena that are of interest and relevant to nursing do not lend themselves to an experimental design. For example, nurses studying the phenomena of pain may be interested in the amount of pain, variations in the amount of pain, and client responses to postoperative pain. The investigator would not design an experimental study that would potentially intensify a client's pain just to study the pain experience from any one of these perspectives. Instead, the researcher would perhaps examine the factors that contribute to the variability in a client's postoperative pain experience. A nonexperimental research design would then be utilized to help answer such questions.

Nonexperimental research also requires a clear, concise problem statement that is based on a theoretical framework. Even though the researcher does not actively manipulate the variables, the concepts of control introduced in Chapter 8 should be followed as much as possible.

Researchers are not in agreement on how to classify nonexperimental studies. For purposes of discussion this chapter will divide nonexperimental designs into **survey studies** and **interrelationship studies** as illustrated in Table 10-1. An overall schema of research design is presented in Fig. 10-1. These categories are some-

EXPERIMENTAL ⟶ QUASIEXPERIMENTAL ⟶ NONEXPERIMENTAL

Fig. 10-1   Continuum of research design.

Table 10-1 Summary of Nonexperimental Research Designs

I. Survey studies
II. Interrelationship studies
   A. Correlational studies
   B. Ex post facto studies
   C. Prediction studies
   D. Developmental studies
      1. Cross-sectional and longitudinal studies
      2. Retrospective and prospective studies

what flexible, and other sources may classify nonexperimental studies in a different way. Some studies fall exclusively within one of these categories, whereas other studies have characteristics of more than one category. This chapter will introduce the reader to the various types of nonexperimental designs, the advantages and disadvantages of nonexperimental designs, the use of nonexperimental research, the issues of causality, and the critiquing process as it relates to nonexperimental research.

SURVEY STUDIES

The broadest category of nonexperimental research is the survey study. Survey studies collect detailed descriptions of existing phenomena and use the data to justify and assess current conditions and practices or to make more intelligent plans for improving them. Data may be collected by either a structured questionnaire or a structured or unstructured interview (see Chapter 13). Survey researchers study either small or large samples of subjects drawn from defined populations. The units of analysis can be either broad or narrow and can be made up of people or institutions. For example, if a primary care rehabilitation unit were to be established in a hospital, a survey might be taken of the prospective applicant's attitudes with regard to primary nursing before the staff of this unit are selected. In a broader example, if a hospital were contemplating converting all client care units to primary nursing, a survey might be conducted to determine the attitudes of a representative sample of nurses in hospital X toward primary nursing. The data may then be the basis for projecting in-service needs of nursing regarding primary care. The scope and depth of a survey are then a function of the nature of the problem.

Surveys are descriptive and exploratory in nature. In descriptive surveys investigators attempt only to relate one variable to another; they do not attempt to determine the cause. The investigators merely search for accurate information about the characteristics of particular subjects, groups, institutions, or situations or about the frequency of a phenomenon's occurrence. The variables of interest can be classified as opinions, attitudes, or facts. An example of an opinion or attitude variable might be the responses of nurses at different educational levels toward abortion (Littlefield-Derby, LoBiondo-Wood, and Olney-Springer, 1981). Another example of a survey is the study conducted by Hendrix, Sabritt, McDaniel, and Field (1988). In this study the researchers surveyed the perceptions and attitudes toward nursing impairment held by 1047 registered nurses.

Examples of facts might include attributes of individuals that are a function of their membership in society, such as sex, income level, political and religious affiliations, ethnic group, occupation, and educational level. Classic examples of survey research may be found in the surveys conducted during political campaigns to determine voter trends. Researchers commonly use demographic variables such as sex, economic status, and geographic location to provide an assessment of voter preference.

There are both advantages and disadvantages of survey research. Two major advantages are that a great deal of information can be obtained from a large population in a fairly economical manner and that survey research information can be surprisingly accurate. If a sample is representative of the population (see Chapter 15), a relatively small number of respondents can provide an accurate picture of the target population.

There are several disadvantages of survey studies. First, the information obtained in a survey tends to be superficial. The breadth rather than the depth of the information is emphasized. Second, conducting a survey requires a great deal of expertise in a variety of research areas. The survey investigator must know sampling techniques, questionnaire construction, interviewing, and data analysis to produce a reliable and valid study. Third, large-scale surveys can be time-consuming and costly, although the use of on-site personnel can reduce costs.

Research consumers should recognize that a well-constructed survey can provide a wealth of data about a particular phenomenon of interest even though relationships between variables are not being examined.

INTERRELATIONSHIP STUDIES

In contrast to investigators who use survey research, other investigators who use nonexperimental designs endeavor to trace interrelationships between variables that will provide a deeper insight into the phenomenon of interest. These studies can be classified as interrelationship studies. The following types of interrelationship studies will be discussed: **correlational studies, ex post facto, prediction,** and **developmental studies.**

Correlational studies

The research consumer will find that an investigator utilizes a correlational design to examine the relationship between two or more variables. The researcher is not testing whether one variable causes another variable but whether the variables covary; that is, as one variable changes does a related change occur in the other variable? The researcher utilizing this design is interested in quantifying the magnitude or strength of the relationship between the variables. The positive or negative direction of the relationship is also a central concern of the researcher (see Chapter 17 for a complete explanation of the correlation coefficient). For example, Newman and Gaudiano (1984) conducted a correlation study that focused on depression as an explanation for the experience of decreased subjective time in the elderly. They defined subjective time as a ratio of awareness to the content of events in an individual's life (Subjective time = Awareness/Content). An analysis of the data showed that there was a positive and significant correlation ($r = 0.35$) between depression and subjective time estimates. This correlation was suggestive to the investigators that higher levels of depression were positively related to decreased subjective time estimation.

It should be remembered that the researchers were not testing a cause-and-effect relationship. All that is known is that the researchers found a relationship and that one variable (depression) varied in a consistent way with another variable (subjective time estimate) for the particular sample studied. When reviewing a correlational study it is important to remember what relationship the researcher is testing and to notice whether the researcher implied a relationship that is consistent with the theoretical framework and hypotheses being tested.

Correlational studies offer researchers and research consumers the following advantages:

◇ An increased flexibility when investigating complex relationships among variables
◇ An efficient and effective method of collecting a large amount of data about a problem area
◇ A potential for practical application in clinical settings
◇ A potential foundation for future, more rigorous research studies
◇ A possible framework for investigating the relationship between variables that are inherently not manipulable

The reader will find that the correlational design has a quality of realism about it and is particularly appealing because it suggests the potential for practical solutions to clinical problems.

The following are disadvantages of correlational studies:

◇ The variables of interest are beyond the researcher's control
◇ The researcher is unable to manipulate the variables of interest
◇ The researcher does not employ randomization in the sampling procedures because of dealing with preexisting groups, and therefore generalizability is decreased
◇ The researcher is unable to determine a causal relationship between the variables because of the lack of manipulation, control, and randomization

One of the most common misuses of a correlational design is the researcher's conclusion that a causal relationship exists between the variables. In the Newman and Gaudiano investigation (1984) the researchers appropriately concluded that a relationship existed between the variables, not that depression in the elderly caused a change in subjective time. The inability to draw causal statements should not lead the research consumer to conclude that a nonexperimental correlational study utilizes a weak design. It is a very useful design for clinical research studies, because many of the phenomena of clinical interest are beyond the researcher's ability to manipulate, control, and randomize. For instance, a researcher interested in studying the grief experiences of women who have recently miscarried could not randomly assign subjects to grief and nongrief groups. Also, the experience of a miscarriage is a naturally occurring process and, as such, cannot be manipulated.

Ex post facto studies

When scientists wish to explain causality or the factors that determine the occurrence of events or conditions, they prefer to employ an experimental design. However, they cannot always manipulate the independent variable X or utilize random assignments. In cases where experimental designs cannot be employed, ex post facto studies may be utilized. *Ex post facto* literally means "from after the fact." Ex post facto studies are also known as explanatory, descriptive studies (Van Dalen, 1979), causal-comparative studies (Van Dalen, 1979), or comparative surveys (Fox, 1982). As we discuss this design further, the reader will see that many elements of ex post facto research are similar to quasiexperimental designs (Campbell and Stanley, 1963).

In ex post facto studies the consumer will find that the researcher hypothesizes, for instance that X (cigarette smoking) is related to and a determinant of Y (lung cancer), but X, the presumed cause, is not manipulated and subjects are not randomly assigned to groups. Rather, a group of subjects who have experienced X (cigarette smoking) in a normal situation is located and a control group of subjects who have not is chosen. The behavior, performance, or condition (lung tissue) of the two groups is compared to determine whether the exposure to X had the effect predicted by the hypothesis. Table 10-2 illustrates a paradigm for ex post facto design. Examination of Table 10-2 reveals that whereas cigarette smoking appears to be a determinant of lung cancer, the researcher is still not in a position to conclude that there is a causal relationship between the variables, because there has been no manipulation of the independent variable or random assignment of subjects to groups.

The advantages of the ex post facto design are similar to those inherent in the correlational design. The additional benefit of the ex post facto design is that it offers a higher level of control than the correlational studies. For example, in the cigarette smoking study a group of nonsmokers' lung tissue samples are compared to samples of smokers' lung tissue. This comparison enables the researcher to establish that there is a differential effect of cigarette smoking on lung tissue. However, the researcher remains unable to draw a causal linkage between the two variables, and this inability is the major disadvantage of the ex post facto design.

Another disadvantage of ex post facto research is the problem of an alternative hypothesis being the reason for the documented relationship. If the researcher obtains data from two existing groups of subjects, such as one that has been exposed to X and one that has not, and the data support the hypothesis that X is related to Y, the researcher cannot be sure whether X or some extraneous variable is the real cause of the occurrence of Y. Finding naturally occurring groups of subjects who are similar in all respects except for their exposure to the variable of interest is very difficult. There is always the possibility that the groups differ in some other way, such as exposure to

Table 10-2 Paradigm for the Ex Post Facto Design

Groups (not randomly assigned)	Independent variable (not manipulated by investigator)	Dependent variable
Exposed group	X	Y_E
Cigarette smokers	Cigarette smoking	Lung cancer
Control group		Y_C
Nonsmokers		No lung cancer

some other lung irritants, which can affect the findings of the study and produce spurious results. Consequently, the critiquer of such a study needs to cautiously evaluate the conclusions drawn by the investigator.

Prediction studies

Researchers in education and management positions at times want to make a forecast or prediction about how successful individuals will be in a particular setting, field of specialty, or circumstance. In this case *prediction studies* are employed. For example, in a study conducted by Bello, Haber, King, and King (1980) an attempt was made to decrease the attrition rate of nursing students in an associate degree nursing program. Retrospective data of past students were used to establish the criteria for success or failure of future students as measured by success on state board exams. Data utilized as criteria were verbal and math scores on the Comparative Guidance and Placement exam; high school algebra, biology, and chemistry grades; as well as demographic factors such as age, marital status, number of children, and related work experience. The goal of the study was to identify preexisting characteristics of the individual that were predictive of a relationship to the dependent variable, success on the state board exams.

In another example, in a study conducted by Johansen, Bowles, and Haney (1988, p. 375) an attempt was made to pilot test a statistical forecasting model and to illustrate its use in "(a) estimating the number of cancer and myocardial infarction patients who are likely to need intermittent skilled home nursing services after discharge; (b) estimating the statewide costs of providing these services after discharge; and (c) incorporating change patterns of hospital length of stay and severity of illness, and reflecting these changes in the estimates of number of patients and costs."

To test the model that the researchers developed they utilized only objectively recorded patient variables; examples are age, marital status, number of critical care days (for patients with myocardial infarction), number of procedures undertaken during hospitalization (for patients with cancer), and number of secondary diagnoses. Variables chosen were based on the literature and clinical experience. The goals of the study were to (1) demonstrate how a model could produce estimates of need and cost and (2) allow simulation of changes in the health care delivery system to assess how these changes are reflected in the estimates. In this study the researchers also utilized retrospective data from two patient groups to forecast needs. It was also hoped that other researchers could use the model to forecast home care needs for other types of patient groups.

The research consumer will find that prediction studies use retrospective data from one group to make predictions about a similar group. This type of design generally employs sophisticated statistical techniques when exploring relationships among variables in one group to make predictions about the behavior of another group.

The major advantage of predictive studies is that they facilitate intelligent decision making, because objective criteria are available to guide the process. This can be particularly important in situations where critical choices, such as student selection, are made. The major disadvantage or limitation of prediction studies is that the design does not imply a cause-and-effect relationship between the chosen independent predictor variables and the dependent criterion variable. In addition, if the predictor variables were not chosen with a sound rationale, then a study may not be valid.

Developmental studies

There are also classifications of nonexperimental designs that use a time perspective. Investigators who utilize *developmental studies* are concerned not only with the existing status and interrelationship of phenomena but also with changes that result from elapsed time. The following four types of developmental study designs will be discussed: cross-sectional, longitudinal, retrospective, and prospective.

Cross-sectional and longitudinal studies

Cross-sectional studies examine data at one point in time; that is, the data are collected on only one occasion with the same subjects rather than on the same subjects at several points in time. An example of a cross-sectional study is Koniak-Griffin's (1988) study, which focused on the relationship between maternal-fetal attachment, social support, and self-esteem in a group of culturally divergent pregnant adolescents. The adolescents filled out three questionnaires at one point in time during their pregnancy. The questionnaires measured the adolescents' perceptions of self-worth, social support, and maternal-fetal attachment.

Another cross-sectional study approach is to simultaneously collect data on the variables of interest from different cohort groups. For example, if an investigator wishes to look at the development of maternal-fetal attachment in relationship to quickening in primiparas, the designated data collection periods may be the twelfth, twenty-fourth, and thirty-sixth weeks of pregnancy. The researcher would then select equivalent groups of primiparas who are at each respective point in their pregnancy. The data from each group would then be compared by use of statistical measures.

In contrast to the cross-sectional design, **longitudinal studies** collect data from the same group at different points in time. For instance, the investigator conducting the same maternal-fetal attachment study could elect to utilize a longitudinal design. In that case the investigator would test the same group of primiparas at each data collection point. By collecting data from each subject at the twelfth, twenty-fourth, and thirty-sixth weeks of pregnancy, a longitudinal perspective of the attachment process is accomplished (LoBiondo-Wood, 1985).

There are many advantages and disadvantages to both designs. When assessing the appropriateness of a cross-sectional study versus a longitudinal study, the research consumer should first assess what the goal of the researcher was in light of the theoretical framework. In the example of the maternal-fetal attachment study, the researcher is looking at a developmental process; therefore a longitudinal design seems more appropriate. However, the disadvantages inherent in a longitudinal design must also be considered. Data collection may be of long duration because of the time it takes for the subjects to progress to each data collection point. In the attachment study it would take each woman 24 weeks to complete the data collection process. It would take the investigator 6 months to complete the data collection *if* all of the subjects were obtained at one time. This does not even account for intervening variables such as attrition, miscarriage, or complications of pregnancy that might occur after the study has begun. These realities make a longitudinal design costly in terms of time, effort, and money. There is also a chance of confounding variables that could affect the interpretation of the results. Subjects in such a study may respond in a socially desirable way that they believe is congruent with the investigators' expectations. This is similar to the Hawthorne effect discussed in Chapters 8 and 9. However, despite the pragmatic constraints imposed by a longitudinal study, the researcher should proceed with this design if the theoretical framework supports a longitudinal developmental perspective.

The advantages of a longitudinal study are that each subject is followed separately and thereby serves as his or her own control; increased depth of responses can be obtained; and early trends in the data can be investigated.

In contrast, cross-sectional studies are less time-consuming, less expensive, and thus more manageable for the researcher. Since large amounts of data can be collected at one point, the results are more readily available. Additionally, the confounding variable of maturation, resulting from the elapsed time, is not present. However, the economic accomplishments are sacrificed in terms of the investigator's lessened ability to establish an in-depth developmental assessment of the interrelationship of the phenomena being studied. Thus the researcher is unable to determine if the change that occurred is related to the change that was predicted by the hypothesis, because the same subjects were not followed over a period of time. In other words, the subjects are unable to serve as their own controls (see Chapter 8).

In summary, it is important for the consumer to realize that longitudinal studies begin in the present and end in the future. Cross-sectional studies look at a broader perspective of a cross section of the population at a specific point in time.

Retrospective and prospective studies

Retrospective studies are basically epidemiological in nature and are essentially the same as an ex post facto study. The term *retrospective* is mainly used by epidemiologists, whereas the term *ex post facto* is preferred by social scientists. Nevertheless the investigator attempts to link present events to events that have occurred in the past. In an example of a retrospective study conducted by Sideleau (1984), data such as sibling position, number of children in the family, and integrity of the family unit were examined in relationship to the diagnosis of mental illness in hospitalized adolescents and adults. The investigator began with a theoretical framework that was derived from a systematic retrospective search to identify the factors related to the development of mental illness. The findings of such retrospective studies can provide the basis for further investigation and require additional research information.

In another example of a retrospective study Shannahan and Cottrell (1985) studied the effect of delivering in a birth chair on the duration of the second stage of labor, fetal outcome (Apgar scores), and maternal blood loss. In order to conduct the study within a retrospective design, the researchers conducted a restrospective chart review of 60 primiparous women at 37 to 41 weeks' gestation within a 2-month period in one hospital setting. All subjects (women and chart data) had a normal pregnancy, spontaneous labor, no augmentation of labor, and admission and postpartum hemoglobin and hematocrit determinations. The data collected from each chart included data on type of delivery, episiotomy, laceration, anesthesia, analgesia, Apgar scores, blood test results, and the duration of the second stage of labor. The researchers found that the birth chair offered no untoward effects on the infant's status, but the mothers who gave birth in birth chairs did have a significantly lower hemoglobin and hematocrit values than the mothers who delivered on tables.

The researchers identified a number of areas for future research in this area. They also noted that they were doing further research and assessing the same variables using a prospective design. This is an excellent example of how researchers develop and expand clinical knowledge by conducting follow-up studies that further test variables.

Prospective studies are also commonly used by epidemiologists. Prospective studies explore presumed causes and then move forward in time to the presumed effect. As such, they are much like longitudinal studies; they start in the present and end in the future. For example, a researcher might want to test the incidence of alcohol consumption during pregnancy in relation to resulting low-birthweight infants. To test this hypothesis the investigator would draw a sample of pregnant women, some who regularly consumed alcohol during their pregnancy and others who did not. The occurrence of low-birthweight infants in both groups would then be analyzed. These data would allow the investigator to assess whether regular alcohol consumption during pregnancy was related to the birthweight of the infant.

In another situation the researcher may wish to study the development of a particular health outcome. In this type of study the investigator selects the participants from a population known to be free of the health outcome under study and classifies the participants according to whether they have one or more factors (independent variables) presumably related to the outcome. These participants, who are frequently referred to as a cohort, are then studied over a period of time, ranging from months to years, to determine who develops the health outcome. The Framingham heart study examined the effect of blood pressure, cholesterol levels, smoking, exercise, and other variables on the development of coronary artery disease in a cohort of healthy men. The subjects were studied at specified intervals over a period of years.

Prospective studies are less common than retrospective studies. This may be explained by the fact that it can take a long time for the phenomenon of interest to become evident in a prospective study. For example, if researchers were studying pregnant women who regularly consume alcohol, it would take 9 months for the effect of low birth weight in the subjects' infants to become evident. The problems inherent in a prospective study are therefore similar to those of a longitudinal study. However, prospective studies are considered to be stronger than retrospective studies because of the degree of control that can be imposed on extraneous variables that might confound the data.

CAUSALITY IN NONEXPERIMENTAL RESEARCH

A great concern of nurses when they are conducting research is the issue of causality. Scientists are interested in explaining cause-and-effect relationships. Historically researchers have said that only experimental research can support the concept of causality. For example, nurses are interested in discovering what causes anxiety in many settings. If we can uncover the causes, we could perhaps develop interventions that would prevent or decrease the anxiety. Causality makes it necessary to order events chronologically; that is, if we find in a randomly assigned experiment that event 1 (stress) occurs before event 2 (anxiety), and that those in the stressed group were anxious whereas those in the unstressed group were not anxious, we can say that the hypothesis of stress causing anxiety is supported by these empirical observations. If these results were found in a nonexperimental study where some subjects underwent the stress of surgery and were anxious and others did not have surgery and were not anxious, we would say that there is an association or relationship between stress (surgery) and anxiety. But on the basis of the results of a nonexperimental study we could not say that the stress of surgery *caused* the anxiety.

Newer methods of stastistical analysis can add to what can be supported with nonexperimental data. Multiple regression techniques allow for the statistical control of many variables (Pedhazur, 1982). Recently researchers have been using sophisticated statistical techniques, such as Path Analysis and LISREL, that analyze nonexperimental data in a way that either supports or does not support the concept of causality.

Critiquing Criteria

1. Which nonexperimental design is utilized in the study?
2. Based on the theoretical framework, is the rationale for the type of design evident?
3. Is the utilized design congruent with the purpose of the study?
4. Is the utilized design appropriate for the research problem?
5. Is the utilized design suited to the data collection methods?
6. Does the researcher present the findings in a manner that is congruent with the utilized design?
7. Does the research go beyond the relational parameters of the findings and erroneously infer cause-and-effect relationships between the variables?
8. Are there any reasons to believe that there are alternative explanations for the findings?
9. Where appropriate, does the researcher discuss the threats to internal and external validity?
10. How does the author deal with the limitations of the study?

CRITIQUING NONEXPERIMENTAL DESIGNS

Criteria for critiquing nonexperimental designs are presented in the box above. When critiquing nonexperimental research designs the consumer should keep in mind that such designs offer the researcher the least amount of control. The first step in critiquing nonexperimental research is to determine which type of design was utilized in the study. Often a statement describing the design of the study appears in the abstract and in the methods section of the report. If such a statement is not present, the reader should closely examine the paper for evidence of which type of design was employed. The reader should be able to discern that either a survey or interrelationship design was used as well as the specific subtype. For example, the reader would expect an investigation of self-concept development in children from birth to 5 years of age to be an interrelationship study utilizing a longitudinal design.

Next, the critiquer should evaluate the theoretical framework and underpinnings of the study to determine if a nonexperimental design was the most appropriate approach to the problem. For example, the numerous mother-infant attachment studies discussed throughout this text are all theoretically suggestive of a nonmanipulable interrelationship between attachment and any of the independent variables under consideration. As such, a nonexperimental correlational, longitudinal, or cross-sectional design is suggested by these studies. Investigators will use one of these designs to examine the relationship between the variables in naturally occurring groups. Sometimes the reader may think that it would have been more appropriate if the investigators had used an experimental or quasiexperimental design. However, the reader must recognize that pragmatic or ethical considerations may also have guided the researchers in their choice of design (see Chapters 3 and 8).

Then the evaluator should assess whether or not the problem is at a level of experimental manipulation. Many times researchers merely wish to examine if relationships exist between variables. Therefore when one critiques such studies, the purpose of the study should be determined. If the purpose of the study does not include describing a cause-and-effect relationship, the researcher should not be criticized for not looking for one. However, the evaluator should be wary of a nonexperimental study in which the researcher suggests a cause-and-effect relationship in the findings.

Finally, the factor(s) that actually influence changes in the dependent variable are often ambiguous in nonexperimental designs. As with all complex phenomena, multiple factors can contribute to variability in the subjects' responses. When an experimental design is not used for controlling some of these extraneous variables that can influence results, the researcher must strive to provide as much control of them as possible within the context of a nonexperimental design. For example, when it has not been possible to randomly assign subjects to treatment groups as an approach to controlling an independent variable, the researcher may use a strategy of matching subjects for identified variables. For example, in a study of infant birth weight, pregnant women could be matched on variables such as weight, height, smoking habits, drug use, and other factors that might influence birthweight. The independent variable of interest, such as the type of prenatal care, would then be the major difference in the groups. The reader would then feel more confident that the only real difference between the two groups was the differential effect of the independent variable, because the other factors in the two groups were theoretically the same. However, the consumer should also remember that there may be other influential variables that were not matched, such as income, education, and diet. Rival factors represent a major influence on the interpretation of a nonexperimental study because they impose limitations on the generalizability of the results.

SUMMARY

Nonexperimental research designs are used in studies that construct a picture or make an account of events as they naturally occur. The major difference between nonexperimental and experimental research is that in nonexperimental designs the independent variable is not actively manipulated by the investigator.

Nonexperimental designs can be classified as either survey studies or interrelationship studies. Survey research collects detailed descriptions of existing phenomena and uses the data either to justify current conditions and practices or to make more intelligent plans for improving them. Survey studies and interrelationship studies are both descriptive and exploratory in nature. Interrelationship studies endeavor to retrace the interrelationships between variables that provide deeper insight into the phenomena of interest. Correlational, ex post facto, prediction, and developmental studies are examples of interrelationship studies. Developmental studies are further broken down into categories of cross-sectional, longitudinal, retrospective, and prospective studies. The advantages and disadvantages of each type of design must be considered by the researcher and critiquer when evaluating the merits of nonexperimental design.

Nonexperimental research designs do not enable the investigator to establish cause-effect relationships between the variables. Consumers must be wary of nonexperimental studies that make causal claims about the findings. Nonexperimental designs also offer the researcher the least amount of control. Rival factors represent a major influence on the interpretation of a nonexperimental study because they impose limitations on the generalizability of the results and as such should be fully assessed by the critical reader.

The critiquing process is directed toward evaluating the appropriateness of the selected nonexperimental design in relation to factors such as the research problem, theoretical framework, hypothesis, methodology, and the data analysis and interpretation.

References

Bello, A., Haber, J., King, V., and King, R. (1980). Identified factors predicting student success or failure in an associate degree nursing program. In *Teaching tomorrow's nurse: a nurse educator reader,* Wakefield, Mass., Nursing Resources, Inc., pp. 174-182.

Campbell, D.T., and Stanley, J.C. (1963). *Experimental and quasi-experimental designs for research,* Chicago, Rand McNally College Publishing Co.

Fox, D.J. (1982). *Fundamentals of research in nursing,* 4th ed., East Norwalk, Conn., Appleton-Century-Crofts.

Hendrix, M.J., Sabritt, D., McDaniel, A., and Field, B. (1988). Perceptions and attitudes toward nursing impairment, *Research in Nursing & Health,* **10**:323-334.

Johansen, S., Bowles, S., and Haney, G. (1988). A model for forecasting intermittent skilled home nursing needs, *Research in Nursing & Health,* **11**:375-382.

Koniak-Griffin, D. (1988). The relationship between social support, self-esteem, and maternal-fetal attachment in adolescents, *Research in Nursing & Health,* **11**:269-278.

Littlefield-Derby, V., LoBiondo-Wood, G., and Olney-Springer, M. (1981). Changing the system to meet the needs of the patient and nurse, *The American Journal of Maternal Child Nursing,* **6**:225-230.

LoBiondo-Wood, G. (1985). The progression of physical symptoms in pregnancy and the development of maternal-fetal attachment, *Dissertation Abstracts International,* **46**:2625-B. (University Microfilms No. 85-21, 973.)

Newman, M.A., and Gaudiano, J.K. (1984). Depression as an explanation for decreased subjective time in the elderly, *Nursing Research,* **33**:137-139.

Pedhazur, E.J. (1982). *Multiple regression in behavioral research,* New York, Holt, Rinehart, & Winston, Inc.

Shannahan, M.D., and Cottrell, B.H. (1985). Effect of the birth chair on duration of second stage labor, fetal outcome and maternal blood loss, *Nursing Research,* **34**:89-92.

Sideleau, B. (1984). Relationship between birth order and family size constellation and integrity to the development of mental illness in adolescence and adulthood. Unpublished doctoral dissertation, Teachers College, Columbia University, New York.

Van Dalen, D.B. (1979). *Understanding educational research: an introduction,* New York, McGraw-Hill Book Co.

Additional Readings

Huck, S.W., and Sandler, H.M. (1979). *Rival hypotheses,* New York, Harper & Row, Publishers.

Kerlinger, F.H. (1986). *Foundations of behavioral research,* 3rd ed. New York, Holt, Rinehart & Winston, Inc.

Sherwen, L.N., and Toussie-Weingarten, C. (1983). *Analysis and application of nursing research: parent-neonate studies,* Belmont, Calif., Wadsworth Health Sciences Division.

Waltz, C.F., and Bausell, R.B. (1981). *Nursing research: design, statistics and computer analysis,* Philadelphia, F.A. Davis Co.

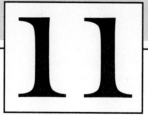

Qualitative Approaches to Research

Carolyn Oiler Boyd

LEARNING OBJECTIVES

After reading this chapter the student should be able to do the following:

◇ Describe distinguishing characteristics of qualitative approaches to research.

◇ Identify the processes of ethnographic, grounded theory, phenomenological, and case study methods.

◇ Recognize critical decision making in qualitative research concerning ethics, reliability, and validity, and level of data analysis.

◇ Use critiquing criteria to evaluate qualitative research reports.

KEY TERMS

case study   lived experience
constant comparative method   phenomenology
ethnography   process consent
grounded theory   theoretical sampling
key informant

In recent years there has been a renewed interest in qualitative approaches to research. There is a growing recognition that qualitative methods are important in the repertoire of tools available for developing knowledge. In nursing we are beginning to explore these methods and their potential for us in our progression as a learned profession. In this chapter, four qualitative approaches will be described: **ethnography, grounded therapy, phenomenology,** and **case study.** The purpose of this chapter is to provide an overview of the qualitative tradition in research so that its distinguishing characteristics are made explicit. Details about the four selected approaches will help to clarify these characteristics and thereby to define the actual and potential usefulness of qualitative studies for nursing.

THE QUALITATIVE TRADITION IN RESEARCH

Baron (1985, p. 606) has illustrated by the following anecdote a confusion physicians often experience in their work: "It happened the other morning on rounds, that while I was carefully auscultating a patient's chest, he began to ask me a question. 'Quiet,' I said, 'I can't hear you while I'm listening.' " One can readily imagine that this kind of confusion can be observed in nursing practice as well. Many nurses report feelings of being torn between the objective and technical aspects of their roles and the subjective and humane aspects. In part, for practicing nurses this tension serves as a stimulus for qualitative research in nursing. Qualitative approaches attend to subjectivities and to our humanistic aims in nursing. There is no question whether nursing needs to be objective and rational as well as technically proficient. However, nurses generally agree that these qualities are insufficient alone. Nursing also intends to provide humanistic care, extracting all that it can from the full nature of being human, inclusive of the complexities, contradictions, and paradoxes that characterize practice situations. For some nursing questions and problems the qualitative approaches to research offer the proper methods and strategies to assist us with making sense out of these practice situations. Collectively, then, the quantitative and qualitative research traditions provide a comprehensive set of tools for the development of knowledge about and for nursing.

Qualitative Research: Orientation and Structure

1. Qualitative research is a holistic approach to questions that recognize that human realities are complex. Research questions tend to be very broad. Some examples are as follows: What are the birth experiences of women in foreign cultures? What is comforting? What is it like to feel lonely when hospitalized?

2. The focus is on human experience. This is a turn toward the subjectivities of people's realities.

3. The research strategies used generally feature sustained contact with people in settings where those people normally spend their time.

4. There is typically a high level of researcher involvement with participants, in which the strategies of participant observation and in-depth, unstructured interviews are often used.

5. The data produced provide a description, usually narrative, of people living through events or situations.

The term *qualitative research* is a very general one that encompasses a variety of research methods. Methods subsumed under this term generally share a common orientation and structure (see box above). In summary, qualitative research involves broadly stated questions about human experiences and realities, studied through sustained contact with people in their natural environments, generating rich, descriptive data that help us to understand their experiences.

Research purposes

The purposes and uses of qualitative data bear a close relationship to the kind of data produced. These purposes may be classified as *instrumentation, illustration, sensitization,* and *conceptualization* (Knafl and Howard, 1986). For example, to serve the purpose of *instrumentation* a researcher might use in-depth, unstructured interviews of wheelchair-bound adults to learn what it is like to live with impaired mobility. The information these adults provide the researcher could then be used to construct an instrument that includes categories based on subjects' actual experiences rather than what we imagine.

The purpose of *illustration* was served in Kramer's study (1968) of reality shock in young baccalaureate graduate nurses. In this study Kramer used qualitative interview data obtained from a sample of graduates to illustrate her quantitative findings about graduates' role orientations. Thus such numerical data as mean scores from quantitative measurement were enriched.

The purpose of *sensitization* is served by qualitative studies to the extent that these studies effectively communicate insights about experiences we need to understand vicariously. For example, Copel (1984) performed a qualitative study of medical-surgical clients' experiences of loneliness in the hospital setting. Learning of these findings functions to sensitize research consumers to their clients and thereby to contribute to the quality of care.

Last, qualitative studies may be undertaken to serve the purpose of conceptualization or theory development. The grounded theory method is the best example of how qualitative study enables us to construct theory that is based on actual human experience. For example, Hutchinson (1986a) used the grounded theory method to learn more about what it is like to be a nurse in a neonatal intensive care unit (NICU). After a protracted period of in-depth observation, participation, and interviews, Hutchinson constructed a theory descriptive of coping strategies of NICU nurses.

Historical perspectives

Bogdan and Biklen (1982, pp. 3-26) provided a description of the historical context of qualitative research. They note that although its recognition as a tool of science is relatively recent, qualitative research has a long and rich tradition. Since the value of qualitative research approaches is debated in nursing as well as in other fields, it is particularly useful to be cognizant of this tradition.

During the late 1800s qualitative methods were used to disclose the rapidly developing social problems in cities subsequent to industrialization, urbanization, and mass immigration. Poverty and crowding created problems with sanitation, health, welfare, and education. Qualitative researchers encouraged social change by making these problems visible to the public through journalistic descriptions of urban conditions. The Pittsburgh survey, for example, provided statistics about the urban poor but also gave us detailed accounts of urban life including photographs, charcoal portraits, and interviews. The statistics were thus cast in human terms by the qualitative data. Although from a later period, *Let Us Now Praise Famous Men* (Agee and Evans, 1941) represents this style of qualitative research extremely well. It is now considered a classic description of the daily life of tenant farmers in the South.

At the time that social surveys were being done at the turn of the century, anthropological field research methods were being developed and taught in universities. The anthropological strategy of participant observation migrated to sociology where it was used along with the case study method to study social problems in communities from a social interaction perspective. During the 1920s and 1930s sociologists used qualitative strategies extensively to study such social phenomena as race relations, ethnicity, and delinquency.

From the 1930s through the 1950s qualitative research waned. Worthy scientific endeavor was defined in accord with the growing expectation that quantitative methods were the means to solutions. Taking the lead primarily from medicine, public health, and sociology, nursing subscribed to this view; and our short history of research activity meshed with the dominant quantitative paradigm in the scientific world.

The 1960s, however, disrupted the scientific world's unquestioning faith in the promise of quantitative methods. A variety of social minority groups clamored to be heard, and there was a renewed interest in the power of qualitative methods to provide us with better understandings of minorities' views and circumstances. During this period grounded theory method was developed (Glaser and Strauss, 1967). In nursing this method was used to study nurses' and clients' experiences with death and dying (Quint, 1967). However, this early endeavor did not flourish nationally. Nurse researchers tended to focus their talents and energies in mastering quantitative methods.

Nevertheless the social unrest of the 1960s, including the feminist movement, stimulated methodological debates in other fields. Education, sociology, and psychology in particular turned toward qualitative methods with renewed interest in the 1970s. These debates surfaced in the literature, in university courses, and at national conferences and gradually engaged nurses in a serious consideration of the merit and prospects of qualitative approaches. Nursing debates occurred in the early 1980s (Oiler, 1982; Munhall, 1982; Tinkle and Beaton, 1983). Today we are in a period of exploring qualitative methods and developing our expertise in their use. Although we continue to rely heavily on direction from other disciplines that have created qualitative approaches for their concerns, we hope to witness nursing's growth toward full maturity as a scientific discipline. Toward this end, we may expect that there will be nursing proposals for new qualitative methods for the investigation of nursing problems.

Characteristics of qualitative approaches

Although qualitative research embraces a number of distinctive methods, each method bears certain general characteristics in common with the others. Collectively the characteristics of qualitative approaches compose a perspective that is founded on select philosophical and theoretical premises. These premises are summarized as leading characteristics of qualitative research (see box on p. 186). In this chapter the qualitative perspective held in common by the various qualitative methods will be described to enhance comprehension of the four methods selected for presentation.

When qualitative researchers speak of *subjectivity*, they are referring to ways people make sense of their experiences and lives. We have accumulated many facts, for example, about menopause, osteoporosis, and pain. However, these facts do not add up to understandings about what it is like to live through menopause or to have osteoporosis or to be in pain. Qualitative researchers are most interested in subjective meanings, not in facts alone. If a client's subjective experience is one of pain, it matters little whether or not the facts about his condition coincide with his experience. Qualitative researchers recognize that human behavior is contingent on human meanings, and they strive to disclose this subjectivity in their studies.

In order to construct methods that disclose subjectivity, qualitative researchers also recognize that people construct meanings in relation to the world in which they live. This is the second leading characteristic of qualitative methods: the natural settings in which people under study live, work, learn, and play are sought for the conduct of the study. The researcher strives to collect data descriptive of the person-environment relationship in the belief that human behavior is best understood

---

Leading Characteristics of Qualitative Research

Inductive reasoning
Focus on human subjectivity
Natural settings
Descriptive data
Process-oriented questions

---

in the context in which it occurs. If a researcher wants to learn about what it is like to live through the menopause, for example, the natural setting would be participants' day-to-day lives. The study design would involve finding ways to be with these women for a time in their lives. A questionnaire, in contrast, would lift participants away from their *natural setting* and experience, and would blind the researcher to such data as participants' interactions with their families and how participants look and behave when they are uncomfortable with physiological responses that are common in menopause.

Since the aim is to disclose subjectivity, the qualitative researcher strives to locate and collect data that serve to describe the experience under study. Words, in the form of field observation notes and transcripts of interviews, are the most common form of qualitative data. However, photographs, videotapes, and the researcher's perceptions of sounds, tastes, and smells are also sometimes included as data. Similarly, diaries, memos, letters, and art might be included if they contribute to understanding and presenting the human experience under study. Usually, qualitative studies produce *narrative descriptions* rather than numerical summaries. The end product, or findings, represent the researcher's best effort to organize and present an accurate "picture" of what he or she has learned by going to people in their natural settings and being with them for a time in order to see as much as he or she can about their lives. The "pictures" that qualitative research produces are distillations of large amounts of various kinds of data that are tracked down by maintaining a research focus on process. For example, a qualitative researcher might study whether or not nursing home residents are lonely, and to what extent, using a scale that measures loneliness. The qualitative researcher on the other hand would pursue the question of *how* do these residents experience loneliness. Other examples of *process questions* are as follows: "What does being a nurse mean to you?" "How are attitudes about women expressed in the physician-nurse relationship?" "What happens to families when there is sudden death of a member?" Such process questions guide the qualitative researcher in a rigorous search for elusive data that help to disclose complex human experiences that often defy attempts simply to report them in interviews or on questionnaires.

The organization and distillation of data that the researcher performs in order to present a picture of the experience under study is an essentially *inductive reasoning process.* Many instances of an event, process, or perception are grouped together to generate a characteristic that is then represented in the picture the researcher provides in the report of the findings. This inductive approach to building knowledge is sometimes referred to as theory development from the bottom up. For example, in Copel's study (1984) of loneliness she identified "problems with relationships" as a component of loneliness. A few of the instances that were grouped together to form this component were clients' statements of feeling unloved, isolated, and secluded and of having a sense of loss and lack of support.

Although this overview of characteristics of qualitative research is not inclusive of all significant features that distinguish qualitative from quantitative approaches, it does provide the reader with a foundation for the remainder of the chapter, in which more detail will unfold. To date, nurses pursuing qualitative research have made use primarily of methods developed in other disciplines. These are ethnography (anthropology), grounded theory (sociology), and phenomenology (philosophy and psychology). Nursing literature is beginning to reflect these nurse researchers' productivity in applying these methods to nursing concerns. Each of these methods as they are interpreted and used in nursing research will be described. In addition, the case study method is described in view of a renewed interest in its potential for contributing to knowledge development in nursing.

ETHNOGRAPHY

The qualitative method of ethnography is one of the research approaches developed by anthropologists to guide inquiry that is designed to produce cultural theory. Ethnography features two major procedures that have been adopted by other qualitative methods: interviewing of **key informants** and participant observation. These two procedures are used by the researcher during an extensive period of time in physical association with people under study in their setting. The researcher participates in the events of the culture under study in a search for patterns or themes that constitute the culture. Germain (1986, p. 148) explains: "These themes include but are not limited to the shared knowledge, norms (rules of behavior), values, belief systems, language, rituals, economics, role behaviors, or patterns of social interaction among members of the subculture."

Cultural units selected for study vary in size and complexity and determine the scope of ethnography. Fig. 11-1 illustrates the continuum of scope in ethnographic studies from long-term study of very complex cultures such as the Aborigines, Aztecs, or Samoans to shorter-term study of subunits of single social institutions such as a group home for retarded adults, a women's shelter, or a nursing unit in a hospital. As the illustration indicates, an ethnographic researcher might select a cultural unit that falls between these two extremes, such as the American Nurses' Association and an apartment complex.

The example of variation in scope of ethnography includes cultural units that would be of interest to nurse researchers. Ethnography is used by a variety of disciplines, including nursing. Germain (1982) has used ethnography to study a cancer

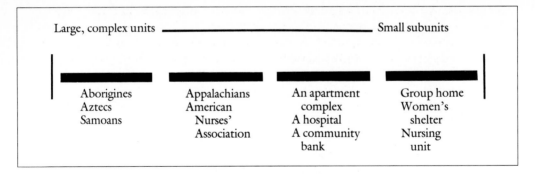

Fig. 11-1   Scope of ethnography.

unit, Kayser-Jones (1981) to study the aged, Aamodt (1986) to study the child's view of chemically induced alopecia, and Kroska (1985) to study the role of "granny" midwives in health services. Many other ethnographic nursing studies have been conducted, and the ethnographic method has been established as an important one for some nursing research questions.

Ethnographic questions and research process

Ethnography is a method used to develop theories of culture, and it produces descriptions of the ways of life in cultures or subcultures. The research questions "take the form of questions such as 'What is this?' or 'What's happening here in this subculture?'" (Germain, 1986, p. 149); or "If I am to behave as a member of this culture, what must I do?" and "What are the rules for appropriate behavior?" (Aamodt, 1982, p. 210). Ethnographic studies are guided by the cultural perspective learned in anthropology. Ethnographic nursing studies thus address those questions that concern how cultural knowledge, norms, values, and the like influence our own and our clients' behaviors. In addition to the examples of ethnographic nursing research just cited, some possible research questions for this method follow:

  ◇ "What does caring mean in Hispanic families?"
  ◇ "What does it mean to be an adolescent in a rural community?"
  ◇ "What is the life-style of multigenerational families?"
  ◇ "What are patient and nurse roles like in long-term care institutions?"
  ◇ "What are the meanings of nursing unit routines and rituals to nurses and to patients?"

In conjunction with formulating the research question, the ethnographic researcher reviews relevant literature to ascertain the need for as well as to conceptualize the significance of the study for nursing. An extensive review of literature is usually not performed, because a lack of descriptive literature on the culture under study is part of the stimulus for the research. The researcher thus enters the cultural setting relatively naive, and uses this naiveté to observe intensely.

Because the researcher is a stranger to the culture under study, he or she seeks to identify members of the culture with whom collaborative relationships can be developed. Referred to as *key informants,* these members are purposely selected for their knowledge about their culture and willingness to share it. A long period of time is usually required for the researcher to locate data sources and build relationships that will yield information to satisfy the research questions. Over time, through participant observation and informal and structured interviews, the researcher amasses data. These data are analyzed to explain the meaning of behavior in the culture, from the members' point of view. To some extent the researcher must become part of the culture for a time in order to gain access to this type of data and to generate insights that will constitute the resultant cultural theory. Aamodt (1982), for example, sang in the church choir and attended devotions at the senior citizen center in her participant observation of Norwegian-American women. Kroska (1985) used her identity as a certified nurse-midwife to help her establish rapport with the "granny" midwives she was studying, and she notes that her clinical experience enabled her to include direct participant experience as a means of gaining access to data.

Throughout the ethnographer's field work, detailed notes are made to preserve observations. Interviews are sometimes tape-recorded, and artifacts are often reviewed to supplement observations. The ethical principles that direct us to ensure informed consent and the rights to privacy and freedom from harm must be adhered to in the research process. It is not at all unusual for ethical dilemmas to arise periodically in the course of the field work. Aamodt (1986, p. 167), for example, reported that in her study of children in a pediatric oncology unit, interviewers often had to abandon their research roles in order to respond humanistically to the children's expressed needs. Other unique features of ethical concerns in qualitative research will be addressed later in this chapter.

The analysis of data in ethnographic research proceeds concurrently with data collection. The researcher's experiences in the field prompt him or her to develop hunches that, in turn, serve to guide in the selection of subsequent experiences that may shed light on the hunches. The researcher concludes data collection when experiences become redundant, yielding no new information. Final analysis of the data to produce cultural theory is an intellectually demanding process in which data are compared, contrasted, and grouped into categories. Readers are encouraged to consult Spradley (1979 and 1980) or Leininger (1985) for detailed descriptions of the analytic process. In effect, in analyzing ethnographic data the researcher casts all the data gathered from the experiences in the field into a cultural perspective that provides description and explanation of that way of life. This final product, when done well, is enjoyable reading and often is in book form. Findings are also sometimes communicated through films that entertain as well as educate. Although article formats are also used, they tend to constrict descriptions sharply. This is a limitation shared by formats of most conferences at which research is presented. Qualitative research findings in general require generous formats for the rich detail that characterizes this kind of research.

To give some indication of the nature of ethnographic findings, the following themes were extracted from Aamodt's investigation (1986, p. 169) of the question "What cultural knowledge influences the behavior of children with chemically induced hair loss?":

1. "There's nothing to be done" portrays the sense of helplessness and fatalism that characterized the responses of the children. Accepting the loss, making the best of it, and then waiting for their hair to grow back was the best they could do.
2. "Loss of hair and loss of friends" illustrates the social stigma associated with hair loss and the persistent cruelty in the social world of children. Forced absence from school coupled with loss of hair meant that all but closest friends disappeared. Upon returning to school, children with hair loss were made fun of and lost more friends.

The third and fourth themes are "Getting used to it" and "Treat me as normal." Collectively these cultural themes serve to communicate the essence of the culture; that is, to inform us about the children's point of view. Aamodt's full report of her study is of course needed to accomplish this.

GROUNDED THEORY METHOD

Grounded theory methodology was developed in the 1960s by two sociologists, Glaser and Strauss (1967). Many nurses have learned this method in Glaser and Strauss' classes and from their publications. A number of grounded theory studies in nursing have been produced (Davis, 1977; Hutchinson, 1986a; Wilson, 1986; Quint, 1966).

The term *grounded* means based on the actual, concrete realities of people as they live through their experiences. Coupled with the word *theory,* grounded theory, then, refers to theory that is constructed from a base of observations of the world as it is lived by people. This is the inductive process described as one of the leading characteristics of qualitative research in general and the from-the-bottom-up approach cited in the discussion of ethnography. As will be seen, grounded theory and ethnography bear multiple similarities, differing primarily in the theoretical perspectives of the disciplines from which they come.

As one might expect, grounded theory method is concerned with social pressures, because it was developed by sociologists to study questions in their discipline. The social nature of nursing has prompted nurse researchers to apply grounded theory method to study certain nursing questions from a social interaction perspective. The specific theoretical framework associated with grounded theory is symbolic interactionism. Consequently the aim in grounded theory is to understand how various groups of people define reality through their associations with one another and to communicate this in the form of theory.

Research purposes

Stern (1980, p. 20) writes that there are two main uses for grounded theory—in investigations of relatively uncharted waters or to gain a fresh perspective in a familiar situation. One purpose of grounded theory, then, is to construct theory where no theory exists. Stern cites her own research as an example. As stepfamilies have increased in number, their unique problems and circumstances have increasingly come to health care providers' attention. Stern's study concerned learning how a stepfather is integrated into the existing family system made up of mother and child "so that other such families could try out strategies which seem to influence successful outcomes" (1980, p. 20).

A second purpose for grounded theory is to construct theory for familiar situations when existing theory fails to resolve persistent problems. Quint's study (1966 and 1967) of nurses' coping difficulties with the emotional strain of caring for dying clients is an example of research designed to serve this purpose. Stern (1980, p. 20) cites a study of hospital personnel's criteria for controlling the client's pain as another example of this research purpose in grounded theory:

> It becomes clear that nurses and doctors administer pain-relieving medication according to their own value system rather than on the basis of what the patient is feeling . . . the nurse or doctor decides good from bad pain.

Researching the familiar with the aim of producing a fresh view of a situation often has immediate and direct implications for practice. In this last example, merely reading the findings could prompt nurses to attend more carefully to their patients' reports of pain.

Grounded theory questions and process

In general, the theoretical perspective for grounded theory directs the researcher to pose questions about a group's social processes. Hutchinson (1986b, p. 114) explains:

> People sharing common circumstances, such as neonatal intensive care unit (NICU) nurses, experience shared meanings and behaviors that constitute the substance of grounded theory. Grounded theorists base their research on the assumption that each such group shares a specific social psychological problem that is not necessarily articulated. This fundamental problem is resolved by means of social psychological processes.

To formulate a grounded theory question, then, one selects a social unit (group of people) of interest, recognizing that in order to understand human behavior, interactions with others must be the contextual focus. In Hutchinson's study of NICU nurses the informal questions were "What is it like to be an NICU nurse? How do they do their work and how do they get satisfaction from it?" Formally the question was "What is the social psychological problem and process of NICU nurses?"

The grounded theory research process is, like enthnography, field research in which participant observation and interview are the primary procedures. In Hutchinson's study of NICU nurses she spent 20 hours a week for 4 months observing NICU activities, interacting with nurses informally, conducting formal interviews, attending workshops on neonatal care, and going along on helicopter and ambulance runs to pick up critically ill newborns (Hutchinson, 1986a, p. 192). From this array of field activities it can be seen that *participant observation* is a very broad term. The participant observer role may be thought of on a continuum from passive to active. The researcher's role in the research setting may fluctuate along this continuum depending on opportunities for participation as well as research objectives. The passive end of the continuum is characterized by noninteractive observational activity and is illustrated in such activity as Hutchinson's attendance at a workshop on neonatal care. The active end of the continuum is characterized by concealing the research role in order to fully assume a group member role. If Hutchinson had accepted a staff patient care assignment in the NICU, for example, her primary role would have been nurse. This would alter the kind of data accessible to her, and this is regarded by most to be an unethical research strategy. Most nursing research using participant observation features strategies that allow the researcher to become involved with others in the setting while maintaining a researcher role. One of the research objectives of participant observation is to become accepted by members of the group under study. The length of the field work will thus depend in part on the researcher's skill in developing rapport and the members' openness to strangers.

Field notes are maintained to record data, and systems for developing ideas about the data are established concurrently with the data collection. In this way the researcher directs activities in the field by pursuing hunches and hypotheses about the data as they are collected. The technique of **theoretical sampling** is used to select experiences that will help the researcher test ideas (hypotheses) in the time-consuming process of searching for completeness in the data. In order to investigate an idea about nurses' coping strategies, the researcher, for example, might arrange a formal interview with a head nurse to elicit views about why staff nurses resign. Or the researcher may elect to study nurses' notes in the chart in order to investigate an idea about nurses' values and priorities in care. Thus the researcher's observational activity becomes increasingly goal-directed as he or she develops the theory.

Data analysis in grounded theory is called the **constant comparative method** and is a search for the main theme or core variable of the people in the setting. Hutchinson (1986b, p. 118) explains that the core variable has three characteristics: ". . . it recurs frequently in the data, it links the various data together, and it explains much of the variation in the data. . . ." This core variable becomes the focus for the theory the researcher develops to explain the group's social process. For example, in Hutchinson's study of NICU nurses (1986a) the core variable was identified as creating meaning as a response to the problem of horror. In Wilson's study of an unconventional treatment modality for schizophrenic patients (1986, p. 134), she identified presencing as one social process used by the group to control behavior.

The constant comparative method involves comparing incidents in the data to identify similarities and differences; this in turn enables the researcher to create categories for the data. Incidents are repeatedly examined for their "fit" in categories, and categories are compared to other categories.

As the researcher continues to conceptualize what is going on in the setting, theoretical constructs are articulated in the progress toward a theory that describes and explains relationships among individual incidents and among the categories and constructs used to organize and make sense of these incidents. Each element of the resultant theory must be thoroughly supported by multiple instances of observed incidents to produce a *grounded* theory. The constant comparative method is an inductive process in which multiple observations are collapsed into categories. These are further collapsed into theoretical constructs created by the researcher to account for the patterns and themes discerned in the data.

To illustrate this process a category of nonprofessional behavior might be developed to group and account for such observations of staff as rough handling of a client, calling a client "honey," talking about a client without including the client, and scolding a client. This category of nonprofessional behavior would then be compared to other categories that the researcher has developed such as staff members' job dissatisfaction, their attitudes toward dependency of patients, and knowledge about patient care. The researcher expresses his or her thinking about the relationship among these categories in theoretical constructs such as, for example, in the statement, "Inability to develop a personal philosophy of care that emphasizes hope, potential, and quality of life results in staff burnout, which in turn produces poor client care" (Hutchinson, 1986b; Davis, 1977).

Related literature may be reviewed continuously from the onset of the study and includes literary works such as novels that may shed light on the phenomenon under study. All literature is treated as data, rather than as conceptualizations about the phenomenon (Chenitz and Swanson, 1986, p. 44). In this way ideas in the literature are compared with the researcher's developing theory as it progresses. At the end of the study the researcher's grounded theory is formally related to and incorporated with existing knowledge.

As with ethnographic findings, excerpts from grounded theory studies cannot communicate the depth and detail that are produced. However, one study will be described in overview to provide an indication of the kinds of concepts and the theory the researcher presents as findings. Davis (1977) studied two skilled-nursing facilities to examine why rehabilitative care goals were impeded. Two kinds of constraints were identified: (1) conflicting perceptions and expectations between clients and staff and (2) incongruities between client needs and the ward routines. Davis' findings are presented in a discussion of how organization (elements of the care structure), interaction, and ward staff philosophy generated these constraints. One concept developed is termed *information exchange*. This category includes the observation that there was a lack of positive association between routine assignment and rehabilitative objectives. Davis cites a nursing entry on the chart, "Got patient up," as a specific incident supportive of this finding. Davis (1977, p. 24), states that

> Comments on the patient's progress in helping himself were usually not recorded. This highly circumscribed emphasis in the assignment and charting stripped the act of its rehabilitative intent, producing an isolated mechanical task supporting the fragmented, compartmentalized perspective on patient care.

Readers are encouraged to read Davis' full report for a complete description of the theory produced in this study.

PHENOMENOLOGY

Phenomenology is a philosophic method that has been adapted for use by social scientists. Its appeal to social sciences resides in the philosophic themes concerning the nature of reality. These themes converge with the general characteristics of qualitative research that were described earlier in this chapter. Like the other methods, phenomenology bears its own unique features, however, as well as several interpretations of its use as a research method in social science.

Phenomenology regards human reality as contingent on the individual perspective in the world; this perspective is formed by one's location in it, one's personal history, and one's voluntary adoption of any of an array of possible points of view. These possible points of view include looking at things scientifically, historically, esthetically, and spiritually. They include human capabilities of perceiving things imaginatively, empathetically, and intuitively. All these ways of looking at things are possible, and each gives its own perspective on reality and what is true. For example, a family member who visits a relative in an intensive care unit will experience a different reality in that environment than the nurse experiences. If each were asked to describe the unit, we could expect quite different accounts of it based on the differences in their knowledge of it, their roles in it, their remembered relationship with the client, their past experiences with the unit, and their learned ways of being a part of this environment. In short, both family member and nurse have individual perspectives in the situation that determine the nature of the reality they experience. There is not one truth about the unit; there are instead perspectives on the truth. Phenomenology's interest and focus are on human perspectives: how they emerge and how they constitute realities.

By definition, phenomenology concerns the study of experience as it is lived. Strictly speaking, the term *experience* in phenomenology refers to human involvement in a situation before interpretation of the experience. For the intensive care nurse, for example, an experience in the unit is routinely and automatically interpreted in terms of his or her scientific knowledge and technical proficiency. Experienced nurses are aware, however, of deeper layers of their experiences, in which perspectives other than the scientific are present. Phenomenology aims to forage through the layers of interpretation to disclose experience as it unfolds relatively naively, in one's initial contact and involvement in a situation. The purposes of such an ambition are (1) to clarify the nature of being human, (2) to expand awareness, (3) to foster human responsibility in the construction of realities, and (4) to tighten the bond between experiences and the concepts and theories we use to refer to and explain those experiences. Phenomenology, then, aims to disclose and describe **lived experiences** (Munhall and Oiler, 1986).

Phenomenological questions and research process

"What is it like to grow old?" "What is it like to have a mastectomy?" "What is it like to be a student nurse?" This form of questioning characterizes phenomenological studies. In psychology, phenomenology has been interpreted in methods designed to answer such questions as "What is the experience of 'really feeling understood?' " (Van Kaam, 1959). The overlap in research concerns between psychology and nursing has prompted nurse researchers to explore the use of phenomenological method as it has been interpreted in psychology. In addition, Paterson and Zderad (1976) have described a uniquely nursing interpretation of phenomenology that differs substantially from the interpretation offered by psychology. Keeping this variety in phenomenological method in mind, three styles of phenomenological research will be briefly noted. Major features of these three styles are summarized in Table 11-1.

In general, phenomenology is concerned with meaning-conferring acts rather than with the specific contents of experience. Phenomenological questions then address acts of consciousness such as perceiving, intuiting, empathizing, and the like. In Van Kaam's study of "really feeling understood" there is a shift to psychological phenomena in the belief that there are basic human experiences that are common to us all. Van Kaam's interpretation of this method calls for an effort to disclose, in this example, the *core* of really feeling understood.

The research process in Van Kaam's phenomenology requires posing the research question to a large number of participants who are asked to respond by writing a description of their experience. It is presumed that people can express lived experience in such a manner and that analysis of their descriptions will reveal the core or essential structure of the human experience under study. Once the researcher obtains the descriptions from willing participants, the analysis proceeds as follows:

1. Each expression (word or phrase) that describes some aspect of the experience is listed separately from the others.
2. Similar expressions are grouped together and labeled.
3. Irrelevant expressions are eliminated.
4. Expressions that bear close relationship to one another are grouped and labeled.
5. The identified core of common elements is checked against a random sample of original descriptions by participants. Discrepancies at this point direct the researcher to start again with the analysis.
6. The steps of analysis (1 to 5) are performed independently by judges to check the reliability of the results.

In Van Kaam's study (1959, p. 69) the essential structure of "really feeling understood" was reported in the following statement:

> The experience of really feeling understood is a perceptual-emotional gestalt: a subject, perceiving that a person co-experiences what things mean to the subject and accepts him, feels, initially, relief from experiential loneliness, and, gradually, safe experiential communion with that person and with that which the subject perceives this person to represent.

The full report includes justification and explanation of each phrase of the description.

A few published nursing studies have used Van Kaam's approach to phenomonology, often with some modification of the process. These modifications usually are reduced sample size and/or the substitution or addition of interview for the written description. Sandelowski and Pollock (1986), for example, interviewed 48 women to identify recurring themes in their experiences of infertility treatment. They were

Methodologist	Data source	Data form	Analysis and product
Table 11-1 **Three Styles of Phenomenological Research**			
Van Kaam	Large sample	Written descriptions	Categorization Identification of "core" of human experience Validation of sample of descriptions with core Cross-analysis by judges
Colaizzi	Small sample	Transcripts of interviews	Categorization Identification of essential meaning of experience Validation with participants
Paterson and Zderad	Researcher's nursing practice	Nursing assessment and process data	Thematic classification Conceptualization of the experience

ambiguity, temporality, and otherness. The description of the experience of infertility pivots around these three themes (elements) and includes elaboration on varying expressions of them (Sandelowski and Pollock, p. 142).

The use of interview in phenomenological study is pointedly included in Colaizzi's (1978) interpretation of the method. Lengthy and repeated interviews often are necessary to facilitate participants' descriptions of their experiences. Interviews have the advantage over a written description of providing the researcher with nonverbal as well as verbal data and of enabling the researcher to use interpersonal skills to encourage participants' efforts to articulate experience. Because such interviews are time-consuming and yield extremely large amounts of narrative data, usually fewer participants are sought for studies featuring interview as the primary data-generating strategy.

Haase's study (1987) of chronically ill adolescents' experiences of courage used the Colaizzi method. Haase interviewed nine chronically ill, hospitalized adolescents and analyzed transcripts of these interviews in a process similar to the process of Van Kaam described above. To illustrate this process of searching for themes in interview data, Haase (p. 67) reported the following example of abstractions from participants' words:

Subject: "My mom just held my hand and talked to me. That made it better."

Researcher's abstractions:
1. Mother holding hand and talking improved situation.
2. Touch and verbal expressions of caring by mother decreased feelings of despair to a tolerable level.

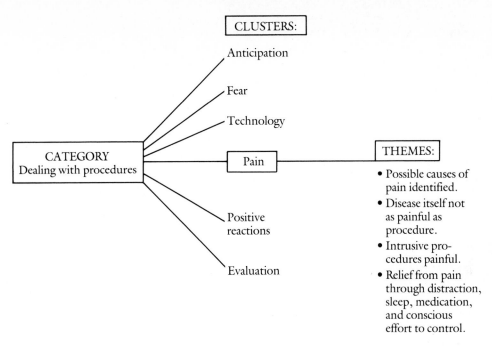

Fig. 11-2   Example of theme categories created from *Theme and Theme Clusters* (Haase, 1987, pp. 77-78).

It can be seen from this example that the process of analysis is one of abstracting from participants' words to formulate an essential meaning in the experience. Such meanings are grouped to constitute themes, themes are grouped into clusters, and clusters into categories. Haase found nine categories, 30 clusters, and an even larger number of descriptive themes within those clusters. Fig. 11-2 provides an example of Haase's inductive ordering of the data in this study.

Paterson and Zderad (1976, pp. 76-81) have proposed a different way for nurses to apply phenomenology in the study of nursing questions. Their interpretation of the method adheres more precisely to phenomenological philosophy and to nursing process. The phases are as follows:

1. Preparation of the researcher: The researcher needs to be an open, self-aware person. These qualities can be nurtured especially well by ongoing study in the humanities.
2. Primary data collection: Observations are made from *within* the situation under study. The researcher must therefore be a practicing nurse rather than an outside observer of nursing. Data will include firsthand observations inclusive of intuitive insights and empathic awarenesses.
3. Scientific analysis: The researcher conceptualizes and expresses his understanding in a reflective turn toward the data collected from clinical experience.
4. Scientific synthesis: The researcher locates other related or similar situations (from past experience and in the literature) to compare and contrast the data with other known

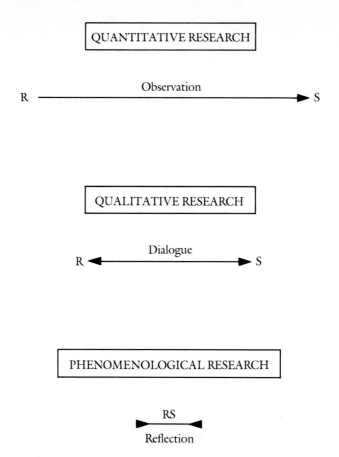

Fig. 11-3   Comparison of researcher-subject relationships.

realities. This is an interpretive activity performed to sort and classify the data thematically.

5. Abstraction: The experience is finally conceptualized to account for its relatedness to other knowledge and its variations. Nursing knowledge is thus expanded, and the researcher as clinician is transformed in perspective.

Paterson and Zderad's study of comfort (1976, pp. 111-122) was accomplished by using these phases as a guide. Primary data were collected and recorded over several months from weekly interactions with 15 hospitalized, psychiatric patients. Through reflective analysis and synthesis of these data, they identified 12 nurse behaviors aimed toward patient comfort, four criteria for estimating the degree of a patient's comfort, 52 items of knowledge needed by a nurse when the aim is to comfort, and a theoretical construct of comfort. Paterson and Zderad's interpretation of phenomenology in nursing is a more faithful reflection of philosophical themes in phenomenology. The primary concern in phenomenology with lived experience requires the researcher to design ways of transcending the automatic interpretation people customarily adopt and accept as the truth. Reflection and intuition are processes emphasized in phenomenological writings and hence are considered strategic in gaining insight about experiences.

Fig. 11-3 presents a comparison of researcher-subject relationships in quantitative research, qualitative research, and phenomenological method. As has been presented, qualitative approaches in general feature high researcher involvement with participants in their settings. This is in contrast to the relatively remote research role in quantitative research. In qualitative research the researcher's relationship with participants is characterized by dialogue and collaboration. For the quantitative researcher the aim is objectivity, and the researcher maintains a stance of observation of participants as objects. Phenomenology, on the other hand, turns the researcher on himself; that is, on his reflective and intuitive grasp of experience. The researcher's direct experience is the source of the data whether immediate or vicarious. As Van Manen (1984, pp. 50-59) states, generating data in phenomenological research includes exploring personal experience and experiential descriptions in the arts as well as descriptions from participants.

As more nurse researchers become learned in phenomenological philosophy, there may be more exploration of the potential for theory development through a combined nurse-researcher role in which there is full use of data generated through clinical practice. In addition to Paterson and Zderad's study, readers are referred to Benner's (1983) proposal for investigating actual nursing practices for valuable knowledge.

CASE STUDY

Case studies are in-depth investigations of one or a few participants to provide detailed descriptions that may satisfy any of the general purposes of qualitative research. As a general strategy for research, the case study may be essentially quantitative rather than qualitative, depending on the researcher's theoretical and philosophical orientation, the selection of design features, and the purpose of the study. Subjects for a case study may include a single individual, a group, a family, an institution, or a social unit such as a neighborhood or a nursing department. For the purpose of this chapter the case study will be discussed solely in relation to its use and potential as a qualitative method.

Research purposes

The case study method is a relatively unexplored approach in nursing research to date. Its primary advantage is the depth and breadth of information that can be collected and analyzed, because the focus is on a single case or a small number of cases. This focus facilitates the researcher's ability to track many details in the aim to disclose complexity and context in human affairs. Yin (1984, p. 23) lists the critical features of the case study strategy:

1. It investigates a contemporary phenomenon within its real-life context.
2. It is indicated as a strategy of choice when the boundaries between phenomenon and context are not clearly evident.
3. It uses multiple sources of data.

Thus the case study can be considered a research design option when the question or problem is so little understood that the relevant variables cannot be readily identified or ordered. In such circumstances the case study would be exploratory in nature. In addition, the detail that is produced in case studies can serve the interest of explaining relationships that might not surface in other types of designs. Like other qualitative approaches, the commitment to preservation of context directs the researcher to multiple sources of data and to the task of field study over a protracted period of time.

Research questions and process

The case study approach to teaching and learning in nursing provides a familiar point of departure for specifying the kinds of questions that might be addressed by the case study design. Areas of general interest that lead to selection of case study method would include those troublesome situations that have evaded satisfactory solutions. Some examples are long-term home care of a chronically ill person, maintenance of persons with schizophrenia in the community, preservation of quality of life for aged persons, and assisting people to make life-style changes in the interests of health. The kinds of questions these situations evoke typically have to do with processes: "How do families cope with chronic illness at home?" "Why do persons with schizophrenia require repeated hospitalizations?" "How is quality of life maintained for the aged in nursing homes?" "How do people comply with prescriptions for life-style changes?" The questions are broad, focus on how and why circumstances occur, and may use a single individual, family, or other social group as the unit of analysis. Thus, to study the effects of chronic illness on a family, a case study might focus, for example, on one family's coping strategies.

Yin (1984) suggests that rationale for selection of a single case for the unit of analysis may be based on any of three considerations. First, the case study may be critical to testing a theory. The case study in this circumstance would be essentially a quantitative design. A second rationale is when a case represents an extreme or unique case. This rationale would apply when the circumstance or situation under study is rare. A third rationale is the relevatory case that has previously been inaccessible to investigators. In nursing, many clinical situations can be conceptualized as unique or revelatory based on their having been inaccessible to quantitative methods. If nurses used case study techniques to perform research concurrently with the nursing care process, significant insights about patients and their circumstances as well as about nursing care might emerge.

Benner (1983), a nurse theorist and qualitative researcher, is an advocate of the case study approach as a means of articulating and formalizing nursing expertise. She believes a wealth of knowledge is embedded in clinical practice that can be explicated through qualitative methods, including the case study. Such knowledge is generalizable in the sense that in the practice world an experience with one patient is used as a kind of building block when the practitioner moves forward to care for others in similar circumstances. Case studies are one way to formalize this kind of experiential knowledge so that it can be communicated and used to promote quality nursing care. Benner (1983, pp. 36-41) suggests that there are six kinds of experiential knowledge to uncover through qualitative research:

1. Graded qualitative distinctions in physiological changes, such as signs of impending shock
2. Common meanings about helping, recovering, and coping resources in health and illness
3. Assumptions, expectations, and sets underlying nursing interventions
4. Paradigm cases that guide nurses' perceptions and actions
5. Maxims or cryptic instructions based on a thorough understanding of a situation
6. Unplanned practices or interventions that have developed with technology and delegated care

Once the researcher identifies the unit of analysis and states the research question, a plan for data collection is formulated. Yin (1984, p. 30) proposes that the plan be guided by stated propositions that express theoretical relationships expected in the data. A more open approach, however, can be adopted, particularly when existing theory is inadequate. In either case the researcher will need to plan both the kinds of data to be collected and timing of the data collection. In common with other qualitative approaches, data sources and strategies include interviews, participant observation, written materials, and physical artifacts. In addition, nurse researchers might include in their case study designs participant observation that coincides with their roles as caregivers and strategies that capitalize on the data that become available through the caregiving role.

Analysis of case study data includes content analysis in a search for patterns and themes. Some techniques listed by Yin (1984) include organizing data in categorical matrices, flow charts, and frequency tables. If propositions are stated at the onset of the study, these guide the researcher's analysis. If propositions are not stated, the researcher might develop a topical outline suggested by the data or the nursing context. For example, a case study of a surgical client's care might be arranged in terms of preoperative, postoperative, and discharge phases. Delineation of phases of the nurse-client relationship is another organizational option that might be used to assist with ordering the data.

The case study report may take a variety of forms, but generally it is written to provide a thorough description of the case. One purpose served by such a description is that the case then can be compared to other cases. Such comparisons may be included in the analysis or the discussion sections. As in other qualitative approaches, the report should relate the case to existing theory in the discussion, with a disciplined effort made to allow the data to guide the conceptualizations. Over time, individual case studies can be analyzed collectively, by means of the same kinds of techniques as in analysis of a single case. In this way nursing can look to the case study method as a means for acquiring knowledge through experience.

ISSUES AND PROBLEMS IN QUALITATIVE RESEARCH

Qualitative research approaches represent a shift in thinking from the more commonly used quantitative approaches. This shift involves embracing a different set of expectations and criteria; this is not easy for many of us who have learned that the scientific method is quantitative in nature. Many of the issues and problems discussed in the literature reflect this struggle with orientation rather than with the limits of qualitative approaches as such. There are nevertheless concerns about qualitative research that need to be addressed as we consider actual and potential uses for qualitative approaches in nursing. In this section, selected issues and problems will be discussed: ethical concerns unique to qualitative approaches, reliability and validity, and combining qualitative and quantitative approaches.

Ethical considerations

Munhall (1988, p. 151) has succinctly stated ethical guidelines for qualitative researchers. These arise primarily from the nature of the researcher's involvement with people in qualitative studies that feature field work and participant observations. They are as follows:

1. The therapeutic imperative of nursing (advocacy) takes precedence over the research imperative (advancing knowledge) if conflict develops.
2. Consent to participate in research is interpreted to mean that individuals are collaborators in the research enterprise.
3. Ongoing negotiation is required to protect collaborators' rights.

In essence then qualitative researchers must attend carefully to their relationships with people observed or interviewed and with whom they might otherwise be involved in the course of field work. Plans for initiating, maintaining, and terminating these relationships are concerns not only for data collection but also for preservation of valued human rights.

The caregiving mission of nursing is maintained as a primary allegiance in the researcher's involvement with others in the field. In designing studies, then, researchers must attempt to anticipate role conflicts and at times may need to compromise the research project in the interest of the client's need for nursing intervention. Often, conflict is avoided when the researcher's nursing identity is carefully suspended from the researcher role. In some cases, however, particularly in research that involves one's own practice, conflict may not be avoidable. Mentors or research colleagues may be indispensable in such research to assist with conflict resolution that is faithful to nursing's professional values.

The qualitative researcher's orientation to participants as collaborators is usually interpreted to mean that the researcher is responsible for the ongoing negotiating, disclosing, and sharing information and decision making with participants. This is known as **process consent**. At the very least, research findings are made readily available to participants whose expertise is recognized and valued in the project. Consent is a dynamic concept in the recognition of changing circumstances and need for ongoing development of data-collection plans. The researcher's provisions for participants' rights, then, are integrated throughout the research process and can be reported in full only after the project is completed.

Reliability and validity

The meaning of *reliability* and *validity* in qualitative research is different from that in quantitative studies. Kirk and Miller (1986, p. 21) suggest that the issue of validity in qualitative research is "a question of whether the researcher sees what he or she thinks he or she sees." Rigor in the standards that guide the process of data collection in the field is identified as the best check of validity. Among these standards a long period of time in the field is often cited as a critical condition to ensure validity. The researcher is the instrument in qualitative studies, and as such, findings are filtered through his or her perceptions and perspectives. Thus the researcher's background and customary ways of processing sensory input are important pieces of information to take into account when reading a qualitative research report. Coinvestigators, mentors, supervisors, judges, and participants themselves are often incorporated into research designs as a check on biased observation. Although distortion or biased observation needs to be controlled, the researcher as an interpretive instrument is acknowledged as an inherent feature in qualitative approaches. All instruments, however, are considered by qualitative researchers to be bound by perspectives or points of view.

Qualitative researchers monitor carefully the effects of their presence on people and events in research settings. Some common strategies to minimize reactivity are to increase the length of time in the field, to assume unobtrusive roles in the field or roles that help the researcher to blend in with others, and to develop trusting relationships with informants and others who are sources of data. Two researchers studying the same topic in the same or different settings are not likely to arrive at exactly the same findings. Replication in the quantitative sense is not possible. However, findings from studies on the same topic would not contradict each other if the researchers are successful in observing and reporting without distortion. Reliability, then, is the fit between the researcher's findings and what actually occurs in the situation under study. The estimation of reliability is based on two points of reference: the researcher's perspective and the context of the observations. One would not expect a single study to account for all perspectives on what actually occurs.

Data are generally collected in qualitative research until it becomes redundant or until no new information appears. Multiple sources of data are used in part as a means of cross-checking information and thereby checking both reliability and validity. Research teams may be used to accomplish this as well. Both the large volume of data and the length of data collection serve to increase reliability and validity. Validating findings with participants is a key strategy in this process.

Combining qualitative and quantitative approaches

Duffy (1987) describes four ways in which qualitative and quantitative methods may be combined. *Triangulation* is a term used to refer to these four combinations: theoretical, data, investigator, and generic triangulations. In order, they involve the use of several perspectives in analysis of data, the use of multiple sources of data, the use of multiple observers, and the use of two or more methods of data collection. Copel's study (1984) of loneliness is an example of combining features of quantitative and qualitative research. She measured loneliness on a scale, thus generating quantitative data, and also interviewed the same participants. The two sets of data were consulted in the analysis.

Others argue against combining approaches based on the divergent philosophies of the two approaches to research. Moccia (1988, p. 8) states,

> For nurse scientists, as for other scientists, choosing between quantitative and qualitative methods therefore means choosing to work either with a closed-system or open-system view of the world, choosing to seek either absolute or relative and contextual knowledge and to develop either a definitive or dynamic science; and choosing to learn how to predict and control phenomena with more reliability and validity or to understand and explain phenomena more fully.

From this point of view the philosophical and theoretical foundations of the quantitative and qualitative research approaches are contradictory and mutually exclusive.

Consumers of research will find that some researchers do combine approaches, using qualitative strategies and data to promote the development of theory that enables us to predict and control nursing phenomena. Consumers will also find "pure" qualitative research that provides depth of understanding that has a direct and immediate effect on practice. Whether or not quantitative and qualitative approaches should be combined is an issue that will continue to be debated. In the meantime consumers need to be aware of the differences between approaches and to look for researchers' rationales for selecting one approach over the other or choosing to combine them.

CRITERIA FOR CRITIQUING OF QUALITATIVE RESEARCH

Each qualitative method has some criteria that are unique to that method. In grounded theory, for example, the research product is a theory that needs to be evaluated by criteria for theories. Based on their commonalities, some criteria proposed here apply to all qualitative studies (see box on p. 205).

Broadly stated research questions are typical of qualitative studies. They reflect either a lack of theory in the areas under investigation or a need to take a fresh approach to a situation that is inadequately described and explained by existing theory. Qualitative approaches are indicated when the question concerns complex human phenomena about which we need detailed description and explanation for genuine insight. To warrant the use of nursing expertise the questions must bear relevance to health and to the knowledge needed by nurses to make their contributions to health care. It is not unusual for the qualitative researcher to modify the question as the study proceeds. This is an expected consequence of venturing into ambiguous territory.

Background information is critical to a research reviewer's ability to evaluate the merit of a qualitative study. In addition to providing a rationale for the study, background information describes the researcher as instrument. The researcher's

Critiquing Criteria

The Research Question

1. Is the question stated broadly enough to preserve an orientation to phenomena in their natural contexts?
2. Does the question concern some aspect of human experience that bears on health?
3. Is the research focused on the subjective nature of human realities?
4. Is the study significant for nursing?

Background

1. Is nursing's need for study of the phenomenon documented?
2. Is a rationale provided for selecting the qualitative method used in the study?
3. Is the researcher's interest described and his or her perspective made explicit?
4. Are presuppositions articulated?

Method

1. Is research process as a human experience described? This should include a description of
   a. Source of data and how obtained
   b. Strategies for recording data
   c. Course of data collection period including ethical concerns and decisions
   d. Method of analysis with rationale
2. Are decisions about method and design features adequate for the research question?
3. Is attention to concerns for validity and reliability adequate?
4. Is data collection exhaustive?

Findings

1. Were plans for analysis implemented faithfully?
2. Are findings descriptive, enabling the reader to "grasp" the phenomenon?
3. Are conceptualizations supported by the data? Is there a balance between concepts and descriptive data?
4. Is the level of analysis consistent with the aim of the study?

Conclusions

1. Are findings related to existing theory?
2. Are findings related to similar studies?
3. Are recommendations formulated?

perspective must be known to appreciate fully the profile of reality disclosed in the study. However, as noted in the discussion of presentation of ethnographic findings, journal and conference formats usually limit researchers to page or time frames that require exclusion of many details; thus background information and detailed accounts of the research process are often necessarily omitted.

As has been seen in the description of the various methods available to qualitative researchers, numerous strategies and techniques may be used in qualitative studies. The research process is fluid and must be responsive to events and circumstances that arise during the data collection period. Thus reviewers must examine studies for description of the research process. Such standards as logical decision making and human sensitivity apply. Throughout the process, reviewers need to be satisfied that the types and amounts of data were adequate, that the means of securing the data were ethical and efficacious, and that the analysis of data was systematic and disciplined.

Essentially, findings in a qualitative study are evaluated in terms of how well conceptualizations are supported by the data. The reviewer should expect to see examples from the data and then must make a judgment about how convincing the researcher's conceptualizations are. When findings are presented well, the reviewer has a sense of understanding the phenomenon under study from the researcher's perspective. This may complement, supplement, coincide with, or contradict the reviewer's experiential knowledge of the phenomenon. Findings that are contradictory to existing theory or to common-sense knowledge would warrant an explanation from the researcher.

Ideally, qualitative research reports should relate findings to existing theory and to similar studies. This criterion does not deviate from that for quantitative studies. However, qualitative findings typically are linked to nursing knowledge at the end of the study rather than in the beginning development of a conceptual framework. Qualitative studies are not conceived and implemented without frameworks, but there is a deliberate attempt to maintain an unbiased, atheoretical stance in relation to the phenomena under study. Consequently, references to existing theory and other studies are made after the data are analyzed, creatively and freshly by the researcher.

SUMMARY

In this chapter, qualitative approaches to research have been described by identifying the distinguishing characteristics of these approaches. Commonalities of the various approaches have been emphasized to clarify the philosophical and theoretical premises that constitute a qualitative tradition in the social sciences that dates to the 19th century. Nursing's uses of qualitative research have been cited in an explication of the actual and potential value of qualitative approaches in the development of nursing knowledge. The methods of ethnography, grounded theory, phenomenology, and case study were explained to reveal the nature of the research process and outcome in qualitative inquiry. General criteria for critiquing qualitative studies were proposed to facilitate reviewers' discriminatory consideration of qualitative research projects.

This has been an introductory chapter with many necessary omissions of details about methodology. Qualitative research in nursing is a relatively new activity with only partial acceptance by the nursing community of researchers and scholars. It is nevertheless a promising and an engaging development in our ongoing search for innovative and productive approaches to constructing knowledge for the practice of nursing. The reader is invited to join with others in this period of scholarly exploration and expansion of qualitative approaches to knowing.

References

Aamodt, A. (1982). Examining ethnography for nurse researchers, *Western Journal of Nursing Research,* **4**:209-221.

Aamodt, A. (1986). Discovering the child's view of alopecia: doing ethnography. In P. Munhall and C. Oiler, eds.: *Nursing research: a qualitative perspective,* Norwalk, Conn., Appleton-Century-Crofts, pp. 163-172.

Agee, J., and Evans, W. (1941). *Let us now praise famous men,* New York, Houghton Mifflin Co.

Baron, R. (1985). An introduction to medical phenomenology: I can't hear you while I'm listening, *Annals of Internal Medicine,* **103:** 606-611.

Benner, P. (1983). Uncovering the knowledge embedded in clinical practice, *Image,* **19**:36-41.

Bogdan, R.C., and Biklen, F.K. (1982). Qualitative research for education: an introduction to theory and method.

Chenitz, W., and Swanson, J. (1986). *From practice to grounded theory,* Menlo Park, Calif., Addison-Wesley Publishing Co.

Colaizzi, P. (1978). Psychological research as the phenomenologist views it. In Vaile, R., and King, M., eds.: *Existential phenomenological alternatives for psychology,* New York, Oxford University Press.

Copel, L. (1984). Loneliness: a clinical investigation (unpublished doctoral dissertation), Texas Women's University.

Davis, M. (1977). Rehabilitative care in the skilled nursing facility: the mismatch of organizational structure and patient needs, *Journal of Nursing Administration,* **7**:22-27.

Davis, M. (1986). Observation in natural settings. In W. Chenitz and J. Swanson, eds.: *From practice to grounded theory,* Menlo Park, Calif., Addison-Wesley Publishing Co., pp. 48-65.

Duffy, M. (1987). Methodological triangulation: a vehicle for merging quantitative and qualitative research methods, *Image,* **19**:130-133.

Germain, C. (1982). *The cancer unit: an ethnography,* Rockville, Md., Aspen.

Germain, C. (1986). Ethnography: the method. In P. Munhall and C. Oiler, eds.: *Nursing research: a qualitative perspective,* Norwalk, Conn., Appleton-Century-Crofts, pp. 147-162.

Glaser, B., and Strauss, A. (1967). *The discovery of grounded theory,* Chicago, Aldine Publishing Co.

Haase, J. (1987). Components of courage in chronically ill adolescents: a phenomenological study, *Advances in Nursing Science,* **9**:64-80.

Hutchinson, S. (1986a). Creating meaning: grounded theory of NICU nurses. In W. Chenitz and J. Swanson, eds.: *From practice to grounded theory,* Menlo Park, Calif., Addison-Wesley Publishing Co., pp. 191-204.

Hutchinson, S. (1986b). Grounded theory: the method. In P. Munhall and C. Oiler, eds.: *Nursing research: a qualitative perspective,* Norwalk, Conn., Appleton-Century-Crofts, pp. 111-130.

Kayser-Jones, J. (1981). *Old, alone, and neglected,* Los Angeles, University of California Press.

Kirk, J., and Miller, M. (1986). *Reliability and validity in qualitative research.* In Sage University Paper Series on Qualitative Research Methods, vol. 1, Beverly Hills, Sage Publications.

Knafl, K., and Howard, M. (1986). Interpreting, reporting and evaluating qualitative research. In P. Munhall and C. Oiler, eds.: *Nursing research: a qualitative perspective,* Norwalk, Conn., Appleton-Century-Crofts, pp. 265-277.

Kramer, M. (1968). Role models, role conception, and role deprivation, *Nursing Research,* **17**:115-120.

Kroska, R. (1985). Ethnographic research method: a qualitative example to discover the role of "granny" midwives in health services. In M. Leininger, ed.: *Qualitative research methods in nursing,* New York, Grune & Stratton, Inc.

Leininger, M. (1985). *Qualitative research methods in nursing*, New York, Grune & Stratton, Inc.

Lynch-Sauer, J. (1985). Using a phenomenological research method to study nursing phenomena. In M. Leininger, ed.: *Qualitative research methods in nursing*, New York, Grune & Stratton, Inc., pp. 93-107.

Moccia, P. (1988). A critique of compromise: beyond the methods debate, *Advances in Nursing Science*, **10**:1-9.

Munhall, P. (1982). Nursing philosophy and nursing research: in apposition or opposition? *Nursing Research*, **31**:176-177, 181.

Munhall, P. (1988). Ethical considerations in qualitative research, *Western Journal of Nursing Research*, **10**:150-162.

Munhall, P., and Oiler, C. (1986). *Nursing research: a qualitative perspective*, Norwalk, Conn., Appleton-Century-Crofts.

Oiler, C. (1982). The phenomenological approach in nursing research, *Nursing Research*, **31**:178-181.

Paterson, J., and Zderad, L. (1976). *Humanistic nursing*, New York, John Wiley & Sons.

Quint, J. (1966). Awareness of death and the nurse's composure, *Nursing Research*, **15**:49-55.

Quint, J. (1967). *The nurse and the dying patient*, New York, Macmillan Publishing Co.

Riemen, D. (1986). The essential structure of a caring interaction: doing phenomenology. In P. Munhall and C. Oiler, eds.: *Nursing research: a qualitative perspective*, Norwalk, Conn., Appleton-Century-Crofts, pp. 85-108.

Sandelowski, M., and Pollock, G. (1986). Women's experiences of infertility, *Image*, **18**:140-144.

Spradley, J. (1979). *The ethnographic interview*, New York, Holt, Rinehart & Winston.

Spradley, J. (1980). *Participant observation*, New York, Holt, Rinehart & Winston.

Stern, P. (1980). Grounded theory methodology: its uses and processes, *Image*, **12**:20-23.

Tinkle, M., and Beaton, J. (1983). Toward a new view of science: implications for nursing research, *Advances in Nursing Science*, **5**:27-36.

Van Kaam, A. (1959). Phenomenal analysis: exemplified by a study of the experience of "really feeling understood," *Journal of Individual Psychology*, **15**:66-72.

Van Manen, A. (1984). Practicing phenomenological writing, *Phenomenology and Pedagogy*, **2**:36-69.

Wilson, H. (1986). Presencing—social control of schizophrenics in an antipsychiatric community: doing grounded theory. In P. Munhall and C. Oiler, eds.: *Nursing research: a qualitative perspective*, Norwalk, Conn., Appleton-Century-Crofts, pp. 131-144.

Yin, R. (1984). *Case study research*, Beverly Hills, Sage Publications.

12

Additional Types of Research

Geri LoBiondo-Wood

LEARNING OBJECTIVES

After reading this chapter the student should be able to do the following:

◇ Identify the historical, methodological, and evaluative types of research.

◇ Describe each of these types of research.

◇ Distinguish and differentiate between each of these types of research.

◇ Identify the purposes of each of these types of research.

◇ Describe the general format of each of these types of research.

◇ Evaluate each of these types of research by applying the critiquing principles relevant to each type.

KEY TERMS

evaluative research   methodological research
external criticism   primary source
historical research   psychometrics
internal criticism   secondary source

The major types of quantitative and qualitative designs have been introduced in previous chapters. Although they are very important to the development of a scientific knowledge base, these designs are not the sum total of all research designs. Other types of designs that complement the science of research utilize a different perspective to identify research problems or topics, form hypotheses, and collect, analyze, and interpret data. These additional types of designs are valid and useful and may be considered for special areas of investigation. They may be experimental, nonexperimental, or qualitative. They lend another means of viewing and interpreting phenomena that gives further breadth and knowledge to nursing science and practice. Additional types of research are utilized to evaluate the past, develop measurement tools, and evaluate programs. These types of research, although less frequently encountered in journals and as frameworks of studies, are important links in the development of nursing research. The types are **historical research, methodological research,** and **evaluative research.** The purpose of this chapter is to present a brief description of each of these types and their respective goals. The principles for evaluating each type and its contribution to nursing within a consumer perspective are also presented.

HISTORICAL RESEARCH

History, as we experience it in the form of written and verbal communication, is an account of past events. The reconstruction of history in writing or historiography allows us to view the occurrences of the past and to visualize the shaping of events, eras, and people. Unlike historiography, *historical research* is the systematic compilation of data and the critical presentation, evaluation, and interpretation of facts regarding people, events, and occurrences of the past. Its process is not the mere writing or chronicling of historical events as in a term paper, but like other research designs, it is based on the gathering of data related to either research questions or hypotheses. Unlike other previously discussed design types (see Chapters 9 and 10), in historical research, data are not manipulated and new data are not generated. Historical research is basically a qualitative method of research, but there are instances in which historical researchers have analyzed historical data using quantitative methods (Kalish, Kalish, and Clinton, 1982). When reading historical research the consumer should note that whether qualitative or quantitative methods were used, the rules of scientific rigor were applied. The data are facts from the past that are judged for authenticity. The goal of such research is to interpret the facts of the past to gain a clearer understanding of contemporary practice and issues. An example of historical research is *Hospitals, Paternalism and the Role of the Nurse* (Ashley, 1976). In this extensive study Ashley traced the factors that contributed to the current role of the nurse and the roots of paternalism in hospitals.

The idea has been previously stressed that when a piece of research is reviewed, it should be obvious to the reader that the researcher is widely read and prepared in the specific and related topics of the study (see Chapter 5). This principle also applies in historical research because the investigation requires not only an understanding of a specific person or historical event but also the context of the time and place of the occurrence. This broad knowledge and data base are present in Ashley's study.

The design of historical research may seem to be more flexible because statistics generally are not used, but this is not the case. Historical research must pass tests of validity and reliability in a process as carefully prescribed as those delineated for any other form of research (Christy, 1975). Hockett (1955) stated that the aim of historical research was to make use of raw statements to arrive at facts. A statement is defined as being nothing more than what someone has said. In light of the possibility of error when judging statements, it becomes the duty of the historian to doubt every statement until it is critically tested (Hockett, 1955, p. 13).

Problem identification

One of the first steps in historical research is to identify the problem area and the purpose of the study. As with other research designs, the historical investigation should reflect the delimitations of study. The period, patterns, or population to be studied should be limited. This provides a researcher with the opportunity for in depth research that can unfold new dimensions of an issue, relationship between events, or parallel developments or factors inherent in attitude or value formation (Krampitz, 1981). For example, O'Brien (1987) explored nursing's journey from domesticity to profession in Philadelphia, Pennsylvania, in her study entitled "All a Woman's Life Can Bring: The Domestic Roots of Nursing in Philadelphia, 1830-1885." Even though the exploration of 55 years of nursing in one city may seem very limited, O'Brien needed to narrow her problem area. Throughout the introduction to the study the reader can see how the final research area was delimited through statements such as the following:

> Traditionally, the written history of modern nursing in the United States begins with the heroic achievements of Florence Nightingale and continues. . . . The history of nursing in Philadelphia could be written as one such story. This study begins in the 1830s, a time when nursing was seen as an innate and lovingresponsibility of women and mothers, and traces through the years the way these domestic roots shaped contemporary thinking.

This case study, then, is a vehicle for developing two interrelated theses. The first addresses the essentially domestic roots of modern nursing and attempts to provide a theoretical context for the recurring tensions nurses today feel. . . .

The second thesis attempts to move the history of nursing from its more traditional focus on its own institutional development; in the broader realm of the history of women, particularly wage-earning women (p. 12).

What the researcher's problem statement or intent was is clearly drawn for the consumer.

In addition to making a statement of the problem, a historical investigation may identify research questions. Inherent in these questions are implied and not always explicitly stated hypotheses (Best, 1970). The following are examples from a study by Wheeler (1985) that explored the editorial position and content of each issue of the first 20 years of the *American Journal of Nursing* in relation to the emergence of nursing as a profession.

⋄ What professional issues captured the attention of nurses during this period, and how were they conceptualized?

⋄ How was the socialization of nurses into the profession presented?

⋄ Who were the major contributors to the journal, and what disciplines or occupations did they represent?

⋄ To what extent did the journal's content attempt to define and influence "professionalism in nursing?"

⋄ To what extent did the journal's content reflect an awareness of and influence by the major social or political movements of the time?

The specific research questions provide the investigator with a direction derived from the identified problem area. The questions provide not just for the mere chronicling of the journal's content, but more important, they set the stage for the interpretive study of the journal to investigate the emergence of professional issues.

Another example of a historical study with specific problem identification and research questions was done by Kalish, Kalish, and Clinton (1982). To answer the following questions these investigators focused on prime-time television programs that were broadcast during the period of 1950 to 1980:

⋄ What is the scope of nursing practice portrayed on television?

⋄ What specific nursing actions are most commonly shown on television, and has their emphasis changed over time?

⋄ What factors are associated with the nurses and nursing actions shown on television?

⋄ Are certain aspects of professional nursing more highly exposed than others to the viewing public?

The studies cited are only three of a slowly growing number of interesting historical research studies. The identification of historical studies as a design and method of research has only recently become more widely accepted. Christy (1975) believed this was because of nursing's need to provide answers to immediate clinical, educational, or administrative problems, and nurses may have thought of historical research as more of a search than research. From the scope of the research questions delimited in these two studies, it becomes obvious not only that these studies are interesting but that negative portrayals of nurses and nursing may have influenced the public's views of the profession and its members.

Data collection

After the research problem and questions have been delimited, the investigator needs to locate and identify data sources. This may not be easy in a historical investigation. Depending on the period of investigation and the location of the needed documents, data may be difficult to locate. It has been said that historical researchers should be free of allergies to dust because they may spend much of their time searching archival literature.

There are two categories of data sources: primary and secondary. Whenever possible, data should include primary sources. **Primary sources** are original documents, films, letters, diaries, records, artifacts, periodicals, tapes, or eyewitness accounts (see Chapter 5). In other words, in historical research the reviewer should be able to identify the use of firsthand information. In the Wheeler study (1985) the *American Journal of Nursing* represents a primary source. In the study by Kalish, Kalish, and Clinton (1982) the films of television shows represent a primary source. An example of an eyewitness account may be found in the New York State Nurses' Association Archives. The Association is compiling videotaped oral histories of nursing leaders. The gathering and use of primary sources are necessary to confirm events or statements in a historical investigation.

Secondary sources are accounts of events written by someone other than the person involved (see Chapter 5). They are used when primary documents are missing or limited. Secondary sources represent a summation or interpretation of events by others. Secondary sources provide a view of an event by someone other than a participant in that event. It is important to remember when critiquing and assessing data sources that the further the review of an event moves from the originator, the greater the risk of error and distortion. Examples of secondary sources are verbal or written secondhand accounts, textbooks, reference books, and encyclopedias. At times, gathering primary data may be highly difficult, but the goal of the historian is to provide primary documentation. Primary documentation provides stronger reliability and validity in the study's data analysis.

Data analysis

Historiographers have developed two processes of data evaluation: **external criticism** and **internal criticism.** The critiquer of a historical study should be able to recognize the researcher's attempts at interpretation of data based on these processes. *External criticism* establishes the validity of the data: Is the document what it seems to be? External criticism is therefore the researcher's evaluation of the credibility and authenticity of the document. In the studies by Wheeler (1985) and Kalish, Kalish, and Clinton (1982) the external criticism applied by the investigators and the reviewer can be easily assessed. In the case of a primary source that is a handwritten letter or document, external criticism may be more difficult to assess. For example, Palmer (1983) conducted a study that looked at Florence Nightingale's life. In the study she used documents that were handwritten by Nightingale. To use these as primary sources Palmer needed to establish that the handwriting was Nightingale's and that the documents were therefore authentic primary sources. The researcher also needed to validate the age of the paper as well. Unsigned letters or memos may present problems for historical researchers. Other aspects of external criticism are ghostwriting and time: Was the document written by an assistant? Was the document dated or, if undated, has the time of writing been established?

The test of reliability for the historical researcher is internal criticism. *Internal criticism* establishes the reliability or consistency of the information within the document. In this process the researcher moves from the document itself to the content of the document. This may be the most difficult step for the historical researcher. During this process the researcher needs to determine whether or not the data regarding the event or occurrence are unbiased. The primary need of the researcher is to understand the document. This means not reading *into* the work and understanding the meaning of the words and colloquialisms of the time. Therefore the researcher needs to avoid taking statements out of context, be aware of historical nuances that may have affected the statements, compare the statements or data with other accounts of the same event, and be aware of possible biases of the document's originator. These steps for weighing and judging the data are critical to the soundness and usefulness of the investigation. The historical researcher accomplishes them as judiciously and carefully as one who is doing an empirical study.

Most historical research does not utilize statistical measures. Examples of exceptions to this are the works of Kalish, Kalish, and Clinton (1982) and Kalish, Kalish, and Young (1983). In these studies the investigators used methods of coding and content analysis to statistically review the data gathered.

Synthesis and the research report

The historical researcher analyzes and then synthesizes the data to form a cohesive picture that addresses the research questions or hypotheses. Synthesis of the data for the final research report requires a great deal of selection based on expert judgment. The raw data are generally massive and require careful selection by the researcher to avoid bias and still portray a representative and appealing piece. The final written report therefore differs from an empirical research report. It may also seem more like a literary piece of work than a research study. The written report seen in a journal does not cite for the reader which statements or data are from primary and secondary sources. Nor do the investigators specifically relate the measures of external and internal criticism. The historical research accomplishes these steps in the analysis and presents an unbiased account of the research questions.

There is the problem of subjective analysis in historical research. Because of this, the "how" of the incident frequently takes precedence over the "why" questions (Krampitz, 1981). It is therefore the critiquer's responsibility to use her knowledge of the historical research process to infer and judge the merits of the piece, its usefulness, and generalizability. Historical research thus becomes an important link for learning about past roles, events, and occurrences. By learning from the past we can avoid repeating its negative aspects and build on its positive aspects. Nursing needs to understand its history and scrutinize its past through historical research to build on its strengths. Understanding the purposes and format of historical research is an important goal of the research consumer.

METHODOLOGICAL RESEARCH

Methodology is a general term and has many meanings. It may mean different ways of doing research for different purposes, ways of stating hypotheses, methods of data collection and measurement, and techniques of data analysis. Methodology also includes aspects of the philosophy of science as an overall critical approach to research (Kerlinger, 1979). As you will find in succeeding chapters (see Chapters 13 and 14), methodology influences research strongly. *Methodological research* is the controlled investigation of the theoretical and applied aspects of mathematics, statistics, measurement, and the means of gathering and analyzing data (Kerlinger, 1979).

The most significant and critically important aspect of methodological research that is addressed in measurement and statistics is called **psychometrics.** Psychometrics deals with the theory and development of measurement instruments or measurement techniques through the research process. Psychometrics thus deals with the measurement of a concept, such as anxiety or interpersonal conflict, with reliable and valid tools (see Chapter 14 for a discussion of reliability and validity). Psychometrics is a most critical issue for nurse researchers. Many of the tools utilized by nurse researchers have been developed by other disciplines, such as psychology and sociology, and may not necessarily be totally appropriate for nursing's use. Since nurses have become more sophisticated in their investigations and knowledge of research, the development of appropriate tools to measure phenomena of interest has increased. Methodological research is critical to the reliability and validity of a study. For example, Klein (1983) conducted a study on the use of contraceptives in women seeking abortion and their perception of the chance and ability to conceive. Although the study's purpose and problems were clear, the tool that was developed and used by the author exhibited various psychometric problems. When studies have inherent psychometric problems, they render the findings questionable or limited.

The main problem for nurse researchers is locating appropriate measurement tools. In the Klein study an important concept, risk-taking behavior, may impinge on contraceptive use and thereby clinical practice, and so it needed to be measured. The appropriate tool was lacking, so the author developed one. Many of the phenomena of interest to nursing practice and research are intangible, such as interpersonal conflict and maternal-fetal attachment. The intangible nature of various phenomena, yet the recognition of the need to measure them, places methodological research in an important position.

Methodological research differs from other designs of research. First, it does not include all of the research process steps as discussed in the introduction to Part II: The Research Process. Second, to implement its techniques the researcher must have a sound knowledge of psychometrics or must consult with a researcher knowledgeable in psychometric techniques. The methodological researcher is not interested in the interrelationship of the independent variable and dependent variable, or in the effect of an independent variable on a dependent variable. The methodological researcher is interested in identifying an intangible construct and making it tangible with a paper-and-pencil tool or observation protocol.

Basically a methodological study includes the following steps:

1. Defining the construct or behavior to be measured
2. Formulating the items
3. Developing instructions for users and respondents
4. Testing the tool's reliability and validity

These steps require a sound, specific, and exhaustive literature review to identify the theories underlying the construct. The literature review provides the basis of item formulation. Once the items have been developed, the researcher assesses the tool's reliability and validity (see Chapter 14). Various aspects of these procedures may differ according to the tools's use, purpose, and stage of development.

Examples of methodological research can be found in the studies done by Bergstrom, Braden, Laguzza, and Holman (1987) and by Braden and Bergstrom (1987). In these studies the researchers identified the construct of pressure sore etiology and defined it conceptually and operationally. Common considerations that researchers incorporate into methodological research are outlined in Table 12-1. Many more examples of methodological research can be found in nursing research literature (Waltz and Strickland, 1988; Strickland and Waltz, 1988). Psychometric or methodological studies are found primarily in journals that report research. The specific procedures of methodological research are beyond the scope of this book, but the reader is urged to look closely at the tools used in studies. References of psychometric or methodological research are provided in the Additional Readings in this chapter.

EVALUATIVE RESEARCH

Recently increased emphasis has been placed on the evaluation of the services and methods of care. Health care consumers and their supporting agencies need and rightfully require documentation of the effectiveness of care. Therefore nursing is becoming increasingly more accountable for its practice (see Chapter 1). This emphasis requires the use of research that can help to validate the use of treatments and programs. Evaluative research provides the needed approach. *Evaluative research* is the utilization of scientific research methods and procedures to evaluate a program, treatment practice, or policy; therefore it utilizes analytic means to document the worth of an activity. Evaluative research is not a separate design; it may be implemented with either an experimental or nonexperimental approach. As a type of research, it impinges directly on practice as an applied method. Bigman (1961) further delineates the following purposes and uses of evaluative research:

1. To discover whether and how well the objectives are being fulfilled
2. To determine the reasons for specific successes and failures

Table 12-1 **Common Considerations in the Development of Measurement Tools**

Consideration	Example
The well-constructed scale, test, interview schedule, or other form of index should consist of an objective standardized measure of samples of a behavior that has been clearly defined. Observations should be made on a small but carefully chosen sampling of the behavior of interest, thus permitting us to feel confident that the samples are representative.	In their study of pressure sore risk Bergstrom et al. (1987) selected six factors that were assessed as being representative of "pressure sore risk" as it had been defined. The basis for the decision was findings from a thorough review of previous theoretical and research literature.
The tool should be *standardized;* that is, a set of uniform items and response possibilities that are uniformly administered and scored.	In the studies by Bergstrom et al. (1987) the evaluation of pressure sore risk consisted of objective assessment by research nurses in various settings. Without specific criteria and ratings for the observed behaviors, the evaluations would be based on the nurses' subjective impressions, which may have varied significantly between observers and conditions.
The items of a measurement tool should be unambiguous; they should be clear-cut, concise, exact statements with only one idea per item. Negative stems or items with negatively phrased response possibilities result in a double negative and ambiguity in meaning and scoring.	In constructing a tool to measure job satisfaction, a nurse-scientist writes the following items, "I never feel that I don't have time to provide good nursing care." The response format consists of "Agree," "Undecided," and "Disagree." It is very likely that a response of "Disagree" will not reflect the respondent's true intent because of the confusion that is created by the double negatives.
The type of items used in any one test or scale should be restricted to a limited number of variations. Subjects who are expected to shift from one kind of item to another may fail to provide a true response as a result of the distraction of making such a change.	Mixing true-or-false items with questions that require a yes-or-no response and items that provide a response format of five possible answers is conducive to a high level of measurement error.
Items should not provide irrelevant clues. Unless carefully constructed, an item may furnish an indication of the expected response or answer. Furthermore the correct answer or expected response to one item should not be given by another item.	An item that provides a clue to the expected answer may contain value words that convey cultural expectations, such as, "A good wife enjoys caring for her home and family."

Continued.

Table 12-1 Common Considerations in the Development of Measurement Tools—cont'd	
Consideration	**Example**
The items of a measurement tool should not be made difficult by requiring unnecessarily complex or exact operations. Furthermore, the difficulty of an item should be appropriate to the level of the subjects being assessed. Limiting each item to one concept or idea helps to accomplish this objective.	A test constructed to evaluate learning in an introductory course in research methods may contain an item that is inappropriate for the designated group, such as, "A nonlinear transformation of data to linear data is a useful procedure before testing a hypothesis of curvilinearity."
The diagnostic, predictive, or measurement value of a tool depends on the degree to which it serves as an indicator of a relatively broad and significant area of behavior known as the universe of content for the behavior. As already emphasized, a behavior must be clearly defined before it can be measured. The definition is developed from the universe of content; that is, the information and research findings that are available for the behavior of interest. The items should reflect that definition. To what extent the test items appear to accomplish this objective is an indication of the validity of the instrument.	Two nurse researchers, A and B, are studying the construct of client satisfaction. Each has defined this construct in a different way. Consequently, the measurement tool that each nurse devises will include different questions. The questions on each tool will reflect the universe of content for client satisfaction as defined by each researcher.
The instrument should also adequately cover the defined behavior. The primary consideration is whether the number and nature of items in the sample are adequate. If there are too few items, then the accuracy or reliability of the measure must be questioned. In general, there should be a minimum of 10 items for each independent aspect of the behavior of interest.	Very few people would be satisfied with an assessment of such traits as intelligence if the scales were limited to three items.
The measure must prove its worth empirically through tests of reliability and validity.	A researcher should demonstrate to the reader that scale is accurate and measures what it purports to measure (see Chapter 14).

3. To direct the course of experiment with techniques for increasing effectiveness

4. To uncover the principles underlying a successful program

5. To base further research on the reasons for the relative success of alternative techniques

6. To redefine the means to be used for attaining objectives and even to redefine subgoals, in the light of the research findings

These purposes, although general, are applicable to evaluative research in nursing. Evaluative research in nursing has mainly been applied to educational program evaluation and not to clinical practices. Evaluation therefore involves more than judging; it also includes understanding and redefining (Suchman, 1967; Twain, 1975). Within an evaluative study the reviewer should be able to note the following steps (U.S. Department of Health, Education, and Welfare, 1955):

1. Identify the goals to be evaluated

2. Analyze the problems that the activity must manage

3. Describe and standardize the activity

4. Measure the degree of change that takes place

5. Determine whether the observed changes are a result of the activity or some other cause

6. Indicate some of the effects

Evaluative studies may incorporate either an experimental or a nonexperimental design depending on the purposes of the evaluation. Evaluative research can be either formative or summative. Formative evaluation refers to an ongoing assessment of a program's success in meeting needs, and it also can target areas for improvement. Summative evaluation refers to the evaluation process that is conducted after completion of the program. An example of a summative evaluation research project was conducted by Nettles-Carlson, Field, Friedman, and Smith (1988). The researchers compared two methods of breast self-examination (BSE) teaching. They assessed whether an individualized program or a routine teaching program improved the frequency of BSE, and they also assessed perceived barriers and benefits to performing BSE. This study utilized an experimental design and was a summative evaluation.

Another example of an evaluative nursing study that used random subject assignment was done by Oberst, Graham, Geller, Stearns, and Tiernan (1981). In this study the investigators compared the effectiveness of two approaches to urinary catheter management in controlling postoperative urinary function in 110 clients after an abdominoperineal resection or a low anterior bowel resection. The researchers evaluated the effectiveness of a straight gravity drainage system and a 6-day progressive catheter clamping program. Within the literature review and introduction to the study, the authors analyzed the problems of postoperative urinary function. The method and procedures sections of this study clearly and specifically outlined the descriptions and standardization procedures of the activity. This study also meets the criteria of measuring the degree of change by gathering baseline data on such variables as the voiding history of each client; the presence or absence of prostatism, cystocele, or rectocele; and the type and extent of surgery. The researchers measured the differences

Critiquing Criteria

Historical Research

1. Does the historical study overall isolate a specific event, occurrence, person, or time frame and do the following:
   a. Identify the problem area, research questions, and the purpose of the study?
   b. Discuss the occurrence within the context of its time and place?
   c. Set limitations with a rationale?
   d. Present the use of primary sources as well as secondary sources?
   e. Reflect the use of external criticism as well as internal criticism in the analysis?
   f. Critically present and evaluate the occurrence in an attempt to answer the question of how the occurrence evolved?

Methodological Research

1. Does the methodological study identify a specific construct or phenomenon that the developed tool will measure?
2. Is the construct defined?
3. Can the investigator's methods of item formulation be recognized? (Examples are client records, literature review, clinical experience, related research, and theory.)
4. Did the investigator perform reliability and validity tests, and which specific types were used?
5. Did the investigator omit a specific type of reliability or validity test? If so, which one was omitted?

Evaluative Research

1. Does the study identify a specific program or treatment that it will evaluate?
2. Are the goals to be evaluated identified?
3. Is the problem(s) analyzed and described?
4. Is the program to be analyzed described and standardized?
5. Is measurement of the degree of change that occurs identified?
6. Is there a determination of whether the observed change is related to the activity or to some other causes?

in observed dysfunction rates with preset guidelines and through the use of statistical measures. The determination of what the observed differences were related to, and the durability of the effects, are dealt with in the results and discussions sections of the investigation. This study is an excellent example of an evaluative approach to a clinical problem because of the systematic investigative approach to the problem and the researchers' ability to present the basis for further research.

When evaluative research is applied to the functioning of a specific program, problems may arise. Individuals in the programs undergoing evaluation may perceive the evaluation as threatening, and this may lead to a lack of cooperation. There may also be a problem when deciding how to measure a program's effectiveness, especially if the program is complex and has many broad goals. Nursing research related to program evaluation is conducted mainly on educational programs. An example of a program evaluation was done by Griggs (1977). In this study Griggs evaluated the effectiveness of an autotutorial minicourse for nurses and hospital personnel that dealt with nosocomial infections and diseases related to the use of respiratory therapy equipment. Prospective payment systems, third party reimbursement criteria, and the need to document the effectiveness of care may contribute to an increase in evaluative research.

CRITIQUING ADDITIONAL TYPES OF RESEARCH

The criteria for critiquing the types of research presented in this chapter are given in the box on p. 222. From your review of this chapter you have found additional means of investigating phenomena related to nursing practice and theory. When critiquing these additional types of research it is important for the consumer to first identify the type of research that was employed in the investigation. Once the type of research is identified, its specific purpose and format need to be understood by the consumer. Understanding the format of a specific type allows the reviewer to apply the relevant principles of critiquing to the respective study. The format and methods of each type of research will vary. Knowing how they vary allows a consumer to assess if the most appropriate design was utilized, and even though the format and methods vary it is important to remember that all research has a central goal: to answer questions scientifically. Therefore, when critiquing one of the additional types of research outlined in this chapter, it is important for the consumer to determine if the question or problem being posed is consistent with the purpose of the research. The study's format should then meet the criteria of the specific research. Finally, the merits of the study should be determined by how well the investigator applied the format at each step in the study. It is within the steps and the format of a particular study that the consumer should find how well the investigator applied the research process.

SUMMARY

It is obvious that researchers have many types of research to choose from when addressing a research problem. The choice of one of the additional research types depends not only on the level of a problem but also on the type of the problem. When the researcher or consumer wishes to explore relationships and facts of the past, the historical design should be utilized. When addressing the need or when searching for reliable and valid measurement tools, the methodological approach is the most appropriate type of research, whereas the evaluation of how well a program or practice functions requires the use of evaluative research. Each type of research can and does answer nursing questions related to the science of nursing. The research consumer should be aware of the purpose of each type when deciding the overall appropriateness, usefulness, and generalizability of the study.

References

Ashley, J. (1976). *Hospitals, paternalism and the role of the nurse,* New York, Teachers College Press.

Bergstrom, N., Braden, B.J., Laguzza, A., and Holman, V. (1987). The Braden Scale for predicting pressure sore risk, *Nursing Research,* **36:**205-210.

Best, J.W. (1970). *Research in education,* Englewood Cliffs, N.J., Prentice-Hall, Inc.

Bigman, S.K. (1961). Evaluating the effectiveness of religious programs, *Review of Religious Research,* **2:**99-110.

Braden, B.J., and Bergstrom, N. (1987). A conceptual schema for the study of the etiology of pressure sores, *Rehabilitation Nursing,* **12:**8-12, 16.

Brody, E.B. (1981). Research design: general introduction. In S.D. Krampitz and N. Pavlovich, eds.: *Readings from nursing research,* St. Louis, The C.V. Mosby Co., pp. 40-48.

Christy, T.E. (1975). The methodology of historical research: a brief introduction, *Nursing Research,* **24:**189-192.

Gordon, M. (1982). *Nursing diagnosis: process and application,* New York, McGraw-Hill Book Co.

Griggs, B.M. (1977). A systems approach to the development and evaluation of a minicourse for nurses, *Nursing Research,* **26:**34-41.

Hockett, H.C. (1955). *Critical method in historical research and writing,* New York, Macmillan Publishing Co., Inc.

Hoskins, C.N. (1981). Psychometrics in nursing research: construction of an interpersonal conflict scale, *Research in Nursing and Health,* **4:**243-249.

Hoskins, C.N. (1983). Psychometrics in nursing research—further development of the interpersonal conflict scale, *Research in Nursing and Health,* **6:**75-83.

Kalish, B.J., Kalish, P.A., and Young, R.L. (1983). Television news coverage of nurse strikes: a resource management perspective, *Nursing Research,* **32:**175.

Kalish, P.A., Kalish, B.J., and Clinton, J. (1982). The world of nursing on prime time tele-

vision, 1950 to 1980, *Nursing Research,* **31:**358-363.

Kerlinger, F. (1979). *Behavioral research: a conceptual approach,* New York, Holt, Rinehart, & Winston, Inc.

Kerlinger, F. (1986). *The foundations of behavioral research,* New York, Holt, Rinehart, & Winston, Inc.

Klein, P.M. (1983). Contraceptive use and perceptions of chance and ability of conceiving in women electing abortion, *Journal of Obstetrics and Gynecology,* **12:**167-171.

Krampitz, S.D. (1981). Research design: Historical. In S.D. Krampitz and N. Pavlovich, eds.: *Readings for nursing research,* St. Louis, The C.V. Mosby Co., pp. 54-58.

Nettles-Carlson, B., Field, M.L., Friedman, B.J., and Smith, L.S. (1988). Effectiveness of teaching breast self-examination during office visits. *Research in Nursing and Health,* **11:**41-50.

Oberst, M.T., Graham, D., Geller, N.L., Stearns, M.W., and Tiernan, E. (1981). Catheter management programs and postoperative urinary dysfunction, *Research in Nursing and Health,* **4:**175-181.

O'Brien, P. (1987). All a woman's life can bring: the domestic roots of nursing in Philadelphia, 1830-1885, *Nursing Research,* **36:**12-15.

Palmer, I.S. (1983). Nightingale revisited, *Nursing Outlook,* **31:**229-233.

Paterson, J., and Zderad, L. (1976). *Humanistic nursing,* New York, John Wiley & Sons, Inc.

Psathas, G. (1973). *Phenomenological sociology: issues and applications,* New York, John Wiley & Sons, Inc.

Rees, B.L. (1980). Measuring identification with the mothering role, *Research in Nursing and Health,* **3:**49-56.

Stevens, B. (1971). A phenomenological approach to understanding suicidal behavior, *Journal of Psychiatric Nursing,* **9:**33-35.

Strickland, O.L., and Waltz, C.F. (1988). *Measurement of nursing outcomes: measuring client outcomes,* vol. 1, New York, Springer Publishing Co.

Suchman, E.A. (1967). *Evaluative research,* New York, Russell Sage Foundation.

Twain, D. (1975). Developing and implementing a research strategy. In E.L. Struening and M. Guttentag, eds.: *Handbook of evaluation research,* Beverly Hills, Sage Publication.

U.S. Department of Health, Education and Welfare. (1955). *Evaluation in mental health,* Publication No. 413, Washington, Government Printing Office.

Waltz, C.F., and Strickland, O.L. (1988). *Measurement of nursing outcomes: measuring client outcomes,* vol. 2, New York, Springer Publishing Co.

Wheeler, C.E. (1985). The American Journal of Nursing and the socialization of a profession, 1900-1920, *Advances in Nursing Science,* 7:20-34.

Additional Readings

Anastasi, A. (1982). *Psychological testing,* New York, Macmillan, Inc.

Barzun, J., and Reaff, H.E. (1977). *The modern researcher,* Chicago, Harcourt Brace Jovanovich, Inc.

Campbell, D., and Fiske, D. (1959). Convergent and discriminant validation by the multitrait-multimethod matrix, *Psychological Bulletin,* 56:81-105.

Hersen, M., and Barlow, D.H. (1977). *Single-case experimental designs,* New York, Pergamon Press.

Kalish, B.J., and Kalish, P.A. (1976). Is history of nursing alive and well? *Nursing Outlook,* 24:362-366.

Kratochwill, T.R. (1978). Single subject research, New York, Academic Press.

Matejski, M.P. (1979). Humanities: the nurse and historical research, *Image,* 11:80-85.

Newton, M.E. (1965). The case for historical research, *Nursing Research,* 14:20-26.

Norman, E.M. (1981). Who and where are nursing's historians? *Nursing Forum,* 20:138-152.

Nunnally, J. (1978). *Psychometric theory,* New York, McGraw-Hill Book Co.

Perry, D.S. (1983). The early midwives of Missouri, *Journal of Nurse-Midwifery,* 28:15-28.

13

Data Collection Methods

Margaret Grey

LEARNING OBJECTIVES

After reading this chapter the student should be able to do the following:

◇ Define the types of data collection methods utilized in nursing research.

◇ List the advantages and disadvantages of each of these methods.

◇ Critically evaluate the data collection methods utilized in published nursing research studies.

KEY TERMS

close-ended item   operational definition
concealment   operationalization
content analysis   reactivity
intervention   scale
objective   systematic
open-ended item

Nurses use all of their senses when collecting data from the clients for whom they provide care. Nurse researchers also have available many ways to collect information about their research subjects. The major difference between the data collected when performing client care and the data collected for the purpose of research is that the data collection methods employed by researchers need to be **objective** and **systematic.** By *objective,* we mean that the data must not be influenced by anyone who collects the information; by *systematic,* we mean that the data must be collected in the same way by everyone who is involved in the collection procedure.

The methods that researchers use to collect information about subjects are the identifiable and repeatable operations that define the major variables being studied. **Operationalization** is the process of translating the concepts that are of interest to a researcher into observable and measurable phenomena. There may be a number of ways to collect the same information. For example, a researcher interested in measuring anxiety physiologically could do so by measuring sweat gland activity or by administering an anxiety **scale** such as the State-Trait Anxiety Scale. The researcher could also observe clients to see if they displayed anxious behavior. The method chosen by the researcher would depend on a number of decisions regarding the problem being studied, the nature of the subjects, and the relative costs and benefits of each method.

This chapter's purpose is to familiarize the student with the various ways that researchers collect information from and about subjects. The chapter will provide nursing research consumers with the tools for evaluating the selection, utilization, and practicality of the various ways of collecting data.

MEASURING VARIABLES OF INTEREST

To a large extent the success of a study depends on the quality of the data collection methods chosen and employed. Researchers have many types of methods available for collecting information from subjects in research studies. Determining what measurement to utilize in a particular investigation may be the most difficult and time-consuming period in study design. In addition, since nursing research is still relatively young, researchers do not have a plethora of quality instruments with adequate reliability and validity (see Chapter 14) from which to choose. This aspect of the research process demands painstaking efforts on the part of the researcher. Thus the process of evaluating and selecting the available tools to measure variables of interest is of critical importance to the potential success of the study. In this section we will discuss the selection of measures and the implementation of the data collection process.

There are many different ways to collect information about phenomena of interest to nurses. We are interested in biological and physical indicators of health, such as blood pressure and heart rates, but nurses are also interested in complex psychosocial questions presented by clients. Psychosocial variables may be measured by several different techniques, such as observation of behavior or self-reports of feelings or attitudes by means of instruments or questionnaires. Researchers may also use data that have already been collected for another purpose, such as records, diaries, or other media, to study phenomena of interest.

As you can surmise, choosing the most appropriate method and instrument is difficult. The method must be appropriate to the problem, the hypothesis, the setting, and the population. For example, if a researcher is interested in studying the behavior of 3-year-old children in day-care, it is unlikely to make much sense to provide the children with some kind of paper-and-pencil test. Whereas the children might be able to draw on the paper, they would not be likely to answer questions appropriately.

Selection of the data collection method begins during the literature review. In Chapter 5 one purpose of the review noted was to provide clues to instrumentation. As the literature review is conducted the researcher begins to explore how previous investigators defined and operationalized variables similar to those of interest in the current study. The researcher uses this information to define conceptually the variables to be studied. Once a variable has been defined conceptually, the researcher returns to the literature to define the variable operationally. This **operational definition** translates the conceptual definition into behaviors or verbalizations that can be measured for the study. In this second literature review the researcher searches for measuring instruments that might be utilized as is or adapted for use in the study. If instruments are available, the researcher needs to obtain permission for their use from the author.

An example may illustrate the relationship of the conceptual and operational definitions. Stress research is popular with researchers from many disciplines, including nursing. Definitions of stressors may be psychological, social, or physiological. If a researcher is interested in studying stressors, the researcher needs first to define what he or she means by the concept of stressor. For example, Holmes and Rahe (1967) defined the stressful life event as any occurrence that required change or adaptation. This definition implies that it is the event that is stressful, not how the individual appraises the event. According to this conceptual definition, the researcher could use a Life Event Checklist (operational definition) to determine the degree of stress encountered by subjects in the study. If the researcher disagreed with this definition and supported the definition that events are stressful only when individuals appraise them as such, then another approach to measurement would be consistent with that view.

It is often the case that no suitable measuring device exists, so then the researcher needs to decide if the variable is important to the study and if a new device should be constructed. This is often a problem in nursing research, as many variables of interest have not been studied. The construction of new instruments for data collection that have reasonable reliability and validity (see Chapter 14) is a most difficult task. Sometimes researchers decide not to study a variable if no suitable measuring device exists; at other times the researcher may decide to invest time and energy in tool development (Chapter 12). Either decision is acceptable depending on the goals of the study and the goals of the researcher.

Whether the researcher uses available methods or creates new ones, once the variables have been operationally defined in a manner consistent with the aims of the study, the population to be studied, and the setting, the researcher will determine how the data collection phase of the study will be implemented. This decision deals with how the instruments for data collection will be given to the subjects. Consistency is the most important issue in this phase.

Consistency means that the way data are collected from each subject in the study must be exactly the same or as close to identical as possible. Thus the researcher must consider ways to minimize subjects' anxiety, maintain their motivation to complete the data collection process, and make the procedures as similar as possible for all participants. Those who collect the data must be very carefully trained in the procedures to be used, and interviewers must be carefully trained and supervised (Collins, Given, Given, and King, 1988). For example, a researcher interested in blood pressure must be sure that each person responsible for taking and recording the blood pressure measurements takes them at the same anatomical location, uses the same type of equipment, and records the same information. This information will be included in a kind of "cookbook" for the research project that will tell those who are gathering the data exactly how their tasks are to be completed. A researcher may spend several months training research assistants to collect data systematically and reliably. If data collectors are used, the reader should expect to see some comment about their training and the consistency with which they collected the data for the study.

DATA COLLECTION METHODS

In general, data collection methods can be divided into the following five types: physiological, observational, interviews, questionnaires, and records or available data. Each of these methods has a specific purpose as well as certain pros and cons inherent in their use. We will discuss each type of data collection method and then compare their respective uses and problems.

Physiological or biological measurement

In everyday practice, nurses collect physiological data about clients, such as their temperature, pulse rate, and blood pressure. Such data are frequently useful to nurse researchers as well. Consider the study by Kunnel, O'Brien, Hazard Munro, and Medoff-Cooper (1988), which is reprinted in Appendix C. The purpose of this study was to compare four sites for temperature recording in the neonate. To study this problem it was important for the researchers to measure temperature similarly in all subjects except that the site varied. Refer to the sections *Instruments* and *Procedures*. Note that the researchers used identical glass mercury thermometers with known accuracy. The procedures used in determining temperature are carefully described.

The study by Kunnel et al. is an excellent example of the use of a particular type of data collection method—physiological. Physiological and biological measures involve the use of specialized equipment to determine the required information. Frequently such measures also require specialized training. Such measures can be physical, such as weight or temperature; chemical, such as blood glucose level; microbiological, as with cultures; or anatomical, as in radiological examinations. What separates these measurements from others used in research is that they require the use of special equipment to make the observation. We can say, "This subject feels warm," but to determine how warm the infant is requires the use of a sensitive instrument, a thermometer.

Physiological or biological measurement is particularly suited to the study of several types of nursing problems. The aforementioned example is typical of studies dealing with ways to improve the performance of certain nursing actions, such as measuring and recording of clients' physiological data. Physiological measures may be important criteria for determining the effectiveness of certain nursing actions. A study by Wolfer and Visintainer (1975) was one of the first true experimental studies to examine the impact of two approaches to preoperative preparation for preschool and school-aged children's recovery from surgery. These researchers used both physiological and psychological measures to compare the recovery of the children. The physiological measures included pulse, respirations, and time to awaken from anesthesia.

Another type of study that uses physiological or biological measures is one of the priorities of the National Center for Nursing Research. The Center has determined that studies of the interrelationships of the physiological and the psychosocial are a priority in nursing research. Such studies are illustrated by an investigation by Hayman, Meininger, Stashinko, Gallagher, and Coates (1988) of the relationship of the type A behavior pattern and its components to the physiological cardiovascular disease risk factors of blood pressure, obesity, lipids, and lipoproteins in school-aged children. By using both psychological (type A behavior pattern) and physiological measures, these researchers were able to demonstrate that no relationship existed between type A behavior and biological risk factors for cardiovascular disease in children, unlike the relationships that have been found in adults. Studies such as this one are important for determining the physiological rationale for certain nursing actions. In this case the results of the study have implications for health education for children.

The advantages of utilizing physiological data collection methods include their objectivity, precision, and sensitivity. Such methods are generally quite objective, because unless there is a technical malfunction, two readings of the same instrument taken at the same time by two different nurses are likely to yield the same result. Since such instruments are intended to measure the variable being studied, they offer the advantage of being precise and sensitive enough to pick up subtle variations in the phenomenon of interest. It is also unlikely that a subject in a study can deliberately distort physiological information.

Physiological measurements are not without inherent disadvantages, however. Some instruments, if they are not available through a hospital, may be quite expensive to obtain. In addition, such instruments often require specialized knowledge and training to be used accurately. Another problem with such measurements is that just by using them, the variable of interest may be changed. Although some researchers think of these instruments as being nonintrusive, the presence of some types of devices might change the measurement. For example, the presence of a heart rate monitoring device might make some clients anxious and increase their heart rate. In addition, nearly all types of measuring devices are affected in some way by the environment. Even a simple thermometer can be affected by the subject drinking something hot immediately before the temperature is taken. Thus it is important to consider whether the researcher controlled such environmental variables in the study. Finally, there may not be a physiological way to measure the variable of interest. Occasionally researchers try to force a physiological parameter into a study in an effort to increase the precision of measurement. However, if the device does not really measure the phenomenon of interest, the validity of its use is suspect.

Observational methods

Sometimes nurse researchers are interested in determining how subjects behave under certain conditions. For example, a researcher might be interested in whether subjects actually comply with certain recommendations about their health, such as stopping smoking. We might ask such subjects about their behavior, but they may distort their responses to please the researcher. Therefore observing the subject may give a more accurate picture of the subject's behavior than asking.

Although observing the environment is a normal part of living, scientific observation places a great deal of emphasis on the objective and systematic nature of the operation. To be scientific, observations must fulfill the following four conditions (Seaman and Verhonick, 1982):

1. The observations are undertaken with certain objectives in mind.
2. The observations are systematically planned and recorded.
3. All of the observations are checked and controlled.
4. The observations are related to scientific concepts and theories.

Thus the researcher is not merely looking at what is happening but rather is watching with a trained eye for certain specific events.

Observation is particularly suitable as a data collection method in complex research situations that are best viewed as total entities and that are difficult to measure in parts, such as studies dealing with the nursing process, parent-child interactions, or group processes. In addition, observational methods can be the best way to operationalize some variables of interest in nursing research studies, particularly individual characteristics and conditions, such as traits and symptoms, verbal and non-verbal communication behaviors, activities and skill attainment, and environmental characteristics.

We have discussed a study by Hayman et al. (1988) of the relationship of type A behavior pattern and cardiovascular risk factors. The type A behavior pattern consists of (1) higher levels of the behaviors of impatience and aggression, (2) underreporting of fatigue, and (3) making greater efforts to excel under certain conditions. Although several methods are available to measure this behavior pattern in adults, with children the most successful method has been the MYTH (Matthews Youth Test for Health). This observational tool is used by teachers to rate the children on the characteristics of the type A behavior pattern. Since the tool requires the recording of observations, it is an excellent example of the use of structured observations in describing characteristics of subjects.

Observational methods can also be distinguished by the role of the observer. This role is determined by the amount of interaction between the observer and those being observed. Each of the following four basic types of observational roles is distinguishable by the amount of **concealment** or **intervention** implemented by the observer:

1. Concealment without intervention
2. Concealment with intervention
3. No concealment without intervention
4. No concealment with intervention

Concealment refers to whether or not the subjects know that they are being observed, and *intervention* deals with whether or not the observer provokes actions from those who are being observed. When a researcher is concerned that the subjects will change the behavior being observed, the type of observation most commonly employed is that of concealment without intervention. In this case the researcher watches the subjects without their knowledge of the observation but does not provoke them into action. Often such concealed observations utilize television cameras, audiotapes, or one-way mirrors. An important ethical problem is created by this type of observation strategy, since observing subjects without their knowledge violates assumptions of informed consent (see Chapter 3).

When the observer is neither concealed nor intervening, the ethical question is not a problem. Here the observer makes no attempt to change the subjects' behavior and informs them that they are to be observed. Because the observer is present, this type of observation allows a greater depth of material to be studied than if the observer is separated from the subjects by an artificial barrier such as a one-way mirror. Participant observation is a commonly used observational technique where the researcher functions as a part of a social group to study the group in question. The problem with this type of observation is **reactivity,** or the distortion created when the subjects change behavior because they are being observed.

Hinds and Martin (1988) studied the process through which adolescents with cancer move to achieve hopefulness. They used a variety of approaches to data collection to construct a model of this process. The methods used included interviews and observations. In this case the observations were of the adolescents' interactions with hospital staff. These researchers used unconcealed observation, because the adolescents in the study had given fully informed consent. These data were used by the researchers to help determine how the children felt about their illness. No intervention was applied, however.

The two other types of observations involve some kind of intervention by the observer. No concealment with intervention is employed when the researcher is observing the effects of some intervention introduced for scientific purposes. Since the subjects know that they are participating in a research study, there are few problems with ethical concerns, but reactivity is a problem with this type of study. Gill, Behnke, Conlon, McNeely, and Anderson (1988) studied the effect of nonnutritive sucking on behavioral state of preterm infants. Since infants cannot report their behavior, they must be observed. The researchers were not hidden from the infants, so the observation was not covert, but they did intervene by providing some infants with pacifiers (nonnutritive sucking). By using the Anderson Behavioral State Scale, a structured tool for observing infant behavior, the researchers found that nonnutritive sucking was an effective modulator of behavioral state.

Concealed observation with intervention involves staging a situation and observing the behaviors that are evoked in the subjects as a result of the intervention. Because the subjects are unaware of their participation in a research study, this type of observation has fallen into disfavor and is rarely used in nursing research.

Observations may be structured or unstructured. Unstructured observational methods, such as those employed by Hinds and Martin (1988), are not characterized by a total absence of structure but usually involve collecting descriptive information about the subjects of interest. In participant observation the observer keeps field notes that record the activities as well as the observer's interpretations of these activities. Field notes are not usually restricted to any particular type of action or behavior; rather, they intend to paint a picture of a social situation in a more general sense. Another type of unstructured observation is the use of anecdotes. Anecdotes are not necessarily funny but usually focus on the behaviors of interest and frequently add to the richness of research reports by illustrating a particular point.

On the other hand, structured observations, such as the MYTH and the Anderson Behavioral State Scale, involve specifying in advance what behaviors or events are to be observed and preparing forms for record keeping, such as categorization systems, checklists, and rating scales. Whichever system is employed, the observer watches the subject and then marks on the recording form what was seen. In any case, the observations must be similar among the observers (see Chapter 14 for a detailed explanation of interrater reliability). Thus it is important that observers be trained to be consistent in their observations and ratings of behavior.

Scientific observation has several advantages as a data collection method, the main one being that observation may be the only way for the researcher to study the variable of interest. For example, what people say that they do is often not what they really do. Therefore, if the study is designed to obtain substantive findings about human behavior, observation may be the only way to ensure the validity of the findings. In addition, no other data collection method can match the depth and variety of information that can be collected when utilizing these techniques. Such techniques are also quite flexible in that they may be used in both experimental and nonexperimental designs and in laboratory and field studies.

As with all data collection methods, observation also has its disadvantages. We mentioned the problems of reactivity and ethical concerns when we discussed the concealment and intervention dimensions. In addition, data obtained by observational techniques are vulnerable to the bias of the observer. Emotions, prejudices, and values can all influence the way that behaviors and events are observed. In general, the more that the observer needs to make inferences and judgments about what is being observed, the more likely it is that distortions will occur. Thus, in judging the adequacy of observational methods, it is important to consider how observational tools were constructed and how observers were trained and evaluated.

Interviews and questionnaires

Subjects in a research study often have information that is important to the study and that can be obtained only by asking the subject. Such questions may be asked orally by a researcher in person or over the telephone in an interview, or they may be asked in the form of a paper-and-pencil test. Both interviews and questionnaires have the purpose of asking subjects to report data for themselves, but each has unique advantages and disadvantages as well.

Survey research relies almost entirely on questioning subjects with either interviews or questionnaires, but these methods of data collection can also be utilized in other types of research. No matter what type of study is conducted, the purpose of questioning subjects is to seek information. This information may be of either direct interest, such as the subject's age, or indirect interest, such as when the researcher uses a combination of items to estimate to what degree the respondent has some trait or characteristic. An intelligence test is an example of how an individual item is combined with several others to develop an overall scale of intelligence. When items of indirect interest are combined to obtain an overall score, the measurement tool is called a *scale*.

The investigator determines the content of an interview or questionnaire from the literature review (see Chapter 5). When evaluating these methods the reader should consider the content of the schedule, the individual items, and the order of the items. The basic standard for evaluating the individual items in an interview or questionnaire is that the item must be clearly written so that the intent of the question and the nature of the information sought are clear to the respondent. The only way to know if the questions are understandable to the target respondents is to pilot test them in a similar population. Items must also ask only one question, be free of suggestion, and use correct grammar. Items may also be **open-ended items** or **close-ended items.** *Open-ended* items are used when the researcher wants the subjects to respond in their own words or when the researcher does not know all of the possible alternative responses. *Close-ended* items are used when there are a fixed number of alternative responses. Many scales use a fixed response format called a Likert scale. Likert scales are lists of statements on which respondents indicate whether they "strongly agree," "agree," "disagree," or "strongly disagree." Structured, fixed-response items are best utilized when the question has a fixed number of responses and the respondent is to choose the one closest to the right one. Fixed-response items have the advantage of simplifying the respondent's task and the researcher's analysis, but they may miss some important information about the subject. Unstructured response formats allow such information to be included but require a special technique to analyze the responses. This technique is called **content analysis** and is a method for the objective, systematic, and quantitative description of communications and documentary evidence.

The box on p. 237 shows a few items from a survey of pediatric nurse practitioners (Grey, 1988). The first items are taken from a list of similar items, and they are both closed and of a Likert-type format. Note that respondents are asked to choose how strongly they agree with each item. In using these questions in the survey we are forcing the respondent to choose from only these answers, because we think that these will be the only responses. The only possible alternative response is to skip the item and leave it blank. On the other hand, sometimes we have no idea or we have only a limited idea of what the respondent will say, or we want the answer in the respondent's own words, as with the second set of items. Here, the respondent may also leave the item blank, but we are not forcing the subject to make a particular response.

Interviews and questionnaires are commonly utilized in nursing research. Both are strong approaches to gathering information for research, because they approach the task directly. In addition, both have the ability to obtain certain kinds of information, such as the subjects' attitudes and beliefs, that would be difficult to obtain without asking the subject directly. All methods that involve verbal reports, however, share a problem with accuracy. There is often no way to know whether what we are told is indeed true. For example, people are known to respond to questions in a way that makes a favorable impression. This response style is known as *social desirability*. Since there is no way to tell if the respondent is telling the truth or responding in a socially desirable way, the researcher usually is forced to assume that the respondent is telling the truth.

Questionnaires and interviews also have some specific purposes, advantages, and disadvantages. Questionnaires and paper-and-pencil tests are most useful when there is a finite set of questions to be asked and the researcher can be assured of the clarity and specificity of the items. Questionnaires are desirable tools when the purpose is to collect information. Face-to-face techniques or interviews are best utilized when the researcher may need to clarify the task for the respondent or is interested in obtaining more personal information from the respondent. Telephone interviews allow the researcher to reach more respondents than face-to-face interviews, and they allow for more clarity than questionnaires.

Vessey (1988) used a combination of interview and questionnaires to compare the effects of two teaching methods on children's knowledge of internal body parts. Since cognitive level would be a potent influence on learning, the investigator determined each child's cognitive level using the Piagetian Interview, which consisted

Examples of Close-Ended and Open-Ended Questions

Close-ended (Likert-type Scale)

A. How satisfied are you with your current position?
   1. Very satisfied
   2. Moderately satisfied
   3. Undecided
   4. Moderately dissatisfied
   5. Very dissatisfied

B. To what extent do the following factors contribute to your current level of positive satisfaction?

	Not at all	Very little	Somewhat	Moderate amount	A great deal
1. % of time in patient care	1	2	3	4	5
2. Types of patients	1	2	3	4	5
3. % of time in educational activity	1	2	3	4	5
4. % of time in administration	1	2	3	4	5

Close-ended

A. On an average, how many clients do you see in one day?
   1. 1 to 3
   2. 4 to 6
   3. 7 to 9
   4. 10 to 12
   5. 13 to 15
   6. 16 to 18
   7. 18 to 20
   8. More than 20

B. Would you characterize your practice as
   1. Too slow
   2. Slow
   3. About right
   4. Busy
   5. Too busy

Open-ended

A. Are there incentives that National Association of Pediatric Nurse Associates and Practitioners ought to provide for members that are currently not being done?

_____

_____

_____

_____

of 10 tasks measuring preoperational thought. The researcher used a paper-and-pencil test to test the outcome of the two teaching methods. The body outline test consisted of a 10-inch line drawing and colored markers, with which the children drew their body parts and explained them. Note that the researcher, in this study, felt that thought processes were better measured with an interview, whereas knowledge was better measured by a paper-and-pencil test.

Researchers face difficult choices when determining whether to use interviews or questionnaires. The final decision is often based on what instruments are available and their relative costs and benefits.

Both face-to-face and telephone interviews offer some advantages over questionnaires. All things being equal, interviews are better than questionnaires because the response rate is almost always higher and this helps to eliminate bias in the sample (see Chapter 15). Respondents seem to be less likely to hang up the telephone or to close the door in a interviewer's face than to throw away a questionnaire. Another advantage of the interview is that some people, such as children, the blind, and the illiterate, could not fill out a questionnaire, but they could participate in an interview.

Interviews also allow for some safeguards to be built into the interview situation. Interviewers can clarify misunderstood questions and observe the level of the respondent's understanding and cooperativeness. In addition, the researcher has strict control over the order of the questions. With questionnaires, the respondent can answer questions in any order. Sometimes changing the order of the questions can change the response.

Finally, interviews allow for richer and more complex data to be collected. This is particularly so when open-ended responses are sought. Even when close-ended response items are used, interviews can probe to understand why a respondent answered in a particular way.

Questionnaires also have certain advantages. They are much less expensive to administer than interviews, because interviews require the hiring and training of interviewers. Thus, if a researcher has a fixed amount of time and money, a larger and more diverse sample can be obtained with questionnaires. Questionnaires also allow for complete anonymity, which may be important if the study deals with sensitive issues. Finally, the fact that no interviewer is present assures the researcher and the reader that there will be no interviewer bias. Interviewer bias occurs when the interviewer unwittingly leads the respondent to answer in a certain way. This problem is especially pronounced in studies that use unstructured interview formats. A subtle nod of the head, for example, could lead a respondent to change an answer to correspond with what the researcher wants to hear.

Records or available data

All of the data collection methods discussed thus far concern the ways that nurse researchers gather new data to study phenomena of interest. Not all studies, though, require a researcher to acquire new information. Sometimes existing information can be examined in a new way to study a problem. The use of records and available data is frequently considered to be primarily the province of historical research, but hospital records, care plans, and existing data sources, such as the census, can also be utilized for collecting information. What sets these studies apart from a literature review is that these available data are examined in a new way, are not merely summarized, and answer specific research questions.

The use of available data has certain advantages. Since the data collection step of the research process is often the most difficult and time-consuming, the use of available records often allows for a significant savings of time. If the records have been kept in a similar manner over time, as with the National Health and Examination Surveys, analysis of these records allows for the examination of trends over time. The time series study in Chapter 9 (Samet et al., 1988) is an example of this type of study. In addition, the use of available data decreases problems of reactivity and response set bias. The researcher also does not have to ask individuals to participate in the study.

On the other hand, institutions are sometimes reluctant to allow researchers to have access to their records. If the records are kept so that an individual cannot be identified, then this is usually not a problem. However, the Privacy Act, a federal law, protects the rights of individuals who may be identified in records. Another problem that affects the quality of available data is that the researcher has access only to those records that have survived. If the records available are not representative of all of the possible records, then the researcher may have a problem with bias. Often there is no way to tell if the records have been saved in a biased manner, and the researcher has to make an intelligent guess as to their accuracy. For example, a researcher might be interested in studying socioeconomic factors associated with the suicide rate. These data are frequently underreported because of the stigma attached to suicide, and so the records would be biased.

Another problem has to do with the authenticity of the records. The distinction of primary and secondary sources is as relevant here as it was in discussing the literature review (see Chapter 5). A book, for example, may have been ghostwritten but credit accorded to the known author. It may be difficult for the researcher to ferret out these types of subtle biases.

Nonetheless, records and available data constitute a rich source of data for study. Kalish, Kalish, and Clinton (1982) provide an excellent example of the use of available data in studying the image of American nurses on television. In this study the researchers were interested in understanding the public's perception of the nurse. To do so, they reviewed, using standardized recording tools, videotapes of news and popular television shows that dealt with nurses or nursing. They concluded that the media treated nurses as nonprofessionals and that this treatment could have a significant influence on the public perception of nursing.

CONSTRUCTION OF NEW INSTRUMENTS

As already mentioned in this chapter, sometimes researchers cannot locate an instrument or method with acceptable reliability and validity to measure the variable of interest. This is often the case when testing a part of a nursing theory or when evaluating the effect of a clinical intervention. A recent example is provided by Browne, Byrne, Roberts, Streiner, Fitch, Corey, and Arpin (1988), who conducted a clinical trial dealing with adjustment to illness. In the clinical trial the meaning given to illness by subjects was judged to be an important variable. They defined meaning of illness as "the cognitive and behavioral effort to manage specific external or internal demands that are appraised as taxing or exceeding one's resources," or the cognitive appraisal of an illness event (p. 368). The authors used this definition to develop a questionnaire to measure this construct, and they have presented the psychometric information about the tool for other researchers to learn about it.

Tool development is complex and time-consuming. It consists of the following steps:
◇ Define the construct to be measured
◇ Formulate the items
◇ Assess the items for content validity
◇ Develop instructions for respondents and users
◇ Pretest and pilot test the items
◇ Estimate reliability and validity

To define the construct to be measured requires that the researcher develop an expertise in the construct. This will require an extensive review of the literature and of all tests and measurements that deal with related constructs. The researcher will use all of this information to synthesize the available knowledge so that the construct can be defined (see Chapter 12).

Once defined, the individual items measuring the construct can be developed. The researcher will develop many more items than are needed to address each aspect of the construct or subconstruct. The items are evaluated by a panel of experts in the field so that the researcher is assured that the items measure what they are intended to measure (content validity, see Chapter 14). Eventually the number of items will be decreased, because some items will not work as they were intended and they will be dropped. In this phase the researcher needs to ensure consistency among the items as well as consistency in testing and scoring procedures.

Finally, the researcher administers the test to a group of people who are similar to those who will be studied in the larger investigation. The purpose of this analysis to determine the quality of the instrument as a whole (reliability and validity) as well as the ability of each item to discriminate individual respondents (variance in item response). The researcher may also administer a related instrument to see if the new instrument is sufficiently different from the older one.

It is important that researchers who invest significant amounts of time in tool development publish those results. This type of research not only serves to introduce other researchers to the tool but will ultimately enhance the field, because our ability to conduct meaningful research is limited only by our ability to measure important phenomena.

CRITIQUING DATA COLLECTION METHODS

Evaluating the adequacy of data collection methods from written research reports is often problematic for new nursing research consumers. This is because the tool itself is not available for inspection and the reader may not feel comfortable about judging the adequacy of the method without seeing it. However, a number of questions can be asked as you read to judge the method chosen by the researcher. These questions are listed in the box on p. 242.

All studies should have clearly identified data collection methods. The conceptual and operational definitions of each important variable should be present in the report. Sometimes it is useful for the researcher to explain why a particular method was chosen. For example, if the study dealt with young children, the researcher may explain that a questionnaire was deemed to be an unreasonable task, so an interview was chosen.

Once you have identified the method chosen to measure each variable of interest, you should decide if the method utilized was the best way to measure the variable. If a questionnaire was utilized, for example, you might wonder why the decision was made not to use an interview. In addition, consider whether the method was appropriate to the clinical situation. Does it make sense to interview clients in the recovery room, for example?

Once you have decided if all relevant variables are operationalized appropriately, you can begin to determine how well the method was carried out. For studies utilizing physiological measurement it is important to determine if the instrument was appropriate to the problem and not forced to fit it. The rationale for selecting a particular instrument should be given. For example, it may be important to know that the study was conducted under the auspices of a manufacturing firm that provided the measuring instrument. In addition, provision should be made to evaluate the accuracy of the instrument and those who use it.

Several considerations are important when reading studies that utilize observational methods. Who were the observers and how were they trained? Is there any reason to believe that different observers saw events or behaviors differently? Remember that the more inferences the observers are required to make, the more likely there will be problems with biased observations. Also consider the problem of reactivity; in any observational situation, the possibility exists that the mere presence of the observer could change the behavior in question. What is important here is not that reactivity could occur, but rather how much reactivity could affect the data. Finally, consider whether the observational procedure was ethical. The reader needs to consider whether subjects were informed that they were being observed, whether any intervention was performed, and whether subjects had agreed to be observed.

Interviews and questionnaires should be clearly described to allow the reader to decide whether the variables were adequately operationalized. Sometimes the researcher will reference the original report about the tool, and the reader may wish to read this study before deciding if the method was appropriate for the present study. The respondents' task should be clear. Thus provision should be made for the subjects

Critiquing Criteria

1. Are all of the data collection instruments clearly identified and described?
2. Is the rationale for their selection given?
3. Is the method used appropriate to the problem being studied?
4. Is the method used appropriate to the clinical situation?
5. Are the data collection procedures similar for all subjects?

Physiological Measurement

1. Is the instrument used appropriate to the research problem and not forced to fit it?
2. Is a rationale given for why a particular instrument was selected?
3. Is there a provision for evaluating the accuracy of the instrument and those who use it?

Observational Methods

1. Who did the observing?
2. Were the observers trained to minimize any bias?
3. Was there an observational guide?
4. Were the observers required to make inferences about what they saw?
5. Is there any reason to believe that the presence of the observers affected the behavior of the subjects?
6. Were the observations performed utilizing the principles of informed consent?

Interviews

1. Is the schedule described adequately enough to know if it covers the subject?
2. Is there clear indication that the subjects understood the task and the questions?
3. Who were the interviewers and how were they trained?
4. Is there evidence of any interviewer bias?

Questionnaires

1. Is the questionnaire described well enough to know if it covers the subject?
2. Is there evidence that subjects were able to perform the task?
3. Is there clear indication that the subjects understood the questionnaire?
4. Are the majority of the items close-ended?

Critiquing Criteria — cont'd

Available Data and Records
1. Are the records that were utilized appropriate to the problem being studied?
2. Are the data examined in such a way as to provide new information and not summarize the records?
3. Has the author addressed questions of internal and external criticism?
4. Is there any indication of selection bias in the available records?

to understand both their overall responsibilities and the individual items. Who were the interviewers in the interview situation? Does the researcher explain how they were trained to decrease any interviewer bias?

Available data are subject to internal and external criticism. Internal criticism deals with the evaluation of the worth of the records. Internal criticism primarily refers to the accuracy of the data. The researcher should present evidence that the records are genuine. External criticism is concerned with the authenticity of the records. Are the records really written by the first author? Finally, the reader should be aware of the problems with selective survival. The researcher may not have an unbiased sample of all of the possible records in the problem area, and this may have a profound effect on the validity of the results.

Finally, the reader should consider the data collection procedure. Is any assurance provided that all of the subjects received the same information? In addition, it is important to try to determine if all of the information was collected in the same way for all of the subjects in the study.

Once you have decided that the data collection method used was appropriate to the problem and the procedures were appropriate to the population studied, then the reliability and validity of the instruments themselves need to be considered. These characteristics are discussed in the next chapter.

SUMMARY

This chapter's purpose was to familiarize the student with the various methods that researchers utilize to collect information from and about subjects. Data collection methods are described as being both objective and systematic. The data collection methods of a study provide the operational definitions of the relevant variables.

The following five types of data collection methods were described: physiological, observational, interviews, questionnaires, and available data or records. The purposes, advantages, and disadvantages of each method were presented.

Physiological measurements are those methods that use technical instruments to collect data about clients' physical, chemical, microbiological, or anatomical status. Such instruments are particularly suited to the study of the effectiveness of nursing care and the ways to improve the provision of nursing care. Physiological measurements are objective, precise, and sensitive. However, they may be very expensive and they may distort the variable of interest.

Observational methods are frequently utilized in nursing research when the variables of interest deal with events or behaviors. Scientific observation requires preplanning, systematic recording, controlling the observations, and relationship to scientific theory. This method is best suited to research problems that are difficult to view as a part of a whole. Observers may be passive or active and concealed or obvious. Observational methods have several advantages, the most important one being the flexibility of the method to measure many types of situations. In addition, observation allows for a great depth and breadth of information to be collected, depending on the problem being studied. Observation has several disadvantages, too. Reactivity, or the distortion of data as a result of the observer's presence, is a common problem in nonconcealed observations. If the observer is concealed, however, there are ethical considerations. Finally, observations may be biased by the person who is doing the observing.

Interviews and questionnaires are the most commonly utilized data collection methods in nursing research. Both have the purpose of asking subjects to report data for themselves. Items on questionnaire and interview schedules may be of direct or indirect interest and can be combined into scales. Scales provide an estimate of the degree to which the respondent possesses some trait or characteristic. Either open-ended or close-ended questions may be utilized when asking subjects questions. The form of the question should be clear to the respondent, free of suggestion, and grammatically correct.

Questionnaires, or paper-and-pencil tests, are particularly useful when there are a finite number of questions to be asked and the researcher is sure that the questions are clear and specific. Questionnaires are also much less costly in time and money to administer to a large number of subjects, particularly if the subjects are geographically widespread. Another advantage of the questionnaire over the interview is that questionnaires have the potential to be completely anonymous. In addition, there is no possibility of interviewer bias.

Interviews, on the other hand, are best utilized when it is important to have a large response rate and an unbiased sample, because the refusal rate for interviews is much less than that for questionnaires. Interviews also allow for some portions of the population who would be precluded by the use of a questionnaire, such as children and the illiterate, to participate in the study. An interviewer can clarify the questions and maintain the order of the questions for all participants.

Records and available data are also an important source for research data. The use of available data may save the researcher considerable time and money when conducting a study. This data collection method reduces problems with both reactivity and ethical concerns. However, records and available data are subject to problems of availability, authenticity, and accuracy.

Finally, the criteria for evaluating data collection methods utilized in published research studies were presented. A critical evaluation of this aspect of a research study should emphasize the appropriateness, objectivity, and consistency of the method employed.

References

Browne, G.B., Byrne, C., Roberts, J., Streiner, D., Fitch, M., Corey, P., and Arpin, K. (1988) The Meaning of Illness Questionnaire: reliability and validity, *Nursing Research,* **37**:368-73.

Collins, C., Given, B., Given, C.W., and King, S. (1988). Interviewer training and supervision, *Nursing Research,* **37**:122-124.

Gill, N.E., Behnke, M., Conlon, M., McNeely, J.B., and Anderson, G.C. (1988). Effect of nonnutritive sucking on behavioral state in preterm infants before feeding, *Nursing Research,* **37**: 347-150.

Grey, M. (1988). Membership survey of the National Association of Pediatric Nurse Associates and Practitioners. (Unpublished manuscript.)

Hayman, L.L., Meininger, J.C., Stashinko, E.E., Gallagher, P.R., and Coates, P.M. (1988). Type A behavior and physiological cardiovascular risk factors in school-aged twin children, *Nursing Research,* **37**:290-296.

Hinds, P.S., and Martin, J. (1988). Hopefulness and the self-sustaining process in adolescents with cancer, *Nursing Research,* **37**:336-340.

Holmes, T.H., and Rahe, R.H. (1967). The social readjustment rating scale, *Journal of Psychosomatic Research,* **11**:213-218.

Kalish, P.A., Kalish, B.J., and Clinton, J. (1982). The world of nursing on prime time television, 1950-1980, *Nursing Research,* **31**:358-363.

Kunnel, M.T., O'Brien, C., Hazard Munro, B., and Medoff-Cooper, B. (1988). Comparisons of rectal, femoral, axillary, and skin-to-mattress temperatures in stable neonates, *Nursing Research,* **37**:162-164, 189.

Samet, J.M., Wiggins, C.L., Key, C.R., and Becker, T.M. (1988). Mortality from lung cancer and chronic obstructive pulmonary disease in New Mexico, 1958-82, *American Journal of Public Health,* **78**:1182-1186.

Seaman, C.C.H., and Verhonick, P.J. (1982). *Research methods for undergraduate students in nursing,* Norwalk, Conn., Appleton-Century-Crofts.

Vessey, J.A. (1988). Comparison of two teaching methods on children's knowledge of their internal bodies, *Nursing Research,* **37**:262-267.

Wolfer, J.A., and Visintainer, M.A. (1975). Pediatric surgical patients' and parents' stress responses and adjustment as a function of psychological preparation and stress-point nursing care, *Nursing Research,* **24**:244-255.

14

Reliability and Validity

Geri LoBiondo-Wood
Judith Haber

LEARNING OBJECTIVES

After reading this chapter the student should be able to do the following:

◇ Discuss measurement error.

◇ Discuss the purposes of reliability and validity.

◇ Define reliability.

◇ Discuss the concepts of stability, equivalence, and homogeneity as they relate to reliability.

◇ Compare and contrast the estimates of reliability.

◇ Define validity.

◇ Compare and contrast content, criterion-related, and construct validity.

◇ Identify the criteria for critiquing the reliability and validity of measurement tools.

◇ Use the critiquing criteria to evaluate the reliability and validity of measurement tools.

KEY TERMS

chance error	item-total correlation
concurrent validity	Kuder-Richardson coefficient
construct validity	parallel or alternate form
content validity	predictive validity
criterion-related validity	reliability
Cronbach alpha	split-half reliability
equivalence	stability
error variance	systematic error
homogeneity	test
internal consistency	test-retest reliability
interrater reliability	validity

Measurement of nursing phenomena is a major concern of nursing researchers. Unless measurement tools validly and reliably reflect the concepts of the theory being tested, conclusions drawn from the empirical phase of the study will be invalid and will not advance the development of nursing theory. Issues of **reliability** and **validity** are of central concern to the researcher as well as the critiquer of research. From either perspective the measurement tools that are used in a research study must be evaluated in terms of the extent to which reliability and validity have been established. Because many new constructs are relevant to nursing theory and few established measurement instruments are available to researchers, investigators frequently face the challenge of developing new instruments and, as part of that process, establishing the reliability and validity of those tools.

In other contexts investigators use tools that have been developed by researchers in nursing or other disciplines. They must evaluate the tools they select to be certain that they are valid and reliable measures, that they accurately operationalize the constructs being tested.

The critiquer of research, when reading research studies and reports, must assess the reliability and validity of the instruments used in the study to determine the soundness of these selections in relation to the constructs under investigation. The appropriateness of the tools and the extent to which reliability and validity are demonstrated have a profound influence on the findings and the internal and external validity of the study. Invalid measures produce invalid estimates of the relationships between variables, thus affecting internal validity. The use of invalid measures produces inaccurate generalizations to the populations being studied, thus affecting external validity. As such, the assessment of reliability and validity is an extremely important task for the research critiquer.

Regardless of whether a new or already developed measurement tool is being used in a research study, evidence of reliability and validity is of crucial importance to the research investigator and evaluator.

The purpose of this chapter is to examine the major types of reliability and validity and demonstrate the applicability of these concepts to the development, selection, and evaluation of measurement tools in nursing research.

RELIABILITY, VALIDITY, AND MEASUREMENT ERROR

Researchers may be concerned about whether the scores that were obtained for a sample of subjects were consistent, true measures of the behaviors and thus an accurate reflection of the differences between individuals. The extent of variability in test scores that is attributable to error rather than a true measure of the behaviors would be the **error variance.**

An observed test score that is derived from a set of items actually consists of the true score plus error (Fig. 14-1). The error may be either **chance error,** or random error, or it may be what is known as **systematic error.** Validity is concerned with systematic error, whereas reliability is concerned with random error (Waltz, Strickland, and Lenz, 1984). Chance or random errors are errors that are difficult to control, such as a respondent's anxiety level at the time of testing. Random errors are unsystematic in nature. Random errors are a result of a transient state in the subject, in the context of the study, or in the administration of the instrument (Jennings and Rogers, 1989). For example, perceptions or behaviors that occur at a specific point in time, such as anxiety in the example given, are known as a state or transient characteristic and are often beyond the awareness and control of the examiner. Another example of random error would be in a study that measures blood pressure. Random error could occur by misplacement of the cuff, not waiting for a specific time period before taking the blood pressure, and random placement of the arm in relationship to the heart while measuring blood pressure.

Systematic or *constant error* is measurement error that is attributable to relatively stable characteristics of the study population that may bias their behavior and/or cause incorrect instrument calibration. Such error has a systematic biasing influence on the subjects' responses and thereby influences the validity of the instruments. For instance, level of education, socioeconomic status, social desirability, response set, or other characteristics may influence the validity of the instrument by altering measurement of the "true" responses in a systematic way.

For example, a subject who wants to please the investigator may constantly answer items in a socially desirable way, thus making the estimate of validity inaccurate. Systematic error also occurs when an instrument is improperly calibrated. Consider a scale that consistently weighs a person 2 pounds less than the actual body weight. The scale could be quite reliable (that is, capable of reproducing the precise measurement), but the result is consistently invalid.

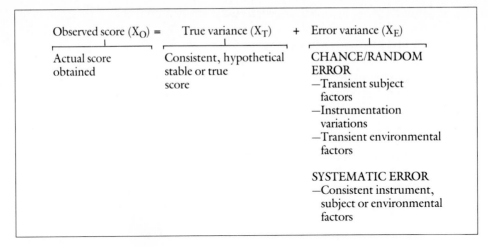

Fig. 14-1   Components of observed scores.

VALIDITY

Validity refers to whether a measurement instrument accurately measures what it is supposed to measure. When an instrument is valid it truly reflects the concept it is supposed to measure.

A valid instrument that is supposed to measure anxiety does so; it does not measure some other construct such as stress. A reliable measure can consistently rank participants on a given construct, such as anxiety, but a valid measure correctly measures the construct of interest. A measure can be reliable but not valid. Let us say that a researcher wanted to measure anxiety in clients by measuring their body temperatures. The researcher could obtain highly accurate, consistent, and precise temperature recordings, but such a measure could not be a valid indicator of anxiety. Thus the high reliability of an instrument is not necessarily congruent with evidence of validity. However, a valid instrument is reliable. An instrument cannot validly be measuring the attribute of interest if it is erratic, inconsistent, and inaccurate.

There are three major kinds of validity that vary according to the kind of information provided and the purpose of the investigator. They are **content validity, criterion-related validity,** and **construct validity.** A critiquer of research articles will want to evaluate whether sufficient evidence of validity is present and whether the type of validity is appropriate to the design of the study and instruments used in the study.

Content validity

Content validity represents the universe of content, or the domain of a given construct. The universe of content provides the framework and basis for formulating the items that will adequately represent the content. When an investigator is developing a tool and issues of content validity arise, the concern is whether the measurement tool and the items it contains are representative of the content domain the researcher intends to measure. The researcher begins by defining the concept and identifying the dimensions that are the components of the concept. Those items that reflect the concept and its dimensions are formulated.

When the researcher has completed this task, the items are submitted to a panel of judges who are considered to be experts about this concept. Researchers typically request that the judges indicate their agreement with the scope of the items and the extent to which the items reflect the concept under consideration.

In the process of developing a tool to measure learned helplessness, Quinless and Nelson (1988) submitted to a panel of three experts a pool of 50 items derived from the literature that reflected the attributional styles theorized to operate within the construct of learned helplessness. The experts were asked the following questions relative to each item: "Do you believe the item measures learned helplessness?" and "How strongly do you feel that the item measures learned helplessness?" Based on the independent reviews of the test items, 20 items were chosen for inclusion in the Learned Helplessness Scale. The items selected were rated as being either strongly indicative of learned helplessness or orthogonal (opposite) to learned helplessness. In addition, several items were modified in accordance with suggestions from the experts.

A subtype of content validity is face validity. *Face validity* is a very rudimentary type of validity that verifies basically that the instrument "looks" like it measures or gives the appearance of measuring the concept. It is an intuitive type of validity in which colleagues or subjects are asked to read the instrument and evaluate the content in terms of whether it appears to reflect the concept the researcher intends to measure. This procedure may be useful in the tool development process in relation to determining readability and clarity of content. However, it should in no way be considered a satisfactory alternative to other types of validity.

Criterion-related validity

Criterion-related validity indicates to what degree the subject's performance on the measurement tool and the subject's actual behavior are related. The criterion is usually the second measure, which assesses the same concept under study.

Two forms of criterion validity are concurrent and predictive. **Concurrent validity** refers to the degree of correlation of two measures of the same concept administered at the same time. A high correlation coefficient indicates agreement between the two measures. **Predictive validity** refers to the degree of correlation between the measure of the concept and some future measure of the same concept. Because of the passage of time the correlation coefficients are likely to be lower for predictive validity studies.

Norbeck, Lindsey, and Carrieri (1981) assessed concurrent validity of the Social Support Questionnaire by correlating scores with those from the Personal Resources Questionnaire, also designed to measure social support. They found that scores on the affect, affirmation, and aid dimensions were significantly and positively correlated with the scores on the Personal Resources Questionnaire.

Stokes and Gordon (1988) assessed predictive validity of the Stokes/Gordon Stress Scale (SGSS), a tool designed to measure stress in adults 65 years of age or older.

Scores on the SGSS were correlated to onset of illness because of the relationship between high stress and onset of illness that had been cited in the literature. The scores on the SGSS at the beginning of a 1-year period correlated significantly with the onset of illness for the total year.

Construct validity

Construct validity is based on the extent to which a test measures a theoretical construct or trait. It attempts to validate a body of theory underlying the measurement and testing of the hypothesized relationships. Empirical testing confirms or fails to confirm the relationships that would be predicted among concepts and, as such, provides greater or lesser support for the construct validity of the instruments measuring those concepts. The establishment of construct validity is a complex process, often involving several studies and several approaches. The hypothesis testing, factor analytic, convergent and divergent, and contrasted-groups approaches will be discussed.

Hypothesis testing approach

When the hypothesis testing approach is employed, the investigator uses the theory or concept underlying the measurement instrument's design to state hypotheses regarding the behavior of individuals with varying scores on the measure, to gather data to test the hypotheses, and to make inferences, on the basis of the findings, concerning whether or not the rationale underlying the instrument's construction is adequate to explain the findings.

For example, Haber (1990) used a hypothesis-testing approach to establish the construct validity of the Level of Differentiation of Self Scale (LDSS), a tool that was theoretically derived from the cornerstone concept of the Bowen Theory (1978) differentiation of self. As illustrated in Table 14-1, Haber derived five hypotheses that represented propositions related to differentiation of self, stress, anxiety, and adult dysfunction. Statistically significant findings provided support for the hypotheses and, as such, for the theoretical basis and conceptual accuracy of the LDSS.

Convergent and divergent approaches

Two strategies for assessing construct validity include convergent and divergent approaches.

Convergent validity refers to a search for other measures of the construct. When two or more tools that theoretically measure the same construct are identified, they are both administered to the same subjects. A correlational analysis is performed. If the measures are positively correlated, convergent validity is said to be supported. In the development of the Miller Hope Scale (MHS) (1988), convergent validity was established by correlating the MHS with the Psychological Well-Being Scale, the Existential Well-Being Scale, and a one-item, 10-point hope self-assessment scale (1, no hope; 10, filled with hope). As illustrated in Table 14-2, the correlation coefficients between the MHS and the other instruments all provide evidence of convergent validity.

Table 14-1 Construct Validity Estimation by Hypothesis Testing Strategy: The LDSS

	Findings	
Hypotheses	F ratio	Pearson *r*
1. Differentiation of self and negative impact ratings of stressful life events will have an additive effect on adult dysfunction.	21.31* 6.44†	
2. There will be a negative relationship between differentiation of self and trait anxiety.		− 0.52*
3. There will be a negative relationship between differentiation of self and state anxiety.		− 0.43*
4. There will be a negative relationship between differentiation of self and adult dysfunction.		− 0.53*
5. Negative impact ratings of stressful life events will have a greater impact than positive impact ratings on adult dysfunction.	58.74* 1.50	

From Haber, J.E. (1990). The Haber Level of Differentiation of Self Scale. In C. Waltz and O. Strickland, eds. *The measurement of educational and clinical outcomes,* New York, Springer Publications.
*$p < 0.001$.
†$p < 0.01$.

Table 14-2 Estimation of Convergent Validity for the MHS

	Psychological well-being scale	Existential well-being scale	One-item hope scale
MHS	0.71*	0.82*	0.69*

*$p < 0.001$.

Divergent validity searches for instruments that measure the opposite of the construct. It refers to the ability to differentiate the construct from others that may be similar. If the divergent measure is negatively related to other measures, validity for the measure is strengthened. In the development of the MHS (1988) divergent validity was established by correlating the MHS with the Hopelessness Scale. A negative correlation, $r = -0.54$, between the MHS and Hopelessness Scale was obtained, thereby lending support to the divergent validity of the MHS.

A specific method of assessing convergent and divergent validity is the *multitrait-multimethod* approach. Similar to the approach described above, this method, proposed by Campbell and Fiske (1959), also involves examining the

relationship between indicators that should measure the same construct and between those that should measure different constructs. However, a variety of measurement strategies are used. For example, anxiety could be measured by
  ◇ Administering the State-Trait Anxiety Inventory
  ◇ Recording blood pressure readings
  ◇ Asking the subject about anxious feelings
  ◇ Observing the subject's behavior
The results of one of these measures should then be correlated with results of each of the others in a multitrait-multimethod matrix (Waltz, Strickland, and Lenz, 1984).

The use of multiple measures of a concept decreases systematic error. A variety of data collection methods such as self-report, observation, interview, and collection of physiological data will also diminish the effect of systematic error.

Contrasted-groups approach

When the *contrasted-groups* approach (sometimes called the known-groups approach) to the development of construct validity is used, the researcher identifies two groups of individuals who are known to score extremely high and low in the characteristic being measured by the instrument. The instrument is administered to both the high- and low-scoring group, and the differences in scores obtained are examined. If the instrument is sensitive to individual differences in the trait being measured, then the *mean performance of these* two groups should differ significantly and evidence of construct validity would be supported. A *t* test or analysis of variance is used to statistically test the difference between the two groups. Hinshaw and Atwood (1982) assessed the validity of a client satisfaction measure by comparing scores across two phases of implementation of care-comfort nursing standards. As predicted, the satisfaction scores improved from the first measurement 1 month before implementation of the standards to the second measure made 6 weeks after the change in standards.

Factor analytic approach

A final approach to assessing construct validity is *factor analysis*. This is a procedure that gives the researcher information about the extent to which a set of items measures the same underlying construct or dimension of a construct. Factor analysis assesses the degree to which the individual items on a scale truly cluster together around one or more dimensions. Items designed to measure the same dimension should load on the same factor; those designed to measure differing dimensions should load on different factors (Nunnally, 1978). This analysis will also indicate whether the items in the instrument reflect a single construct or several constructs.

A factor analysis was carried out by Haber (1990) during the establishment of construct validity of the LDSS. The original scale consisted of a 32-item, two-subscale instrument. Findings from three factor analytic studies indicated that 24 of the 32 items loaded on factor I, only six loaded on factor II, and two did not load significantly on either factor. As a result of these and other findings, a decision was made to revise the LDSS as a 24-item unidimensional scale that measures one rather than two aspects of the concept of differentiation of self.

RELIABILITY

Reliable people are people whose behavior can be relied on to be consistent and predictable. *Reliability* of a research instrument likewise is defined as the extent to which the instrument yields the same results on repeated measures. Reliability is then concerned with consistency, accuracy, precision, **stability, equivalence,** and **homogeneity.** Concurrent with the questions of validity or after they are answered the researcher and the critiquer of research ask the question of how reliable is the instrument? A reliable measure is one that can produce the same results if the individual is measured again by the same scale. Reliability then refers to the proportion of accuracy to inaccuracy in measurement. In other words, if we use the same or comparable instruments on more than one occasion to measure a set of behaviors that ordinarily remain relatively constant, we would expect similar results if the tools are reliable. The three main attributes of a reliable scale are *stability, homogeneity,* and *equivalence.* The stability of an instrument refers to the instrument's ability to produce the same results with repeated testing. The homogeneity of an instrument means that all the items in a tool measure the same concept or characteristic. An instrument is said to exhibit equivalence if the tool produces the same results when equivalent or parallel instruments or procedures are used. Each of these attributes and the means to estimate them will be discussed. Before these are discussed an understanding of how to interpret reliability is essential.

Reliability coefficient interpretation

Since all the attributes of reliability are concerned with the degree of consistency between scores that are obtained at two or more independent times of testing, they often are expressed in terms of a correlation coefficient. The reliability coefficient ranges from 0 to 1. The reliability coefficient expresses the relationship between the error variance, true variance, and the observed score. A zero correlation indicates that there is no relationship. When the error variance in a measurement instrument is low, the reliability coefficient will be closer to 1. The closer to 1 the coefficient is, the more reliable the tool. For example, a reliability coefficient of a tool is reported to be 0.89. This tells the reader that the error variance is small and the tool has little measurement error. On the other hand, if the reliability coefficient of a measure is reported to be 0.49, the error variance is high and the tool has a problem with measurement error. For a tool to be considered reliable, a level of 0.70 or higher is considered to be an acceptable level of reliability. The interpretation of the reliability coefficient depends on the proposed purpose of the measure. There are five major tests of reliability that can be utilized to calculate a reliability coefficient. The test(s) used depend on the nature of the tool. They are known as test-retest, parallel or alternate form, item-total correlation, split-half, Kuder-Richardson (KR-20), Cronbach's alpha, and **interrater reliability.** These tests will be discussed as they relate to the attributes of stability, equivalence, and homogeneity (see box on p. 256). There is no best means to assess reliability in relationship to stability, homogeneity, and equivalence. The critiquer of research should be aware that the method of reliability that the researcher uses should be consistent with the investigator's aim.

Measures Used to Test Reliability
Stability
Test-retest reliability
Parallel or alternate form
Homogeneity
Item-total correlation
Split-half reliability
Kuder-Richardson coefficient
Cronbach's alpha
Equivalence
Parallel or alternate form
Interrater reliability

Stability

An instrument is thought to be stable or to exhibit *stability* when the same results are obtained on repeated administration of the instrument. Researchers are concerned with the stability of an instrument when they want the instrument to be able to measure the concept consistently over a period of time. Measurement over time is important when an instrument is used in a longitudinal study and therefore will be used on several occasions. Stability is also a consideration when the researcher is conducting an intervention study that is designed to effect an alteration in a specific variable. In this case the instrument is administered once and again later after the alteration or change intervention has been completed. The tests that are used to estimate stability are *test-retest* and *parallel or alternate form.*

Test-retest reliability

Test-retest reliability is the administration of the same instrument to the same subjects under similar conditions on two or more occasions. Scores on the repeated testing are compared. This comparison is expressed by a correlation coefficient, usually a Pearson *r.* The interval between repeated administrations varies and is dependent on the phenomenon being measured. For example, if the variable that the test measures is related to the developmental stages in children, then the interval between tests should be short. The amount of time over which the variable was measured should also be recorded in the report. An example of an instrument that was tested for test-retest reliability is the MHS (Miller and Powers, 1988). The Scale was administered on two separate occasions to the same 308 of the original 522 respondents within a 2-week period. The correlation yielded was 0.82, which supports the idea that the instrument has the attribute of stability.

Parallel or alternate form

Parallel or alternate form reliability is applicable and can be tested only if two comparable forms of the same instrument exist. It is like test-retest reliability in that the same individuals are tested within a specific interval, but it differs because a different form of the test is given to the subjects on the second testing. Parallel forms or tests contain the same types of items that are based on the same domain or concept, but the wording of the items is different. The development of parallel forms is desired if the instrument is intended to measure a variable for which a researcher feels that "test-wiseness" will be a problem. For example, there are two alternate forms of the Interpersonal Conflict Scale (Hoskins, 1983) that may be used in a repeated-measures design. An item on one scale ("I am able to tell my partner how I feel") is consistent with the paired item on the second form ("My partner tries to understand my feelings").

Another example of a parallel test is the Multidimensional Health Locus of Control Scale (Wallston, Wallston, and DeVellis, 1978), which was designed to measure three dimensions or sources of reinforcement for health-related behaviors. This scale has parallel forms for studies that incorporate a repeated-measures design. Examples of parallel items are "If I get sick, it is my own behavior that determines how soon I get well." This item compares with "If I get sick, I have the power to make myself well again." As can be seen, the two items, although worded differently, reflect the same idea. Practically speaking, it is difficult to develop alternate forms of an instrument when one considers the many issues of reliability and validity of an instrument. If alternate forms of a test exist, they should be highly correlated if the measures are to be considered reliable.

Homogeneity

Another attribute of an instrument related to reliability is the **internal consistency** or homogeneity with which the items within the scale reflect or measure the same concept. This means that the items within the scale correlate or are complementary to each other. This also means that a scale is unidimensional. A unidimensional scale is one that measures one concept. For example, a scale that is designed to measure anxiety should not be designed to measure depression as well. There are scales, such as the Multidimensional Health Locus of Control Scale (Wallston, Wallston, and DeVellis, 1978), that do contain two or more concepts or dimensions within them. If that is the case, the researcher should identify this for the reader and should also have tested each concept within the scale separately. The internal consistency of items allows the investigator to tally the items and obtain a total score for the concept. The total score is then used in the analysis of data. Homogeneity can be assessed by using one of four methods: **item-total correlations, split-half reliability, Kuder-Richardson (KR-20) coefficient,** or **Cronbach's alpha.**

Item to total correlations

Item to total correlations measure the relationship between each of the items and the total scale. When item to total correlations are calculated, a correlation for each item

Table 14-3 Examples of Item to Total Correlations from Computer-Generated Data

Item	Item to total correlation
1	0.5096
2	0.4455
3	0.4479
4	0.4369
5	0.4139
6	0.4016

on the scale is generated (Table 14-3). Items that do not achieve a high correlation may be deleted from the instrument. Usually in a research study not all the item to total correlations are reported unless the study is a report of a methodological study. Typically the lowest and highest correlations are reported. An example of an item to total correlation report is "The lowest item to total correlation was $r = 14$ for the item, 'Although it is hard to pin down, I feel hopeful.' This item is problematic in that it provides two distinct perceptions. The highest item to total correlation was .68 for the item, 'I am positive about the future'" (Miller and Powers, 1988, p. 8). The investigators are expressing concern that one of the items may have too low a correlation, whereas the others are high enough to be measuring the same concept without being redundant. If item to total correlations are found to be too high, they are considered to be redundant and therefore not complementary to each other (Anastasi, 1982). This is unlike the other errors of reliability in which a higher correlation is generally a better correlation.

Split-half reliability

Split-half reliability involves dividing a scale into two halves and making a comparison. The halves may be odd-numbered and even-numbered items or a simple division of the first from the second half, or items may be randomly selected as to the halves that will be analyzed opposite one another. The split-half provides a measure of consistency in terms of sampling the content. The two halves of the test or the contents in both halves are assumed to be comparable, and a reliability coefficient is calculated. If the scores for the two halves are approximately equal, the test may be considered reliable. A formula called the Spearman-Brown formula is one method used to calculate the reliability coefficient.

Kuder-Richardson (KR-20) coefficient

The Kuder-Richardson (KR-20) coefficient is the estimate of homogeneity utilized for instruments that have a dichotomous response format. A dichotomous response format is one in which the question asks for a yes/no or a true/false response. The technique yields a correlation that is based on the consistency of responses to all the

	Definitely yes	Yes	Uncertain	No	Definitely no
I am uncertain about being pregnant	5	4	3	2	1
The baby seems to know when I feel tense or anxious	5	4	3	2	1

Fig. 14-2 Examples of a Likert scale. (From LoBiondo-Wood, G., O'Rourke Vito, K., and Brage D. [1989]).

items of a single form of a test that is administered one time. Beck, Weissman, Lester, and Trexler (1974) developed the Hopelessness Scale, which is designed to objectively measure an individual's negative expectancies. It utilizes a 20-item true/false format. A Kuder-Richardson reliability was calculated, and a correlation of 0.93 was arrived at, thus establishing that the instrument was internally consistent.

Cronbach's alpha

The fourth and most commonly utilized test of internal consistency is Cronbach's alpha. Many tools utilized to measure psychosocial variables and attitudes have a Likert scale response format. A Likert scale format asks the subject to respond to a question on a scale of varying degrees of intensity between two extremes. The two extremes are anchored by responses such as "strongly agree" to "strongly disagree" or "most like me" to "least like me." The points between the two extremes may range from 1 to 5 or 1 to 7. Subjects are asked to circle the response closest to how they feel. Fig. 14-2 provides examples of items from a tool that uses a Likert scale format. Cronbach's alpha compares each item in the scale simultaneously to each other. Examples of reported Cronbach's alpha are in the box on p. 260.

Equivalence

Equivalence is either the consistency or agreement among observers utilizing the same measurement tool or the consistency or agreement among alternate forms of a tool. An instrument is thought to demonstrate equivalence when two or more observers have a high percentage of agreement of an observed behavior or when alternate forms of a test yield a high correlation. There are two methods to test equivalence: *interrater reliability* and *alternate or parallel form*.

Interrater reliability

Some measuring instruments are not self-administered questionnaires but are direct measurements of observed behavior. Instruments that depend on direct observation of a behavior that is to be systematically recorded need to be tested for interrater reliability. To accomplish interrater reliability there need to be two or more individuals making an observation or one observer observing the behavior on several occasions. The observers need to be trained or oriented to the definition of the behavior to be

Examples of Reported Cronbach's Alpha

Quinless, F.W., and Nelson, M.A. (1988, p. 13): "The alpha reliability coefficient of the Learned Helplessness Scale in the sample was .85."

Miller, J.F., and Powers, M.J. (1988, p. 8): "Cronbach's alpha on the Miller Hope Scale using 522 respondents was .93."

Stokes, S.A., and Gordon, S.E. (1988, p. 17): "Cronbach's alpha for internal consistency was estimated on another, similar, convenience sample of 63. The alpha was .86."

LoBiondo-Wood, G., O'Rourke Vito, K., Brage, D. (1989): "Cronbach's alpha for the 29 items relevant to all stages of pregnancy (N = 650) was .89."

observed. In the method of direct observation of behavior, the consistency or reliability of the observations between observers is extremely important. In the instance of interrater reliability the reliability or consistency of the observer is tested rather than the reliability of the instrument. Interrater reliability is expressed as a percentage of agreement between scorers or as a correlation coefficient between the scores assigned to the observed behaviors.

In the development of the Braden Scale for Predicting Pressure Sore Risk, the researchers conducted three studies to determine interrater reliability of the scale (Bergstrom, Braden, Laguzza, and Holman, 1987). The three studies utilized different levels of nursing personnel to rate the items of pressure sore risk. The report of the interrater reliability assessment in the first study is as follows (p. 207):

> Subjects were rated by both the Registered Nurse (RN) and Graduate Student (GS) for a period of 1 to 7 weeks. Scores on admission ranged from 11 to 15; on discharge, from 11 to 22. There were a total of 86 pairs of RN and GS observations. Pearson product moment correlation between observers was $r = .99$, $p < .001$. The percent agreement, a more conservative measure of reliability than a correlation (Goodwin & Prescott, 1981), was 88%. In no case was the total score by the two raters more than 1 point different.

The researchers further describe the other two studies they conducted to establish interrater reliability. In the other two studies they use both percentage agreement and correlation coefficients. Based on these three studies and others noted by the researchers in the article, they have established that the Braden Scale is a highly reliable instrument when used by registered nurses, primary nurses, and graduate nurses to measure pressure sore risk. But they note that the interrater reliability between licensed practical nurses and nursing assistants was not highly correlated. The researchers review the reasons for this and conclude that the tool should most appropriately be used by caregivers who are registered nurses.

Another example of interrater reliability is given in a study conducted by O'Brien (1980). O'Brien studied parent-child communication and interaction and operationalized parent-child communication by constructing a measurement tool, the Parent-

Child Communication Schedule (PCCS). This tool uses an observational method and therefore needs an assessment of interrater reliability. O'Brien measured interrater reliability using the following procedures (p. 153):

> The reliability of coding observations with the PCCS was assessed through the use of videotaped interactions of five parent-child dyads engaged in tasks similar to those of the proposed study. Following a period of training, the investigator and two observers independently coded the videotaped interactions of the five parent-child dyads. When an identical category was recorded by each observer for the same exchange, it was scored as agreement. The percentage of agreement between the investigator and the two observers was calculated using the formula: Number of agreements/(number of agreements + number of disagreements). The agreement between all ratings made by the investigator and the two observers was 84 percent and 82 percent, respectively.

Parallel or alternate form

Parallel or alternate form has been described previously under the heading Stability. Use of parallel forms is then a measure of stability and equivalence. The procedures for assessing equivalence using parallel forms are the same.

CRITIQUING RELIABILITY AND VALIDITY

Reliability and validity are two crucial aspects in the critical appraisal of a measurement instrument. Criteria for critiquing reliability and validity are presented in the box on p. 262. The reviewer evaluates an instrument's level of reliability and validity and the manner in which they were established. In a research report the reliability and validity of the data for each measure should be presented. If these data have not been presented at all, the reviewer must seriously question the merit and use of the tool and the study's results.

Appropriate reliability tests should have been performed by the developer of the measurement tool and should then have been included by the current user in the research report. If the initial standardization sample and the current sample have different characteristics, the reader would expect (1) that a pilot study for the present sample would have been conducted to determine if the reliability was maintained or (2) that a reliability estimate was calculated on the current sample. For example, if the standardization sample for a tool that measures "satisfaction in an intimate heterosexual relationship" were made up of undergraduate college students and if an investigator plans to use the tool with married couples, it would be advisable to reexamine the reliability for the latter group.

The investigator determines which type of reliability procedures are used in the study, depending on the nature of the measurement tool and how it will be used. For example, if the instrument is to be administered twice, the critiquer might determine that test-retest reliability should have been used. If an alternate form has been developed for use in a repeated-measures design, evidence of alternate form reliability should be presented. If the degree of internal consistency among the items is relevant,

Critiquing Criteria

1. Was an appropriate method used to **test** the reliability of the tool?
2. Is the reliability of the tool adequate?
3. Was an appropriate method(s) used to test the validity of the instrument?
4. Is the validity of the measurement tool adequate?
5. If the sample from the developmental stage of the tool was different from the current sample, were the reliability and validity recalculated to determine if the tool is still adequate?
6. Have the strengths and weaknesses of the reliability and validity of each instrument been presented?

an appropriate test of internal consistency should be presented. In some instances more than one type of reliability will be presented, but the evaluator will want to determine whether all are appropriate. For example, the Kuder-Richardson formula implies that there is a single right or wrong answer, making it inappropriate to use with scales that provide a format of three or more possible responses. In such cases another formula is applied, such as Cronbach's coefficient alpha formula. Another important consideration is the acceptable level of reliability, which varies according to the type of test. Coefficients of reliability of 0.70 or higher are desirable. The validity of an instrument is limited by its reliability; that is, less confidence can be placed in scores from tests with low reliability coefficients.

Satisfactory evidence of validity is probably the most difficult item for the reviewer to ascertain. It is this aspect of measurement that is most likely to fall short of meeting the required criteria. Validity studies are time-consuming as well as complex, and sometimes researchers will settle for presenting minimal validity data. Therefore the critiquer will want to closely examine the item content of a tool when evaluating its strengths and weaknesses and will endeavor to find conclusive evidence of content validity. However, in the body of a research article it is most unusual to have more than a few sample items available for review. Since that is the case, the critiquer will want to determine if the appropriate assessment of construct validity was used to meet the researcher's goal. Such procedures provide the reviewer with assurance that the tool is psychometrically sound and that the content of the items is consistent with the conceptual framework and construct definitions. Construct and criterion-related validity comprise some of the more precise statistical tests of whether the tool measures what it is supposed to measure. Ideally an instrument should provide evidence of content validity as well as criterion-related or construct validity before a reviewer invests a high level of confidence in the tool.

As the reader can see, the area of reliability and validity is complex. These aspects of research reports can be evaluated to varying degrees. The research consumer should not feel inhibited by the complexity of this topic but may use the guidelines presented in this chapter to systematically assess the reliability and validity aspects of a research study. Collegial dialogue is also an approach to evaluating the merits and shortcomings of an existing as well as a newly developed instrument that is reported in the nursing literature. Such an exchange promotes the understanding of methodologies and techniques of reliability and validity, stimulates the acquisition of a basic knowledge of psychometrics, and encourages the exploration of alternative methods of observation.

SUMMARY

Reliability and validity are crucial aspects of conducting and critiquing research.

Validity refers to whether an instrument measures what it is purported to measure, and it is a crucial aspect of evaluating a tool. Three types of validity are content validity, criterion-related validity, and construct validity. The choice of a validation method is important and is made by the researcher on the basis of the characteristics of the measurement device in question and its utilization.

Reliability refers to the accuracy/inaccuracy ratio in a measurement device. The major tests of reliability are the following: test-retest, parallel or alternate form, split-half, item-total correlation, Kuder-Richardson, Cronbach's alpha, and interrater reliability. Again, the selection of a method for establishing reliability will depend on the characteristics of the tool, the testing method that is used for collecting data from the standardization sample, and the kinds of data that are obtained.

References

Anastasi, A. (1982). *Psychological testing,* New York, Macmillan, Inc.

Beck, A.T., Weissman, A., Lester, D., and Trexler, L. (1974). The measurement of pessimism: the hopelessness scale, *Journal of Consulting and Clinical Psychology,* **42:**861-865.

Bergstrom, N., Braden, B.J., Laguzza, A., and Holman, V. (1987). The Braden scale for predicting pressure sore risk, *Nursing Research,* **36:**205-210.

Bowen, M. (1978). On the differentiation of self. In M. Bowen, ed.: *Family therapy in clinical practice,* New York, Jason Aronson, pp.467-528.

Campbell, D., and Fiske, D. (1959). Convergent and discriminant validation by the matrix, *Psychological Bulletin,* **53:**273-302.

Haber, J.E. (1990). The Haber Level of Differentiation of Self Scale. In C. Waltz and O. Strickland, eds: The measurement of educational and clinical outcomes, New York, Springer Publications.

Hinshaw, A.S., and Atwood, J. (1982). A patient satisfaction instrument: precision by replication, *Nursing Research,* **31:**170-175.

Hoskins, C.N. (1983). Psychometrics in nursing research—further development of the interpersonal conflict scale, *Research in Nursing and Health,* **5:**75-83.

Jennings, B.M., and Rogers, S. (1989). Managing measurement error, *Nursing Research,* **38:** 186-187.

LoBiondo-Wood, G., O'Rourke Vito, K., and Brage, D. (1989). *The prenatal maternal attachment scale: a methodological study,* Paper presented at the meeting of the 13th Annual Midwest Nursing Research Society Conference, Cincinnati, Ohio.

Miller, J.F., and Powers, M.J. (1988). Development of an instrument to measure hope, *Nursing Research,* **37:**6-10.

Norbeck, J., Lindsey, A., and Carrieri, V. (1981). The development of an instrument to measure social support, *Nursing Research,* **30**:264-269.

Nunnally, J.C. (1978). *Psychometric theory,* New York, McGraw-Hill Book Co., Inc.

O'Brien, R.A. (1980). Relationship of parent-child communication to child's exploratory behavior and self-differentiation, *Nursing Research,* **29**: 150-156.

Stokes, S.A., and Gordon, S.E. (1988). Development of an instrument to measure stress in the older adult, *Nursing Research,* **37**:16-19.

Quinless, F.W., and Nelson, M.A. (1988). Development of a measure of learned helplessness, *Nursing Research,* **37**:11-15.

Wallston, K.S., Wallston, B.S., and DeVellis, B.S. (1978). Development of the multidimensional health locus of control (MHLC) scales, *Health Education Monographs,* **6**:160-170.

Waltz, C., Strickland, O., and Lenz, E. (1984). *Measurement in nursing research,* Philadelphia, F.A. Davis Co.

15

Sampling

Judith Haber

LEARNING OBJECTIVES

After reading the chapter the student should be able to do the following:

◇ Identify the purpose of sampling.

◇ Define population, sample, and sampling.

◇ Compare and contrast a population and a sample.

◇ Discuss the eligibility criteria for sample selection.

◇ Define nonprobability and probability sampling.

◇ Identify the types of nonprobability and probability sampling strategies.

◇ Compare the advantages and disadvantages of specific nonprobability and probability sampling strategies.

◇ Discuss the factors that influence determination of sample size.

◇ Discuss the procedure for drawing a sample.

◇ Formulate a sampling plan for a research study.

◇ Identify the criteria for critiquing a sampling plan.

◇ Use the critiquing criteria to evaluate the sampling section of a research report.

KEY TERMS

convenience sampling   random selection
cluster sampling   representative sample
delimitation   sample
eligibility criteria   sampling
element   sampling interval
nonprobability sampling   sampling unit
population   simple random sampling
probability sampling   stratified random sampling
purposive sampling   systematic sample
quota sampling

Sampling is the process of selecting representative units of a population for study in a research investigation. Although sampling is a complex process, it is a familiar one. In our daily lives we gather knowledge, make decisions, and formulate predictions based on sampling procedures. For example, nursing students may make generalizations about the overall quality of nursing professors as a result of their exposure to a **sample** of nursing professors during their undergraduate programs. Clients may make generalizations about a hospital's food during a 1-week hospital stay. It is apparent that limited exposure to a limited portion of these phenomena forms the basis of our conclusions and so much of our knowledge and decisions are based on our experience with samples.

Scientists also derive knowledge from samples. Many problems in scientific research cannot be solved without employing sampling measures. For example, when testing the effectiveness of a medication for clients with cardiac disease, the drug is administered to a sample of the population for whom the drug is potentially appropriate. The scientist must come to some conclusions without administering the drug to every known client with cardiac disease or every laboratory animal in the world. But because human lives are at stake, the scientist cannot afford to casually arrive at conclusions based on the first dozen clients available for study. The consequences of arriving at erroneous conclusions or making inaccurate generalizations from a small, nonrepresentative sample are much more severe in scientific investigations than in everyday life. Consequently, research methodologists have expended considerable effort to develop sampling theories and procedures that produce accurate and meaningful information. Essentially, researchers sample representative segments of the population, because it is rarely feasible or necessary to sample the entire population of interest to obtain relevant information.

This chapter will familiarize the research consumer with the basic concepts of sampling as they pertain to the principles of research design, nonprobability and probability sampling, sample size, and the related critiquing process.

SAMPLING CONCEPTS

Population

A **population** is a well-defined set that has certain specified properties. A population can be composed of people, animals, objects, or events. For example, if a researcher is studying undergraduate nursing students, the type of educational preparation of the population must be specified. In this instance the population consists of undergraduate students enrolled in a generic baccalaureate nursing program. Examples of other possible populations might be all male clients admitted for a first myocardial infarction in hospital ABC during the year 1989; all children with Down's syndrome in the state of New York; or all men and women with a diagnosis of unipolar depression in the United States. These examples illustrate that a population may be broadly defined and potentially involve millions of people or narrowly specified to include only several hundred people.

The reader of a research report should consider whether or not the researcher has identified the population descriptors that form the basis for the **eligibility criteria** that are used to select the sample from the array of all possible units, be they people, objects, or events. Let us consider the population previously defined as undergraduate nursing students enrolled in a generic baccalaureate program. Would this population include part-time as well as full-time students? Would it include students who had previously attended another nursing program? How about foreign students? Would freshmen through seniors qualify? Insofar as it is possible, the researcher must demonstrate that the exact criteria used to decide whether an individual would or would not be classified as a member of a given population were specifically delineated. The population descriptors that provide the basis for eligibility criteria should be evident in the sample; that is, the characteristics of the population and the sample should be congruent. The degree of congruence is evaluated to assess the representativeness of the sample. For example, if a population was defined as full-time, American-born, senior nursing students enrolled in a generic baccalaureate nursing program, the sample would be expected to reflect these characteristics.

Eligibility criteria may also be viewed as **delimitations,** or those characteristics that restrict the population to a homogeneous group of subjects. Examples of delimitations include the following: sex, age, marital status, socioeconomic status, religion, ethnicity, level of education, age of children, and diagnosis. In a study comparing rectal, femoral, axillary, and skin-to-mattress temperatures in stable neonates (Kunnel, O'Brien, Hazard Munro, and Medoff-Cooper, 1988), the researchers established several of the following delimitations:

⋄ Full-term neonate — 38 to 40.5 weeks' gestation
⋄ Normal weight — 2750 to 4000 g
⋄ Age — 1 to 4 days
⋄ Abnormalities — none known

These delimitations were selected because their potential effect on temperature would limit the validity of the findings as well as the ability to generalize about the findings. Let us consider the criterion of full-term neonate. If full-term and preterm infants were grouped together in the sample, the researcher would end up with two groups of infants whose temperature patterns may be very different and hence the accuracy of findings may be distorted. The heterogeneity of this sample group would inhibit the researcher's ability to meaningfully interpret the findings and make generalizations. It is much wiser to either study only one homogeneous group or include all three groups as distinct subsets of the sample and study the groups comparatively. The reader should remember that delimitations are not established in a casual or meaningless way, but they are established to control for extraneous variability or bias. Each delimitation should have a rationale, presumably related to a potential contaminating effect on the dependent variable. The careful establishment of sample delimitations will increase the precision of the study and contribute to the accuracy and generalizability of the findings.

The population criteria establish the *target population;* that is, the entire set of cases about which the researcher would like to make generalizations. A target population might include all undergraduate nursing students enrolled in generic baccalaureate programs in the United States. It is often not feasible, because of time, money, and personnel, to pursue utilizing a target population. An *accessible population,* one that meets the population criteria and that is *available,* is used instead. For example, an accessible population might include all full-time generic baccalaureate students attending school in Connecticut. Pragmatic factors must also be considered when identifying a potential population of interest.

The reader should know that a population is not restricted to human subjects. It may consist of hospital records; blood, urine, or other specimens taken from clients at a clinic; historical documents; or laboratory animals. For example, a population might consist of all the urine specimens collected from clients in the Crestview Hospital antepartum clinic or all of the patient charts on file at the Day Surgery Center. It is apparent that a population can be defined in a variety of ways. The important thing to remember is that the basic unit of the population must be clearly defined, since the generalizability of the findings will be a function of the population criteria.

Samples and sampling

Sampling is a process of selecting a portion of the designated population to represent the entire population. A *sample* is a set of elements that make up the population, and an **element** is the most basic unit about which information is collected. The most common element in nursing research is individuals, but other elements can form the basis of a sample or population. A **sampling unit** is the element or set of elements used for selecting the sample. Sometimes the sampling unit and the element represent the same thing, and other times it is more efficient to use a unit larger than the element for sampling purposes. For example a researcher was planning a study that compared the effectiveness of different nursing interventions on the healing rate of decubitus ulcers. Four hospitals, each using a different treatment protocol, were identified as the sampling units rather than the nurses themselves or the treatment alone.

The purpose of sampling is to increase the efficiency of a research study. The novice reviewer of research reports must realize that it would not be feasible to examine each and every element or unit in the population. When sampling is properly done it allows the researcher to draw inferences and make generalizations about the population without examining each and every unit in the population. Sampling procedures that entail the formulation of specific criteria for selection ensure that the characteristics of the phenomena of interest will be, or are likely to be, present in all of the units being studied. The researcher's endeavors to ensure that the sample is representative of the target population put the researcher in a stronger position to draw conclusions from the sample findings that are generalizable to the population.

Evaluators of research studies will find that samples and sampling procedures vary in terms of merit. The foremost criterion in evaluating a sample is its representativeness. A **representative sample** is one whose key characteristics closely approximate those of the population. If 70% of the population in a study of child-rearing practices consisted of women and 40% were full-time employees, then a representative sample should reflect these characteristics in the same proportions.

It must be understood that there is no way to guarantee that a sample is representative without obtaining a data base about the entire population. Since it is difficult and inefficient to assess a population, the researcher must employ sampling strategies that minimize or control for sample bias. If an appropriate sampling strategy is utilized, it is almost always possible to obtain a reasonably accurate understanding of the phenomena under investigation by obtaining data from a sample.

TYPES OF SAMPLES

Sampling strategies are generally grouped into two categories: **nonprobability sampling** and **probability sampling.** In *nonprobability* sampling, elements are chosen by nonrandom methods. The drawback of this strategy is that there is no way of estimating the probability that each element has of being included in the samples. Essentially there is no way of ensuring that every element has a chance for inclusion in the nonprobability sample. *Probability sampling* utilizes some form of random selection when choosing the sample units. This type of sample enables the researcher to estimate the probability that each element of the population will be included in the sample. Probability sampling is the more rigorous type of sampling strategy, because it is more likely to result in a representative sample. The remainder of this section will be devoted to a discussion of different types of nonprobability and probability sampling strategies. A summary of sampling strategies appears in Table 15-1.

Nonprobability sampling

The nonprobability sampling strategy is less rigorous than probability sampling strategy, and it tends to produce less accurate and representative samples. However, most samples, not only in nursing research but in other disciplines as well, are nonprobability samples. Although such samples are more feasible for the researcher to obtain, the use of nonprobability samples does limit the ability of the researcher to make generalizations about the findings. The three major types of nonprobability sampling are the following: convenience, quota, and purposive sampling strategies.

Table 15-1 **Summary of Sampling Strategies**

Nonprobability sampling strategies	Probability sampling strategies
Convenience sampling	Simple random sampling
Quota sampling	Stratified random sampling
Purposive sampling	Cluster sampling
	Systematic sampling

Convenience sampling

Convenience sampling is the use of the most readily accessible persons or objects as subjects in a study. The subjects may include volunteers, the first 25 clients admitted to hospital X with a particular diagnosis, all people who enrolled in program Y during the month of September, or all students enrolled in course Z at a particular university during 1990. The subjects are convenient and accessible to the researcher and are sometimes called an *accidental sample*. For example, a researcher studying marital communication patterns utilized an accidental sample of the first 200 couples meeting the sample criteria and who volunteered to participate in the study. Another researcher studying the effect of group client education on cardiac rehabilitation utilized all clients transferred from the coronary care unit to the intermediate coronary care unit in hospital X between September and December 1989.

The advantage of a convenience sample is that it is easier for the researcher to obtain subjects. All the researcher may have to be concerned with is obtaining a sufficient number of subjects who meet the same criteria.

The major disadvantage of a convenience sample is that the risk of bias is greater than in any other type of sample. The problem of bias is related to the fact that convenience samples tend to be self-selecting; that is, the researcher ends up obtaining information only from the people who volunteer to participate. In this case the following questions must be raised: What motivated some of the people to participate and others to not participate? What kind of data would I have obtained if nonparticipants had also responded? How representative are the people who did participate in relation to the population? For example, a researcher may stop people on a street corner to ask their opinion on some issue; place advertisements in the newspaper; or place signs in local churches, community centers, or supermarkets indicating that volunteers are needed for a particular study. A researcher may even offer to pay the participants for their time. The problem is that those who choose to participate may not be typical of the population with regard to the variables being measured. There is no way to assess the biases that may be operating. In cases where the phenomena under investigation are relatively homogeneous within the population, the risk of bias may be minimal. However, in heterogeneous populations the risk of bias is great.

The evaluator of a research report should recognize that the convenience sample is the weakest form of sampling strategies with regard to generalizability. Its use should be avoided whenever possible. When convenience sample is utilized, caution should be exercised in analyzing and interpreting the data. When critiquing a research study that has employed this sampling strategy, the reviewer will be justifiably skeptical about the external validity of the findings.

Quota sampling

Quota sampling refers to a form of nonprobability sampling in which knowledge about the population of interest is utilized to build some representativeness into the sample. A quota sample identifies the strata of the population and proportionally represents the strata in the sample. For example, the data in Table 15-2 reveal that 40% of the 5000 nurses in city X are diploma graduates, 40% are associate degree graduates, and 20% are baccalaureate graduates. Each stratum of the population should be proportionately represented in the sample. In this case the researcher used a proportional quota sampling strategy and decided to sample 10% of a population of 5000, or 500 nurses. Based on the proportion of each stratum in the population, 200 diploma graduates, 200 associate degree graduates, and 100 baccalaureate graduates were the quotas established for the three strata. The researcher recruited subjects who met the eligibility criteria of the study until the quota for each stratum was filled. In other words, once the researcher obtained the necessary 200 diploma, 200 associate degree, and 100 baccalaureate graduates, the sample was complete.

The researcher systematically ensures that proportional segments of the population are included in the sample. The quota sample is not randomly selected; that is, once the proportional strata have been identified, the researcher obtains subjects until the quota for each stratum has been filled, but it does increase the representativeness of the sample. This sampling strategy addresses the problem of overrepresentation or underrepresentation of certain segments of a population in a sample.

The characteristics chosen to form the strata are selected according to a researcher's judgment based on knowledge of the population and the literature review. The criterion for selection should be a variable that would reflect important differences in the dependent variables under investigation. Age, sex, religion, ethnicity, medical diagnosis, socioeconomic status, level of completed education, and occupational rank are among those variables that are likely to be important stratifying variables in nursing research investigations.

The critiquer of a research study seeks to determine whether or not the sample strata appropriately reflect the population under consideration and whether the stratifying variables are homogeneous enough to ensure a meaningful comparison of differences between strata. Even when the preceding factors have been addressed by the researcher, the evaluator must remember that as a nonprobability sample, the quota strategy contains an unknown source of bias that affects external validity.

Table 15-2 Numbers and Percents of Students in Strata of a Quota
Sample of 5000 Graduates of Nursing Programs in City X

	Diploma graduates	Associate degree graduates	Baccalaureate graduates
Population	2000 (40%)	2000 (40%)	1000 (20%)
Strata	200	200	100

Purposive sampling

Purposive sampling is a strategy in which the researcher's knowledge about the population and its elements is utilized to handpick the cases to be included in the sample. The researcher usually selects subjects who are considered to be *typical* of the population. A purposive sample is also used when a highly unusual group is being studied, such as a population with a rare genetic disease such as Tay-Sachs disease. In this case the researcher would describe the sample characteristics very precisely to ensure that the reader will have an accurate picture of the subjects in the sample.

In another situation the researcher may wish to interview individuals who reflect different ends of the range of a particular characteristic. For example, a researcher investigates attitudes about death in individuals who test positive for the human immunodeficiency virus but have no symptoms, in comparison to individuals who have active disease.

The researcher who utilizes a purposive sample assumes that errors of judgment in overrepresenting or underrepresenting elements of the population in the sample will tend to balance out. However, there is no objective method for determining the validity of this assumption. The evaluator must be aware of the fact that the more heterogeneous the population, the greater the chance of bias being introduced in the selection of a purposive sample. Conscious bias in the selection of subjects remains a constant danger. As such, the findings from a study utilizing a purposive sample should be regarded with caution. As with any nonprobability sample, the ability to generalize is very limited.

The following are several instances when a purposive sample may be appropriate:
1. The effective pretesting of newly developed instruments with a purposive sample of divergent types of people
2. The validation of a scale or test with a known-groups technique
3. The collection of exploratory data in relation to an unusual or highly specific population, particularly when the total target population remains an unknown to the researcher

Even when the use of a purposive sample is appropriate, the researcher as well as the critiquer should be cognizant of the limitations of this sampling strategy.

Probability sampling

The primary characteristic of probability sampling is the **random selection** of elements from the population. *Random selection* occurs when each element of the population has an equal and independent chance of being included in the sample. Four commonly used probability sampling strategies are **simple random sampling, stratified random sampling, cluster sampling,** and **systematic sampling.**

Simple random sampling

Simple random sampling is a laborious and carefully controlled process. Since the more complex probability designs incorporate the principles of simple random sampling in their procedures, the principles of this strategy will be presented.

The researcher defines the population (a set), lists all of the units of the population (a sampling frame), and selects a sample of units (a subset) from which the sample will be chosen. For example, if American hospitals specializing in respiratory problems are the sampling unit, then a list of all such hospitals would be the sampling frame. If certified clinical specialists constituted the accessible population, then a list of those nurses would be the sampling frame.

Once a list of the population elements has been developed, the best method of selecting a sample is to employ a table of random numbers containing columns of digits such as the one appearing in Fig. 15-1. After assigning consecutive numbers to units of the population, the researcher starts at any point on the table of random numbers and reads consecutive numbers in any direction (horizontally, vertically, or diagonally). When a number is read that corresponds with the written unit on a card, that unit is chosen for the sample. The investigator continues to read until a sample of the desired size is drawn.

The advantages of simple random sampling are the following:
1. The sample selection is not subject to the conscious biases of the researcher.
2. The representativeness of the sample in relation to the population characteristics is maximized.
3. The differences in the characteristics of the sample and the population are purely a function of chance.
4. The probability of choosing a nonrepresentative sample decreases as the size of the sample increases.

However, the consumer must remember that despite the utilization of a carefully controlled sampling procedure that minimizes error, there is no guarantee that the sample will be representative. Factors such as sample heterogeneity and subject dropout may jeopardize the representativeness of the sample despite the most stringent random sampling procedure.

The major disadvantage of simple random sampling is that it is a time-consuming and inefficient method for obtaining a random sample. Consider the task of listing all of the baccalaureate nursing students in the United States. In addition, it may be impossible to obtain an accurate or complete listing of every element in the population. Imagine trying to obtain a list of all completed suicides in New York City for the year

```
20 09 54 18 10 49 53 20 29 11 61 32 52 06 56 20 10 38 29 96 05 01 37 99 11 32
37 42 44 92 89 62 39 80 96 99 86 23 14 11 66 63 24 70 34 00 71 99 92 49 13 74
20 80 24 12 87 56 56 05 70 10 46 61 70 51 58 22 96 40 59 60 86 65 36 87 31 10
15 68 56 48 84 93 02 49 15 78 73 46 26 22 37 84 02 31 64 22 73 94 31 90 71 46
93 15 26 67 10 63 99 16 81 49 73 44 24 67 32 47 66 86 08 14 33 44 78 97 18 30
03 71 18 44 50 31 48 18 23 96 48 21 06 89 23 63 00 09 97 85 58 35 66 61 28 25
84 31 97 89 14 96 13 61 83 59 79 12 87 04 18 40 20 11 50 28 61 48 87 44 06 53
26 06 24 52 95 01 65 30 06 10 84 92 93 22 20 56 57 72 57 99 25 70 69 19 98 43
07 09 38 25 04 65 17 20 75 07 69 63 69 10 37 31 44 66 12 39 85 54 52 02 82 33
95 03 87 65 81 03 86 59 16 03 62 88 19 19 63 32 93 05 72 94 52 78 13 63 91 30
61 94 07 43 67 25 66 92 74 77 97 32 69 76 58 25 79 15 44 55 02 38 73 19 96 62
56 81 76 05 32 62 69 99 94 05 05 85 17 10 73 59 62 22 60 68 44 93 55 92 48 59
86 72 78 41 95 08 67 30 65 95 44 50 40 29 08 65 67 45 27 81 33 16 96 58 09 52
54 75 26 06 31 52 40 70 99 12 26 35 99 71 63 18 52 50 09 02 24 57 12 03 02 01
38 94 08 93 95 38 06 71 72 80 30 74 21 08 10 91 85 70 90 68 03 75 10 86 10 78
07 80 46 11 90 58 89 94 97 21 12 25 05 73 71 32 03 11 66 37 44 29 42 75 75 76
88 50 51 24 19 33 41 09 86 10 94 70 74 99 39 58 64 53 70 07 09 62 50 56 67 81
15 97 57 96 75 56 68 65 97 29 19 47 17 22 81 21 35 81 94 46 23 41 39 54 26 78
54 79 88 81 42 21 91 38 47 51 36 25 79 78 24 43 12 59 38 22 80 04 56 74 65 66
75 85 66 33 52 21 89 44 90 49 26 74 40 83 67 37 14 74 66 61 70 22 58 66 18 53
00 13 21 22 16 00 98 72 65 81 58 01 73 67 19 36 06 65 54 55 11 24 37 30 06 11
71 94 55 21 12 81 23 78 46 98 03 40 97 49 61 62 54 35 65 65 36 37 05 82 24 82
57 58 60 36 59 97 02 01 71 64 38 67 03 17 93 92 15 20 68 65 85 27 44 28 04 80
79 79 71 49 24 15 99 69 00 36 20 23 01 29 94 54 29 66 69 26 29 88 91 43 94 34
47 98 26 41 63 08 11 99 04 76 38 61 88 05 66 44 54 92 10 89 39 17 60 78 97 71
05 64 93 40 12 20 75 35 34 63 96 36 93 43 65 14 19 36 54 78 91 51 63 94 01 77
00 84 17 34 41 10 40 47 60 98 94 26 10 54 59 05 66 26 27 72 65 43 49 18 93 76
18 65 50 05 76 03 82 95 54 20 92 77 57 54 38 45 01 73 64 62 05 38 11 51 20 20
60 60 76 75 12 92 87 41 97 28 53 75 19 93 06 08 57 15 31 56 44 15 33 46 55 14
17 67 54 91 82 94 59 46 43 98 77 30 34 89 98 64 61 28 27 25 69 28 71 14 07 16
74 13 15 78 81 02 98 91 18 06 86 15 37 27 96 71 62 44 42 89 89 70 38 37 66 92
32 93 57 33 80 92 07 48 75 39 95 93 81 04 03 75 56 18 67 25 28 08 71 75 01 04
74 01 40 47 25 97 77 31 10 73 78 68 45 55 45 17 59 52 81 94 33 38 46 27 26 30
69 36 01 63 85 62 50 52 53 95 15 76 59 20 79 06 21 23 65 60 34 29 68 18 77 16
01 53 85 65 34 40 65 14 27 22 21 79 68 95 22 20 35 49 26 49 43 20 28 73 79 49
42 55 14 47 79 69 04 42 73 12 76 41 70 23 59 65 03 69 46 59 55 41 12 02 00 14
07 31 98 53 15 89 75 07 05 25 04 14 80 89 30 64 42 85 16 05 57 20 17 22 72 75
61 04 37 16 72 47 78 91 33 70 31 21 95 10 08 23 21 63 35 03 47 19 94 90 28 06
44 96 38 19 06 14 05 56 06 06 92 86
```

Fig. 15-1   A table of random digits. (From Wilson, E. Bright, Jr.: An introduction to scientific research, New York, copyright 1952 by McGraw-Hill, Inc.
Used with permission of McGraw-Hill, Inc.)

1989. It is often the case that although suicide may have been the cause of death,
another cause such as cardiac failure appears on the death certificate. It would be
difficult to estimate how many elements of the target population would be eliminated
from consideration. The issue of bias would definitely enter the picture despite the
researcher's best efforts. Thus the evaluator of a research report must exercise caution

in generalizing from reported findings, even when random sampling is the stated strategy, if the target population has been difficult or impossible to list completely.

Stratified random sampling

Stratified random sampling requires that the population be divided into strata or subgroups. The subgroups or subsets that the population is divided into are homogeneous. An appropriate number of elements from each subset are randomly selected, based on their proportion in the population. This strategy's goal is to achieve a greater degree of representativeness. Stratified random sampling is similar to the proportional stratified quota sampling strategy discussed earlier in the chapter. The major difference is that stratified random sampling utilizes a random selection procedure for obtaining sample subjects. Fig. 15-2 provides an example that illustrates the use of stratified random sampling.

The population is stratified according to any number of attributes such as age, sex, ethnicity, religion, socioeconomic status, or level of completed education. The variables selected to make up the strata should be adaptable to homogeneous subsets with regard to the attributes being studied.

The following criteria can be used for decision making in the selection of a stratified sample:

1. Is there a critical variable or attribute that provides a logical basis for stratifying the sample?
2. Does the population list contain sufficient information about the attributes that will be used to divide the sample into subsets?
3. Is it appropriate for each subset to be equal in size, or is it more appropriate for each subset to be proportionally stratified based on the proportion of each subset in the population?
4. If proportional sampling is being utilized, is there a sufficient number of subjects in each subset for basing meaningful comparisons?
5. Once the subset comparison has been determined, are random procedures used for selection of the sample?

There are several advantages to a stratified sampling strategy: (1) The representativeness of the sample is enhanced. (2) The researcher has a valid basis for making comparisons between subsets if information on the critical variables has been available. (3) The researcher is able to oversample a disproportionately small stratum to adjust for their underrepresentation, statistically weigh the data accordingly, and continue to be able to make legitimate comparisons.

The obstacles encountered by a researcher utilizing this strategy include the following: (1) the difficulty of obtaining a population list containing complete critical variable information, (2) the time-consuming effort of obtaining multiple enumerated lists, and (3) the time and money involved in carrying out a large-scale study utilizing a stratified sampling strategy. The critiquer needs to question the appropriateness of this sampling strategy to the problem under investigation. For example, if the reader refers to Fig. 15-2, it is clear that the study population consisted of diploma, associate degree, and baccalaureate degree nurses, three distinct strata. It is appropriate for the

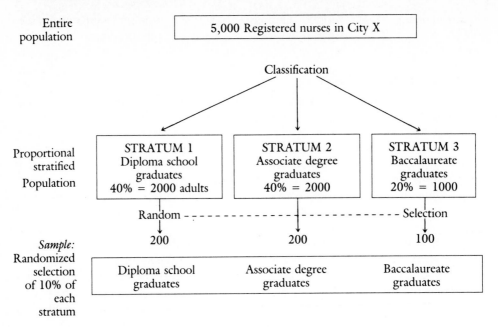

Entire population — 5,000 Registered nurses in City X

Classification

Proportional stratified Population

STRATUM 1
Diploma school graduates
40% = 2000 adults

STRATUM 2
Associate degree graduates
40% = 2000

STRATUM 3
Baccalaureate graduates
20% = 1000

Random - Selection

Sample: Randomized selection of 10% of each stratum

200   200   100

Diploma school graduates   Associate degree graduates   Baccalaureate graduates

Fig. 15-2   Subject selection using a proportional stratified random sampling strategy.

researcher to strive to proportionately represent all three strata in the study sample. This strategy would not be necessary if the researcher were studying only one of the three subsets, unless that subset was being logically divided into strata based on other attributes.

Cluster sampling

Cluster sampling involves a successive random sampling of units that progress from large to small. The first unit consists of large units or "clusters." For example, if a sample of clinical specialists is desired, a random sample of hospitals might make up the cluster. A large-scale national survey would use states as the first unit and proceed to successively smaller units like counties, cities, districts, blocks, and then households.

The clusters are selected by either simple random or stratified random methods. For example, when selecting clusters of hospitals it might be appropriate to stratify by the size of the hospital. The final selection from within a cluster may also be performed by simple random or stratified random sampling. The usual procedure is to begin sampling the large, inclusive unit and proceed to smaller, less inclusive units, and finally to the smallest unit of the population, the individual. This procedure involves successive stages of sampling and so it is called *multistage sampling.*

The main advantage of cluster sampling is that it is considerably more economical in terms of time and money than other types of probability sampling, particularly when the population is large and geographically dispersed. There are two major disadvantages: (1) more sampling errors tend to occur than with simple random or stratified random sampling, and (2) the appropriate handling of the statistical data from cluster samples is very complex.

The reader who is evaluating a research report will need to consider whether the use of cluster sampling is justified in light of the research design as well as other pragmatic considerations such as economy.

Systematic sampling

Systematic sampling refers to a sampling strategy that involves the selection of every "kth" case drawn from a population list at fixed intervals, such as every tenth member listed in the directory of the American Association of Critical-Care Nurses. Systematic sampling might be used to sample every "kth" person to enter a hospital lobby or hospitalized with a diagnosis of acquired immunodeficiency syndrome in 1989. When systematic sampling is used, the population must be narrowly defined as consisting, for example, of all those people entering or leaving in order for the sample to be considered as a probability sample. If senior citizens were sampled systematically on entering a hospital lobby, the resulting sample would not be called a *probability sample,* since not every senior citizen would have a chance of being selected.

However, systematic sampling strategies can be designed to fulfill the requirements of a probability sample. In this case the researcher, who has a list or sampling frame, divides the population *(N)* by the size of the desired sample *(n)* to obtain the sampling interval width *(k)*. The **sampling interval** is the standard distance between the elements chosen for the sample. For example, to select a sample of 50 staff nurses from a population of 500 staff nurses, then the sampling interval would be as follows:

$$k = \frac{500}{50} = 10$$

Essentially, every tenth case (element) on the staff nurse list would be sampled. The first case should be selected by means of a table of random numbers (see Fig. 15-1). In this instance the number 51 is randomly selected from a table. The staff nurses corresponding to numbers 51, 61, 71, and so forth would be included in the sample of 50.

Systematic and simple random sampling are essentially the same type of procedure. The advantage of systematic sampling is that the results are obtained in a more convenient and efficient manner. The disadvantage of systematic sampling is that bias in the form of nonrandomness can inadvertently be introduced to the procedure. This problem may occur if the population list is arranged so that a certain type of element is listed at intervals that coincide with the sampling interval. Let us say that if every tenth nursing student on a population list of all types of nursing students in New York State were a baccalaureate student, and the sampling interval were ten, then baccalaureate students would be overrepresented in the sample. Cyclical fluctuations are also a factor. For example, if a list is kept of nursing students using the college library each day, a biased sample will probably be obtained if every seventh day is chosen as the sampling interval, because fewer and perhaps different nursing students probably study in the library on Sundays than on weekdays. Therefore caution must be exercised about departures from randomness as they affect the representativeness of the sample and, as a result, affect the external validity of the study.

The critiquer will want to note whether or not a satisfactory random selection procedure was carried out. If randomization was not used, the systematic sampling may have become a nonprobability quota sample. It is important to be cognizant of this issue, because the implications related to interpretation and generalizability are drastically altered if the evaluator is dealing with a nonprobability sample.

SAMPLE SIZE

There is no single rule that can be applied to the determination of a sample's size. When arriving at an estimate of sample size, many factors, such as the following, must be considered:

1. The type of sampling procedure being utilized
2. The type of sample estimation formula being used
3. The degree of precision required
4. The heterogeneity of the attributes under investigation
5. The relative frequency of occurrence of the phenomenon of interest in the population; that is, a common versus a rare health problem
6. The projected cost of utilizing a particular sampling strategy

The sample size should be determined before the study is conducted. A general rule of thumb is always to use the largest sample possible. The larger the sample, the more representative of the population it is likely to be; smaller samples produce less accurate results.

The principle of "larger is better" holds true for both probability and nonprobability samples. Results based on small samples (under 10) tend to be unstable; that is, the values fluctuate from one sample to the next. Small samples tend to increase the probability of obtaining a markedly deviant sample. As the sample size increases the mean more closely approximates the population values and thus introduces less sampling error.

An example of this concept is illustrated by a study in which the average monthly sleeping pill consumption is being investigated for clients on a rehabilitation unit after a cerebrovascular accident. The data in Table 15-3 indicate that the population consists of 20 clients whose average consumption of sleeping pills is 15.15 per month. Two simple random samples with sample sizes of two, four, six, and 10 have been drawn from the population of 20 clients. Each sample average in the right-hand column represents an estimate of the population average, which is known to be 15.15. In most cases the population value is unknown to the researchers, but because the population is so small, we could calculate it. As we examine the data in Table 15-3, we note that with a sample size of two, the estimate might have been wrong by as much as eight

Table 15-3 **Comparison of Population and Sample Values and Averages in Study of Sleeping Pill Consumption**

Number in group	Group	Number of sleeping pills consumed (values expressed monthly)	Average
20	Population	1, 3, 4, 5, 6, 7, 9, 11, 13, 15, 16, 17, 19, 21, 22, 23, 25, 27, 29, 30	15.15
2	Sample 1A	6, 9	7.5
2	Sample 1B	21, 25	23.0
4	Sample 2A	1, 7, 15, 25	12.0
4	Sample 2B	5, 13, 23, 29	17.5
6	Sample 3A	3, 4, 11, 15, 21, 25	13.3
6	Sample 3B	5, 7, 11, 19, 27, 30	16.5
10	Sample 4A	3, 4, 7, 9, 11, 13, 17, 21, 23, 30	13.8
10	Sample 4B	1, 4, 6, 11, 15, 17, 19, 23, 25, 27	14.8

sleeping pills in sample 1B. As the sample size increases the averages get closer to the population value and the differences in the estimates between samples A and B get smaller as well. Large samples permit the principles of randomization to work effectively; that is, to counterbalance, in the long run, atypical values.

It is possible to estimate the sample size with the use of a statistical procedure known as *power analysis* (Cohen, 1977). It is beyond the scope of this chapter to describe this complex procedure in great detail, but a simple example will illustrate its use. A researcher wants to determine the effect of nurse preoperative teaching on client postoperative anxiety. Clients are randomly assigned to an experimental group or a control group. How many clients should be used in the study? When using power analysis the researcher must estimate how large a difference will be observed between the groups; that is, the difference in the mean amount of postoperative anxiety following the experimental preoperative teaching program. If a small difference is expected, the sample would need to be large (in this case 196 patients in each group) to ensure that the differences will actually be revealed in a statistical analysis. If a medium-sized difference is expected, the total sample size would be 128, 64 in each group. When expected differences are large it does not take a very large sample to ensure that differences will be revealed through statistical analysis.

Power analysis is an advanced statistical technique that is used increasingly by researchers and is a requirement for external funding. When it is not used, research studies may be based on samples that are too small. When samples are too small, the researcher may have unsupported hypotheses and may commit a type I error of accepting a null hypothesis when it should have been rejected (see Chapter 17).

Despite the principles related to determining sample size that have been identified, the consumer should be aware that large samples do not ensure representativeness or accuracy. A large sample cannot compensate for a faulty research design. The proportion of the population that is sampled does not provide a guarantee of accurate results. It is often possible to obtain accurate results from only a small fraction of a large population. For example, a 10% probability sample of a population containing 1500 elements will yield more precise results than a nonprobability 0.01% sample of a population with 100,000 elements.

The critiquer should evaluate the sample size in terms of whether or not it adequately represents the elements and subsets of the population. Unless representativeness is ensured, all the data in the world become inconsequential.

SAMPLING PROCEDURES

Critera for drawing a sample will vary according to the sampling strategy. Regardless of which strategy is used, it is important that the procedure be systematically organized. This will eliminate the bias that occurs when sample selection is carried out inconsistently. Several general steps can be identified that will ensure a consistent approach by the researcher. Initially the target population must be identified; that is, the entire group of people or objects about whom the researcher wants to draw conclusions or make generalizations. The target population may consist of all male clients with a first-time myocardial infarction, all children with acute leukemia, all pregnant teenagers, or all doctoral students in the United States. Next, the accessible portion of the target population must be delineated. An accessible population might consist of all clinical specialists in the state of California, or all male clients with acquired immunodeficiency syndrome admitted to hospital X during 1989, or all pregnant teenagers in a specific prenatal clinic, or all children with acute leukemia under care at a specific hospital specializing in oncology. Then, once the accessible population has been established, permission is obtained from the institution's research committee. This permission provides free access to the desired population. Finally, a sampling plan or a protocol for actually selecting the sample from the accessible population is formulated. The researcher makes decisions about how subjects will be approached, how the study will be explained, and who will select the sample—the researcher or a research assistant. Regardless of who implements the sampling plan, consistency in how it is done is of paramount importance. The reader of a research study will want to find a description of the sample as well as the sampling procedure in the report. Based on the appropriateness of what has been reported, the critiquer is able to make judgments about the soundness of the sampling protocol, which of course will affect the interpretations made about the findings.

When an appropriate sample size and sampling strategy have been used, the researcher can feel more confident that the sample is representative of the accessible population; however, it is more difficult to feel confident that the accessible population is representative of the target population. Are clinical specialists in California representative of all clinical specialists in the United States? It is impossible to be sure about this. Researchers must exercise judgment when assessing typicality. Unfortunately there are no guidelines for making such judgments, and there is even less basis for the critiquer to make such decisions. The best rule of thumb to use when evaluating the representativeness of a sample and its generalizability to the target population is to be realistic and conservative about making sweeping claims relative to the findings.

CRITIQUING THE SAMPLE

The criteria for critiquing the sampling technique of a study are presented in the box on p. 284. The research consumer approaches the sample section of a research report with a different perspective than does the researcher. The consumer must raise two questions. The first question asks, "If this study were to be replicated, would there be enough information presented about the nature of the population, the sample, the sampling strategy, and sample size for another investigator to carry out the study?" The second question asks, "Are the previously mentioned factors appropriate in light of the particular research design, and if not, which factors require modification, especially if the study is to be replicated?"

Sampling is considered to be one important aspect of the methodology of a research study. As such, data pertaining to the sample usually appear in the methodology section of the research report. The sampling content presented should reflect the outcome of a series of decisions based on sampling criteria appropriate to the design of the study as well as the options and limitations inherent in the context of the investigation. The following discussion will highlight several sampling criteria that the research consumer will want to consider when evaluating the merit of a sampling strategy as it relates to a specific research study.

Initially the parameters or attributes of the study population should clearly specify to what population the findings may be generalized. Generally the target population of the study is not specifically identified by the researcher, but the nature of it is implied in the description of the accessible population and the sample. For example, if a researcher states that 100 subjects were randomly drawn from a population of married primiparas who were vaginally delivered of full-term infants at hospital L during 1989, the critiquer is able to specifically evaluate the parameters of the population. Demographic characteristics of the sample such as age, sex, diagnosis, ethnicity, religion, and marital status should also be presented, since they provide further explication about the nature of the sample and enable the critiquer to evaluate the sampling procedure more accurately. For example, in a study by Krouse and Krouse (1982) titled "Cancer as a Crisis: The Critical Elements of Adjustment," the age range of the subjects was 30 to 60 years of age. Additionally, the subjects were potential candidates for mastectomy or hysterectomy. The subjects were divided into three sample groups according to the diagnosis and the type of treatment. However, age was not a factor in terms of grouping subjects. The evaluator who has this demographic sample information available is able to question the validity of utilizing a sampling strategy that does not also consider the differential effect of age on an individual's adjustment to cancer. It would seem logical that there might be a difference

Critiquing Criteria

1. Do the parameters of the study population specify to what population the findings may be generalized?
2. Is the sample representative of the population as defined?
3. Would it be possible to replicate the study population?
4. Is the method of sample selection appropriate? How was the sample selected?
5. What bias, if any, is introduced by this method?
6. Is the sample size appropriate? How is it substantiated?
7. Are there indications that the human rights of the subjects have been ensured?

in terms of adjustment between a 30-year-old woman and a 66-year-old woman each having a mastectomy.

It is also helpful if the researcher has presented a rationale for having elected to study one type of population versus another. For example, why did the previously cited study focus only on married primiparas who were vaginally delivered of full-term infants, as opposed to unmarried women or women who had had cesarean births? In a research study that utilizes a nonprobability sampling strategy, it is particularly important to fully describe the population and the sample in terms of who the study subjects are, how they were chosen, and why they were chosen. If these criteria are adhered to, the degree of heterogeneity or homogeneity of the sample can be determined. The utilization of a homogeneous sample minimizes the amount of sampling error introduced, a problem particularly common in nonprobability sampling.

Next, the defined representativeness of the population should be examined. Probability sampling is clearly the ideal sampling procedure for ensuring the representativeness of a study population. Utilization of random selection procedures such as simple random, stratified, cluster, or systematic sampling strategies minimizes the occurrence of conscious and unconscious biases, which, of course, would affect the researcher's ability to generalize about the findings from the sample to the population. The evaluator should be able to identify the type of probability strategy utilized and to determine whether the researcher adhered to the criteria for a particular sampling plan. In experimental and quasiexperimental studies the evaluator must also know whether or how the subjects were assigned to groups. If the criteria have not been followed, the reader would have a valid basis for being cautious about the proposed conclusions of the study.

Although random selection is the ideal in establishing the representativeness of a study population, more often realistic barriers, such as institutional policy, inaccessibility of subjects, lack of time or money, and the current state of knowledge in the field, necessitate the utilization of nonprobability sampling strategies. Many important research problems that are of interest to nursing do not lend themselves to experimental design and probability sampling. A well-designed, carefully controlled study utilizing a nonprobability sampling strategy can yield accurate and meaningful findings that make a significant contribution to nursing's scientific body of knowledge. The critiquer needs to ask a philosophical question: "If it is not possible to conduct an experimental or quasiexperimental investigation that utilizes probability sampling, should the study be abandoned?" The answer usually suggests that it is better to carry out the investigation and be fully aware of the limitations of the methodology, than to lose the knowledge that can be gained. The researcher is always able to move on to subsequent studies that either replicate the study or utilize more stringent design and sampling strategies to refine the knowledge derived from a nonexperimental study.

The critiquer of a research study will want to apply the following criteria as a standard for evaluating the sampling plan:

1. Have the population and sample characteristics been completely described?
2. Are criteria for eligibility in the sample specifically identified?
3. Have sample delimitations been established?
4. How was the sample selected?
5. What kinds of bias are inherent in this type of selection procedure?
6. What factors influenced the researcher's choice of a sampling plan?
7. How homogeneous or heterogeneous is the sample?
8. How conservative is the researcher about the inferences and conclusions drawn from the data?
9. Does the researcher identify the limitations in generalizability of the findings from the sample to the population?
10. Does the researcher indicate how replication of the study with new samples would provide increased support for the findings?

The greatest difficulty in nonprobability sampling stems from the fact that not every element in the population has an equal chance of being represented in the sample. Therefore it is likely that some segment of the population will be systematically underrepresented. If the population is homogeneous on critical characteristics, systematic bias will not be very important. However, few of the attributes that researchers are interested in are sufficiently homogeneous to render sampling bias an irrelevant consideration.

Next, the sampling plan's suitability to the research design should be evaluated. Experimental and quasiexperimental designs utilize some form of random selection or random assignment of subjects to groups (see Chapter 9). The critiquer evaluates whether or not the researcher adhered to the principles of random selection and assignment. Lack of adherence to such principles compromises the representativeness of the sample and the external validity of the study. The following are questions the evaluator might pose relative to this issue:

1. Has a random selection procedure been identified, such as a table of random members?

2. Has the appropriate random sampling plan been selected; that is, has a proportional stratified sampling plan been selected instead of a simple random sampling plan in a study where there are three distinct occupational levels that appear to be critical variables for stratification?

3. Has the particular random sampling plan been carried out appropriately; that is, if a cluster sampling strategy was utilized, did the sampling units logically progress from the largest to the smallest?

Random sampling should not be looked on as a cure-all. Sometimes bias is inadvertently introduced even when the principle of random selection is utilized.

Nonexperimental designs often utilize nonprobability sampling strategies. In this instance the question that can be raised by the critiquer is whether or not a nonexperimental design and a related nonprobability sampling plan were most appropriate for this study. It is sometimes true that if the researcher had utilized another type of design or sampling plan, he or she could have constructed a stronger study that would have allowed greater confidence to be placed in the findings and greater generalizability. However, the critiquer is rarely in a position to know what factors entered into the decision to plan one type of study versus another.

Then the evaluator should determine if the sample size is appropriate and whether its size is justifiable. It is unusual for the researcher to indicate in a research article how the sample size was arrived at; this is more commonly seen in doctoral dissertations. However, the method of arriving at the sample size and the rationale should be briefly mentioned. For example, a researcher may state in a very detailed way

> The sample size was set on the basis of a significance level of 0.05, a medium effect of 0.13, and a power of 0.95 in multiple regression analysis (Cohen, 1977). This sample size, $N = 168$, is larger than required for nine predictors with a conventional power of 0.80 ($N = 110$). The sample size was expanded to allow for the shrinkage of R^2.

The importance of this example lies not in understanding every technical word cited but rather in understanding that this type of statement or some abbreviated form of it meets the criteria stated at the beginning of the paragraph and should be evident on the research report.

Other considerations with respect to sample size, especially where the sample size appears to be small or inadequate and there is no stated rationale for the size, are the following:

◇ How will the sample size affect the accuracy of the results?
◇ Are any subsets or cells of the sample overrepresented or underrepresented?
◇ Are any of the subsets so small as to limit meaningful comparisons?
◇ Has the researcher examined the effect of attrition or dropouts on the results?
◇ Has the researcher recognized and identified any limitations posed by the size of the sample?

Essentially, these criteria demand that the critiquer carefully scrutinize several important elements pertaining to sample size that have implications for the generalizability of the findings.

Finally, evidence that the rights of human subjects have been protected should appear in the sample section of the research report. The critiquer will evaluate whether permission was obtained from an institutional review board that reviewed the study relative to the maintenance of ethical research standards (see Chapter 3). For example, the review board examines the research proposal to determine if the introduction of an experimental procedure may be potentially harmful and therefore undesirable. The critiquer also examines the report for evidence of informed consent on the part of subjects as well as protection of confidentiality or anonymity. It is highly unusual for research studies not to demonstrate evidence of having met these criteria. Nevertheless, the careful evaluator will want to be certain that ethical standards that protect sample subjects have been maintained.

It is evident that there are many factors to consider when critiquing the sample section of a research report. The type and appropriateness of the sampling strategy become crucial elements in the analysis and interpretation of data, in the conclusions derived from the findings, and in the generalizability of the findings from the sample to the population. As stated earlier in this chapter, the major purpose of sampling is to increase the efficiency of a research study by utilizing a sample that is representative of the particular population so that every element need not be studied, and yet generalizing the findings from the sample to the population. The critiquer needs to justify that the sampling strategy utilized provided a valid basis for feeling confident of the findings and their generalizability.

SUMMARY

Sampling is a process that selects representative units of a population for study. Researchers sample representative segments of the population, because it is rarely feasible or necessary to sample entire populations of interest to obtain accurate and meaningful information.

A *population* is a well-defined set that has certain specified properties. A population may consist of people, objects, or events. Researchers establish *eligibility criteria;* these are descriptors of the population and provide the basis for selection into a sample. Eligibility criteria, also referred to as *delimitations,* include the following: age, sex, socioeconomic status, level of education, religion, and ethnicity. The researcher must identify the *target population;* that is, the entire set of cases about which the researcher would like to make generalizations. However, because of pragmatic constraints, the researcher usually utilizes an *accessible population,* one that meets the population criteria and is available.

Sampling is a process that selects a portion of the designated population to represent the entire population. A *sample* is a set of elements that comprise the population. A *sampling unit* is the element or set of elements used for selecting the sample. The foremost criterion in evaluating a sample is the *representativeness* or congruence of characteristics with the population.

Sampling strategies consist of nonprobability and probability sampling. In *nonprobability sampling* the elements are chosen by nonrandom methods. Types of nonprobability sampling include convenience, quota, and purposive sampling. *Probability sampling* is characterized by the random selection of elements from the population. In *random selection* each element in the population has an equal and independent chance of being included in the sample. Types of probability sampling include simple random, stratified random, cluster, and systematic sampling.

Sample size is a function of the type of sampling procedure being used, the degree of precision required, the type of sample estimation formula being used, the heterogeneity of study attributes, the relative frequency of occurrence of the phenomena under consideration, and cost.

Criteria for drawing a sample vary according to the sampling strategy. Systematic organization of the sampling procedure minimizes bias. The target population is identified, the accessible portion of the target population is delineated, permission to conduct the research study is obtained, and a sampling plan is formulated.

The critiquer of a research report evaluates the sampling plan for its appropriateness in relation to the particular research design. Completeness of the sampling plan is examined in light of potential replicability of the study. The critiquer evaluates whether the sampling strategy is the strongest plan for the particular study under consideration.

An appropriate systematic sampling plan will maximize the efficiency of a research study. It will increase the accuracy and meaningfulness of the findings and enhance the generalizability of the findings from the sample to the population.

References

Bright, W.E., Jr. (1952). *An introductin to scientific research,* New York, McGraw-Hill Book Co.

Brown, R.C., Jr. (1976). Research Q and A on sampling, *Nursing Research,* **25**:62.

Cohen, J. (1977). *Statistical power analysis for the behavioral sciences* (rev. ed.), New York, Academic Press.

Downs, F.S., and Newman, M.A. (1977). *A source book of nursing research,* Philadelphia, F.A. Davis Co.

Kerlinger, F.N. (1986). *Foundations of behavioral research,* New York, Holt, Rinehart & Winston, Inc.

Krouse, H.J., and Krouse, J.H. (1982). Cancer as a crisis: the critical elements of adjustment, *Nursing Research,* **31**:96-100.

Kunnel, M.T., O'Brien, C., Hazard Munro, B., and Medoff-Cooper, B. (1988). Comparison of rectal, femoral, axillary, and skin-to-mattress temperatures in stable neonates, *Nursing Research,* **37**:162-164.

Levey, P.S., and Lemeshow, S. (1980). *Sampling for health professionals,* New York, Lifetime Learning.

Owens, J.F., McCann, C.S., and Hutelmyer, C.M. (1978). Cardiac rehabilitation: a patient education program, *Nursing Research,* **27**:148-150.

Sudman, S. (1976). *Applied sampling,* New York, Academic Press.

Van Dalen, D.B. (1979). *Understanding educational research,* 4th ed., New York, McGraw-Hill Book Co.

Volicer, B.J. (1984). *Multivariate statistics for nursing research,* Orlando, Fla., Grune & Stratton, Inc.

16

Descriptive Data Analysis

Ann Bello

LEARNING OBJECTIVES

After reading this chapter the student should be able to do the following:

⋄ Define descriptive statistics

⋄ State the purposes of descriptive statistics

⋄ Identify the levels of measurement in a research study

⋄ Describe a frequency distribution

⋄ List measures of central tendency and their use

⋄ List measures of variability and their use

⋄ Critically analyze the descriptive statistics utilized in published research studies

KEY TERMS

descriptive statistics	modality
frequency distribution	mode
interval measurement	nominal measurement
kurtosis	normal curve
levels of measurement	ordinal measurement
mean	percentile
measurement	range
measures of central tendency	ratio measurement
measures of variability	semiquartile range
median	standard deviation
modal percentage	Z score

After carefully collecting data the researcher is faced with the task of organizing the individual pieces of information so that the meaning is clear. It would be neither practical nor helpful to the reader to list individually each piece of data collected. The researcher must choose methods of organizing the raw data based both on the kind of data collected and on the hypothesis that was tested.

Statistical procedures are used to give organization and meaning to data. Procedures that allow researchers to describe and summarize data are known as **descriptive statistics.** Procedures that allow researchers to estimate how reliably they can make predictions based on the data are known as *inferential statistics* (see Chapter 17). Descriptive statistical techniques reduce data to manageable proportions by summarizing them, and they also describe various characteristics of the data under study. Descriptive techniques include **measures of central tendency,** such as **mode, median,** and **mean; measures of variability,** such as **modal percentage, range,** and **standard deviation;** and some correlation techniques, such as scatter plots. The research consumer does not need a detailed knowledge of how to calculate these statistics but does need an understanding of their meaning, use, and limitations.

Measures of central tendency describe the average member of the sample, whereas measures of variability describe how much dispersion is in the sample. If a researcher reported that the average age of one nursing class was 22 years, with the youngest member being 18 and the oldest 25, and that in another nursing class students had an average age of 22 years but the youngest member was 17 and the oldest 45, the reader would form a very different picture of the two classes. In both cases the average member of the sample was the same, but in the second class there was much greater variation or dispersion in the age of the members of the class.

Descriptive statistics may by presented in several ways in a research report. The data may be reported in words in the text of the report or summarized in tables or graphs. Whatever the method of presentation, the report should give the reader a clear and orderly picture of the research results.

This chapter and the next are designed to provide the reader of nursing research with an understanding of statistical procedures. This chapter will focus on the understanding and evaluation of descriptive statistical procedures, and the next chapter will discuss inferential statistical procedures. To evaluate the appropriateness of the statistical procedures used in a study, the research consumer should have an understanding of the **levels of measurement** that are appropriate to each statistical technique.

LEVELS OF MEASUREMENT

Measurement is the assignment of numbers to objects or events according to rules (Kerlinger, 1986). Every event that is assigned a specific number must be similar to every other event assigned that number; for example, male subjects may be assigned the number 1 and female subjects the number 2. The measurement level is determined by the nature of the object or event being measured. Levels of measurement in ascending order are nominal, ordinal, interval, and ratio. The levels of measurement are the determining factors of the type of statistics to be used in analyzing data.

The higher the level of measurement, the greater the flexibility the researcher has in choosing statistical procedures. Every attempt should be made to utilize the highest level of measurement possible so that the maximum amount of information will be obtained from the data (see Table 16-1).

Nominal measurement

Nominal measurement is used to classify objects or events into categories. The categories are mutually exclusive; the object or event either has the characteristic or does not have it. The numbers assigned to each category are nothing more than labels; such numbers do not indicate more or less of a characteristic. Examples of nominal level measurement can be used to categorize a sample on such information as sex, hair color, marital state, or religious affiliation. In Brooten, Kumar, Brown, Butts, Finkler, Bakewell-Sachs, and Delivoria-Papadopoulos' (1986) study of early discharge of low-birth-weight infants from hospitals, there are several examples of nominal level measurement, including the mother's marital status, race, the availability of a telephone in the home, type of health insurance, and the infant's need for an apnea monitor. The nominal level of measurement allows the least amount of mathematical manipulation. Most commonly the *frequency* of each event is counted as well as the *percent of the total* each category represents. In Table 1 of their study Brooten et al. summarize much of the nominal data in their study by reporting first the total number of mothers in each group and then the percent of the mothers who fall into each of the categories, such as marital status, race, and type of hospital insurance (see Appendix A).

Ordinal measurement

Ordinal measurement is used to show relative rankings of objects or events. The numbers assigned to each category can be compared, and a member of a higher category can be said to have more of an attribute that one in a lower category. The

Table 16-1 **Summary Table**

Measurement	Description	Measures of central tendency	Measures of variability
Nominal	Classification	Mode	Modal percentage range
Ordinal	Relative rankings	Mode, median	Range, percentile, semi-quartile range
Interval	Rank ordering with equal intervals	Mode, median, mean	Range, percentile, semi-quartile range, standard deviation
Ratio	Rank ordering with equal intervals and absolute zero	Mode, median, mean	All

intervals between numbers on the scale are not necessarily equal nor is zero an absolute zero. For example, ordinal measurement is used to formulate class rankings where one student can be ranked higher or lower than another. However, the difference in actual grade point average between students may differ widely. Baillie, Norbeck, and Barnes' (1988) study of family caregivers of the elderly measured the level of functioning of the elderly using ordinal level scales. The scale reflected the ability of the elderly individuals to care for themselves. A low number reflected greater self-care ability than a higher number, but it is not possible to say a score of 4 represents four times less self-care ability than a score of 1.

Ordinal level data are limited in the amount of mathematical manipulation possible. In addition to what is possible with nominal data, *medians,* **percentiles,** and *rank order coefficients of correlation* can be calculated.

Interval measurement

Interval measurement shows rankings of events or objects on a scale with equal intervals between the numbers. The zero point remains arbitrary. For example, interval measurements are used in measuring temperatures on the Fahrenheit scale. The distances between degrees are equal, but the zero point is arbitrary. Kunnel, O'Brien, Hazard Munro, and Medoff-Cooper's (1988) study of temperatures in stable neonates illustrates the use of interval measurement.

In many areas in the social sciences, including nursing, there is much controversy over the classification of the level of measurement of intelligence, aptitude, and personality tests, with some regarding these measurements as ordinal and others as interval. The research consumer needs to be aware of this controversy and to look at each study individually in terms of how the data are analyzed (Kerlinger, 1986). Interval level data allow more manipulation of data, including the addition and subtraction

Table 16-2 Frequency Distribution

Individual				Group		
Score	Tally	Frequency		Score	Tally	Frequency
90	ǀ	1		> 89	ǀ	1
88	ǀ	1				
86	ǀ	1		80-89	⽶ ⽶ ⽶	15
84	⽶ ǀ	6				
82	ǁ	2		70-79	⽶ ⽶ ⽶	23
80	⽶	5			⽶ ǀǁǁ	
78	⽶	5				
76	ǀ	1		60-69	⽶ ⽶	10
74	⽶ ǁ	7				
72	⽶ ǁǁǁ	9		< 59	ǁ	2
70	ǀ	1				
68	ǁǁ	3				
66	ǁ	2				
64	ǁǁǁ	4				
62	ǀ	1				
60		0				
58	ǀ	1				
56		0				
54	ǀ	1				
52		0				
50		0				
TOTAL		51				51

Mean, 73.1; standard deviation, +12.1; median, 74; mode, 72; range, 36 (54-90).

of numbers and the *calculation of means.* This additional manipulation is why many want to argue for the higher classification level.

Ratio measurement

Ratio measurement shows rankings of events or objects on scales with equal intervals and absolute zeros. The number represents the actual amount of the property the object possesses. This is the highest level of measurement, but it is usually achieved only in the physical sciences. Examples of ratio level data are height, weight, pulse, and blood pressure. Brooten et al.'s (1986) study (Appendix A) has several examples of ratio data, including infant weight at birth and discharge.

All mathematical procedures can be performed on data from ratio scales. Therefore the use of any statistical procedure is possible as long as it is appropriate to the design of the study (see Chapter 17).

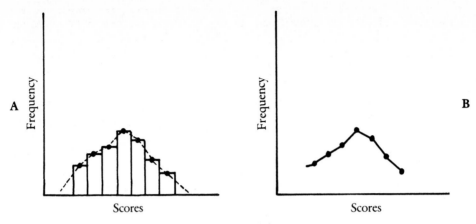

Fig. 16-1 **A,** Histogram and **B,** frequency polygon.

FREQUENCY DISTRIBUTION

One of the most basic ways of organizing data is in a **frequency distribution.** In a *frequency distribution* the number of times each event occurs is counted or the data are grouped and the frequency of each group is reported. An instructor reporting the results of an exam could report the number of students receiving each grade or could group the grades and report the number in each group. Table 16-2 shows the results of an exam given to a class of 51 students. The results of the exam are reported in several ways. The columns on the left give the raw data *tally* and the *frequency* for each grade, whereas the columns on the right give the grouped-data tally and grouped frequencies.

Bliss-Holtz (1988), in her study of "Primiparas' Prenatal Concern for Learning Infant Care," rather than reporting the results for each women for each week of pregnancy, places the women in groups labeled early, middle, and late pregnancy and reports the results for each group.

When data are grouped it is necessary to define the size of the group or the *interval width* so that no score will fall into two groups. The grouping of the data in Table 16-2 prevents overlap; each score falls into only one group. If the grouping had been 70 to 80 and 80 to 90, scores of 80 would have fallen into two categories. The grouping should allow for a precise presentation of the data without serious loss of information. Very large interval widths lead to loss of data information and may obscure patterns in the data. If the test scores in Table 16-2 had been grouped as 40 to 69 and 70 to 99, the pattern of the scores would have been obscured.

Information about frequency distributions may be presented in the form of a table such as Table 16-2 or in graphic form. Fig. 16-1 illustrates the most common graphic forms: the histogram and the frequency polygon. The two graphic methods are similar in that both plot scores or percents of occurrence against frequency. The greater the number of points plotted, the smoother the resulting graph. The shape of the resulting graph allows for observations that will further describe the data.

Table 16-3 Illustration of Data Reporting: Anxiety and Depression in Mothers of Preterm and Term Infants

| | | Preterm infants | | | | | Term infants | | | |
| | | Anxiety | | Depression | | | Anxiety | | Depression | |
Week	N	Mean	SD	Mean	SD	N	Mean	SD	Mean	SD
1	41	37.6	7.1	6.5	3.1	41	31.8	10.6	5.0	2.3
2	16	34.3	6.2	6.2	3.1	10	32.1	5.9	6.6	3.8
3	16	33.5	8.2	6.6	5.1	10	35.6	8.0	6.3	3.5
4	16	32.7	11.7	6.8	5.2	10	36.9	14.2	7.2	6.5
5	16	39.0	15.1	8.7	7.0	10	35.2	10.2	7.0	4.8
6	16	34.1	9.7	6.9	3.8	10	34.8	9.9	6.6	4.4
7	16	34.8	5.9	6.0	3.3	10	35.2	8.6	8.7	5.7

From Gennaro, S. (1988). *Nursing Research,* **37**:2.
SD, Standard deviation.

MEASURES OF CENTRAL TENDENCY

Measures of central tendency answer questions such as, "What does the average nurse think?" and "What is the average temperature of clients on a unit?" They yield a single number that describes the middle of the group. They summarize the members of a sample. Therefore they are known as summary statistics and are sample specific. Since they are sample specific, they will change with each sample. Gennaro (1988, p. 84), in her study of anxiety and depression in postpartum women, lists the mean anxiety and depression scores for each of her groups of mothers for the first 7 weeks post partum (Table 16-3). These scores represent the average amount of anxiety and depression the mothers experienced each week.

The characteristics of a sample in a study are described in terms of summary statistics. The mean test score reported in Table 16-2 is an example of such a statistic. If a different group of students were given the same test, it is likely that the mean would be different.

The term *average* is a nonspecific, general term. In statistics there are three kinds of averages: the mode, the median, and the mean. Depending on the distribution, these may not all give the same answer to the question, "What is the average?" Each type of average has a specific use and is most appropriate to specific kinds of measurement and types of distributions.

Mode

The *mode* is the most frequent score or result, and it can be obtained by inspection of the frequency distribution table or graph. A distribution can have more than one mode. The number of modes contained in a distribution is called the **modality** of the distribution. Figs. 16-2, *A* and *E,* and 16-3 show unimodal or one-peak distributions. Fig. 16-2, *B,* shows a bimodal or two-peaked distribution. Multimodal distributions

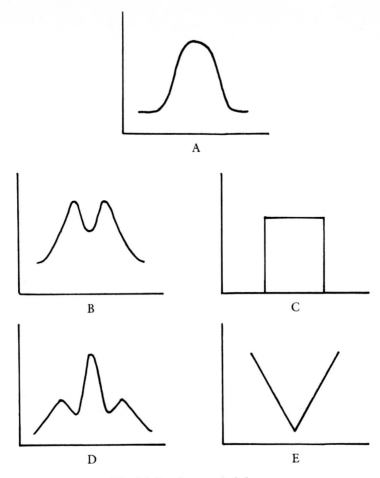

Fig. 16-2 Symmetrical shapes.

having two or more peaks are shown in Fig. 16-2, *B* and *D*. Table 16-4 illustrates how the change in a few scores can change the modality of a distribution from unimodal to bimodal.

The mode is most appropriately used with nominal data. It cannot be used for any subsequent calculations, and it is unstable; that is, the mode can fluctuate widely from sample to sample from the same population. A change in just one score in Table 16-2 would change the mode from 72.

Median

The *median* is the middle score or the score where 50% of the scores are above it and 50% of the scores are below it. The median is not sensitive to extremes in high and low scores. In the series of scores in Table 16-2 the twenty-sixth score will always be the median regardless of how high the highest or low the lowest

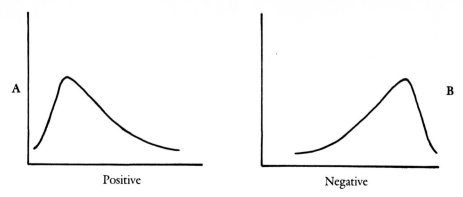

Positive   Negative

Fig. 16-3   **A**, Positive and, **B**, negative skew.

score. It is best used when the data are skewed (see The Normal Distribution in this chapter) and the researcher is interested in the "typical" score. For example, if age is a variable and there is a wide range with extreme scores that may affect the mean, it would be appropriate to also report the median. The median is easy to find by either inspection or calculation.

Mean

The *mean* is the arithmetic average of all the scores. It is what is usually thought of when the term *average* is used in general conversation and is the most widely used measure of central tendency. Most tests of significance use the mean (see Chapter 17). The mean is affected by every score but is more stable than the median or mode, and

Table 16-4 **Measures of Central Tendency**

Score	Frequency	Measure
35	‖‖	
36	‖‖ ‖‖	Mode
37	‖‖‖‖	Median, mean
38	‖‖	
39	‖‖	
40	‖‖ ‖	
35	‖‖	
36	‖‖ ‖‖‖	Mode
37	‖‖‖	Mean
38	‖‖‖‖	Median
39	‖‖ ‖‖‖	Mode
40	‖‖	

of the three measures of central tendency, it is the most constant or least affected by chance. The larger the sample size, the less affected the mean will be by a single extreme score. The mean is generally considered the single best point for summarizing data. In Table 16-4 the mean is the least affected by the change in the distribution from unimodal to bimodal.

When one compares the measures of central tendency, the mean is the most stable and the median the most typical of these statistics. If the distribution is symmetrical and unimodal, the mean, median, and mode will coincide. If the distribution is skewed, the mean will be pulled in the direction of the long tail of the distribution. With a skewed distribution, all three statistics should be reported. For example, national income in the United States is skewed. The mean wage differs from the median wage, because the large salaries are so much greater than the low salaries. The median or the mode would be more representative of the average income. The mean and the median always exist in a sample and are unique; however, there may not be a single mode. The mode is the easiest to calculate, but the mean is the most useful for additional calculations.

THE NORMAL DISTRIBUTION

The concept of the normal distribution is a theoretical one, based on the observation that data from repeated measures of interval or ratio level group themselves about a midpoint in a distribution in a manner that closely approximates the **normal curve** illustrated in Fig. 16-4. In addition, if the means of a large number of samples of the same interval or ratio data are calculated and plotted on a graph, that curve also approximates the normal curve. This tendency of the means to approximate the normal curve is termed the *sampling distribution of the means*. The mean of the sampling distribution of the means is the mean of the population (see Chapter 17).

The normal curve is one that is symmetrical about the mean and is unimodal. The mean, median, and mode are equal. An additional characteristic of the normal curve is that a fixed percentage of the scores fall within a given distance of the mean. As shown in Fig. 16-4, about 68% of the scores or means will fall within ± 1 standard deviation (SD) of the mean, 95% within ± 2 SD of the mean, and 99.7% within ± 3 SD of the mean.

Skewness

Not all samples of data approximate the normal curve. Some samples are *nonsymmetrical* and have the peak off center. If one tail is longer than the other, the distribution is described in terms of *skew*. In a positive skew the bulk of the data are at the low end of the range and there is a longer tail pointing to the right or the positive end of the graph. Worldwide individual income has a positive skew, with most individuals in the low to moderate range and very few in the upper range. The mean in a positive skew is to the right of the median. In a negative skew the bulk of the data are in the high

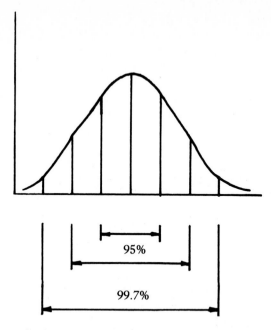

Fig. 16-4 Standard deviation. Normal curve.

range and there is a longer tail pointing to the left or the negative end of the graph. Age at death in the United States has a negative skew, since most deaths occur at older ages. In a negative skew the mean is to the left of the median. Fig. 16-3 illustrates positive and negative skew. In each diagram the peak is off center and one tail is longer.

Symmetry

When the two halves of a distribution are folded over and they can be superimposed on each other, the distribution is said to be *symmetrical.* In other words, the two halves of the distribution are mirror images of each other. The overall shape of the distribution does not affect symmetry. Although the shapes in Fig. 16-2 are different, they are all symmetrical; however, only Fig. 16-2, *A,* approximates the normal curve.

Symmetry and modality are independent. Look at Figs. 16-2, *A,* and 16-3. These are all unimodal, but Fig. 16-3 is skewed, whereas Fig. 16-2, *A,* is symmetrical.

Kurtosis

Kurtosis is related to the peakness or flatness of a distribution. The peakness or flatness of a distribution is related to the spread of the data. The farther the data are spread out on a scale, the flatter the peak. The distribution that peaks sharply is called *leptokurtic,* whereas a broad, flat distribution is *platykurtic.* Fig. 16-5 illustrates kurtosis. Neither the leptokurtic nor the platykurtic distributions approximate the normal curve.

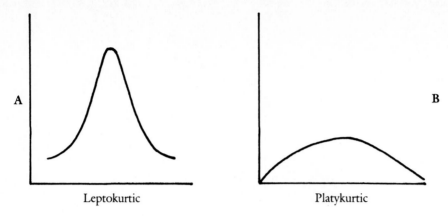

Fig. 16-5   Kurtosis. **A**, Leptokurtosis. **B**, Platykurtosis.

INTERPRETING MEASURES OF VARIABILITY

Variability or dispersion is concerned with the spread of data. Samples with the same mean could differ in both distribution (kurtosis) and skew. Variability measures answer the following questions: "Is the sample homogeneous or heterogeneous?" and "Is the sample similar or different?" If a researcher measures oral temperatures in two samples, one sample drawn from a healthy population and one sample from a hospitalized population, it is possible that the two samples will have the same mean. However, it is likely that there will be a wider range of temperatures in the hospitalized sample than in the healthy sample. Measures of variabiity are used to describe these differences in the dispersion of data.

As with measures of central tendency, the various measures of variability are appropriate to specific kinds of measurement and types of distributions.

Modal percentage is used with nominal data and is the percentage of cases in the mode. A high modal percentage is indicative of decreased variability.

Range

The *range* is the simplest but most unstable measure of variability. Range is the difference between the highest and lowest scores. A change in either of these two scores would change the range. The range should always be reported with other measures of variability. The range in Table 16-2 is 36, but this could easily change with an increase or decrease in the high score of 90 or the low score of 54.

Semiquartile range

The **semiquartile range** (semiinterquartile range) indicates the range of the middle 50% of the scores. It is more stable than the range, since it is less likely to be changed by a single extreme score. It lies between the upper and lower quartiles, the upper quartile being the point below which 75% of the scores fall and the lower quartile being the point below which 25% of the scores fall. The middle 50% of the scores in Table 16-2 lie between 68 and 78, and the semiquartile range is 10.

Percentile

A **percentile** represents the percent of cases a given score exceeds. The median is the 50th percentile, and in Table 16-2 it is a score of 74. A score in the 90th percentile is exceeded by only 10% of the scores. The zero percentile and the 100th percentile are usually dropped (McNemar, 1969).

Standard deviation

The *standard deviation* (SD) is the most frequently used measure of variability and it is based on the concept of the normal curve (see Fig. 16-4). It is a measure of average deviation of the scores from the mean and as such should always be reported with the mean. It takes all scores into account and can be used to interpret individual scores.

Since the mean (X) and standard deviation (SD) for the exam in Table 16-2 was 73.1 ± 12.1, a student should know that 68% of the grades were between 85.1 and 61. If the student received a grade of 88, he would know he did better than most of the class, whereas a grade of 58 would indicate he did not do as well as most of the class. Table 16-3, taken from the study by Gennaro (1988, Table 1), reports the mean and standard deviation for each group of mothers by week post partum. As illustrated in this table, the week 1 mean score for anxiety in mothers of preterm infants is 37.6 and the standard deviation is 7.1. This means that 68% of the week 1 anxiety scores of mothers in the preterm group would be expected to fall between 30.5 and 44.7. This listing allows the reader to inspect the data and get a feel for the variation the data contain.

The standard deviation is used in the calculation of many inferential statistics (see Chapter 17). One limitation of the standard deviation is that it is expressed in terms of the units used in the measurement and cannot be used to compare means that have different units. If researchers were interested in the relationship between height measured in inches and weight measured in pounds, it would be necessary for them to convert the height and weight measurements to standard units or **Z scores.**

Z scores

The *Z score* is used to compare measurements in standard units. Each of the scores is converted to a Z score, and then the Z scores are used to examine the relative distance of the scores from the mean. A Z score of +1.5 means that the observation is 1.5 SD above the mean, whereas a score of −2 means that the observation is 2 SD below the mean. By utilizing Z scores a researcher can compare results from scales that utilize different units, such as height and weight.

Many measures of variability exist. The modal frequency is the easiest to calculate, but the standard deviation is the most useful. The standard deviation and the

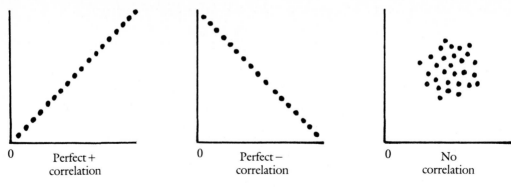

0	0	0
Perfect + correlation	Perfect − correlation	No correlation

Fig. 16-6   Scatter plots.

semiquartile range always exist and are unique for each sample. The standard deviation is the most stable statistic. Transformation of scores to Z scores allows comparison between scores that have different measurement units.

CORRELATION

Correlations are used to answer the question, "To what extent are the variables related?" Correlations are used with ordinal or higher data. Most correlations are discussed in Chapter 17, but here we will briefly mention scatter plots, which are visual representations of the strength and magnitude of the relationship between two variables. The strength of the correlation is demonstrated by how closely the data points approximate a straight line. In a positive correlation the higher the score on one variable, the higher the score on the other. Temperature and pulse are positively correlated; that is, a rise in temperature generally is associated with a rise in the pulse rate. In a negative correlation the higher the score on one measure, the lower the score on the other measure. A decrease in blood volume is generally associated with a rise in the pulse rate. Fig. 16-6 illustrates a perfect positive correlation, a perfect negative correlation, and no correlation. In most research, correlation results lie between these extremes.

CRITIQUING DESCRIPTIVE STATISTICS

Many students who have not had a course in statistics feel that they cannot critique descriptive statistics. However, the student should be able to critically analyze the use of statistics even if the student does not understand the derivation of the numbers presented. What is most important in critiquing this aspect of a research study is that the procedures for summarizing the data make sense in light of the purpose of the study. The criteria for critiquing descriptive statistics are presented in the box on p. 305.

Critiquing Criteria

1. Were appropriate descriptive statistics used?
2. What level of measurement is used to measure each of the major variables?
3. Is the sample size large enough to prevent one extreme score from affecting the summary statistics utilized?
4. What descriptive statistics are reported?
5. Were these descriptive statistics appropriate to the level of measurement for each variable?
6. Are there summary statistics for each major variable?
7. Is there enough information present to judge the results?
8. Are the results clearly and completely stated?
9. If tables and graphs are used, do they agree with the text and extend it or do they merely repeat it?

Before the reader can decide if the statistics employed make sense, it is important to return to the beginning of the paper and determine the purpose of the study. Although all studies use descriptive statistics to summarize the data obtained, many studies go on to use identical statistics to test specific hypotheses (see Chapter 17). If a study is an exploratory one, it is possible that only descriptive statistics will be presented, since their purpose is to describe the characteristics of a population.

Just as the hypotheses should flow from the problem and purpose of a study, so should the hypotheses suggest the type of analysis that will follow. The hypotheses should indicate the major variables that the reader can expect to have presented in summary form. Each of the variables in the hypotheses should be followed in the results section with appropriate descriptive information.

After studying the hypotheses the reader should proceed to the methods section. Using the operational definition provided, the reader identifies the level of measurement employed to measure each of the variables that were listed in the hypotheses. From this information the reader should be able to determine the measures of central tendency and variability that should be employed to summarize the data. For example, you would not expect to see a mean used as a summary statistic for the nominal variable of sex. In all likelihood, sex would be reported as a frequency distribution. The reader should expect that the means and standard deviations will be provided for measurements performed at the interval level. The sample size is another aspect of the methods section that is important when evaluating the researcher's use of descriptive statistics. The larger the sample, the less chance that one outlying score will affect the summary statistics.

Only after these aspects of the study have been examined should the reader should begin to consider the results presented by the researcher. Each important variable should have an appropriate measure of central tendency and variability presented. If tables or graphs are used, they should agree with the information presented in the text. The tables and the charts should be clearly and completely labeled. If the researcher presents grouped frequency data, the groups should be logical and mutually exclusive. The size of the interval in grouped data should not obscure the pattern of the data nor should it create an artificial pattern. Each table and chart should be referred to in the text, but each should add to the text and not merely repeat it. Each table or graph should have an obvious connection to the study being reported. For example, there may be one table that describes the sample and another that presents data relevant to the hypotheses being studied. Table 16-4 illustrates a clearly presented table; each group is mutually exclusive, and the data in the table agree with the data in the text.

The results should be written so that they are understandable to the intended audience. The audience for nursing research is the average practicing nurse. Thus the descriptive information presented should be clear enough that the reader at that level can determine the usefulness of the study in the individual practice situation.

Descriptive statistics cannot be critiqued apart from the study as a whole. Each part of the research paper must make sense in relation to the entire paper. Therefore the reader should evaluate each portion of the paper in relation to what has preceded it. As such, the evaluation of the descriptive statistics must precede the evaluation of the inferential statistics.

The following is a partial critique of Kunnel et al.'s (1988) study of temperature in the stable neonate; only one option is chosen at each step:

Purpose of study:	To determine optimum placement time at the sites	
Hypothesis:	Not stated explicitly but implied—optimum thermometer placement time will vary by site	
Variable:	Time	
Operational definition:	How long it takes for the thermometer to reach maximum temperature at a specific site	
Level of measurement:	Ratio	

	Expected	*Reported*
Summary statistics:	Mean time	In text—rectal, 2.66 min
Measure of variability:	SD	In text— ± 2.2

Sample size:	99 Infants with repeated measures
Conclusion:	Reported statistics are appropriate for the problem, hypothesis, and the level of measurement; sample size is large enough to prevent one score from having a large effect on the mean

SUMMARY

This chapter has introduced the student to the use of descriptive statistics as a means of describing and organizing data gathered in research. The focus has been on the understanding of the techniques rather than on their use.

Basic to the discussion has been an understanding of the levels of measurement utilized in a study. Each level of measurement, such as nominal, ordinal, interval, and ratio, has appropriate descriptive techniques associated with it.

Measures of central tendency describe the average member of a sample. The mode is the most frequent score, the median is the middle score, and the mean is the arithmetic average of the scores. The mean in the most stable and useful of the measures of central tendency, and with the standard deviation it forms the basis for many of the inferential statistics described in Chapter 17.

Three ways of describing and summarizing data have been presented. The frequency distribution presents data in tabular or graphic form and allows for the calculation or observation of characteristics of the distribution of the data, including skewness, symmetry, modality, and kurtosis. In nonsymmetrical distributions the degree and direction of the pull of the peak off center are described in terms of skew. In speaking of modality the number of peaks is described as unimodal, bimodal, or multimodal. The relative spread of the data is described by kurtosis. Each characteristic of the frequency distribution is independent.

Measures of variability reflect the spread of the data. The modal percentage is the percent of the cases in the mode. The ranges reflect differences between high and low scores. The standard deviation is the most stable and useful measure of variability.

The standard deviation is derived from the concept of the normal curve. In the normal curve, sample scores and the means of large numbers of samples group themselves around the midpoint in the distribution, with a fixed percentage of the scores falling within given distances of the mean. This tendency of means to approximate the normal curve is called the *sampling distribution of the means*. A Z score is the standard deviation converted to standard units.

Finally, the concept of correlation was introduced. The scatter plot was discussed as a measure of correlation.

The principles of descriptive statistics were then applied to the critical analysis of published research reports. Special emphasis was given to the relationship of levels of measurement and appropriate descriptive techniques.

References

Baillie, V., Norbeck, J.S., and Barnes, L.E.A. (1988). Stress, social support, and psychological distress of family care-givers of the elderly, *Nursing Research,* **37:**217-222.

Bliss-Holtz, J.V. (1988). Primiparas' prenatal concern for learning infant care, *Nursing Research,* **37:**1.

Brooten, D., Kumar, S., Brown, L.P., Butts, P., Finkler, S.A., Bakewell-Sachs, S., Gibbons, A., and Delivoria-Papadopoulos, M. (1986). A randomized clinical trial of early hospital discharge and home follow-up of very-low-birth-weight infants, *New England Journal of Medicine,* **315:**934-939.

Fox, D.J. (1982). *Fundamentals of research in nursing,* Norwalk, Conn., Appleton-Century-Crofts.

Gennaro, S. (1988). Postpartal anxiety and depression in mothers of term and preterm infants, *Nursing Research,* **37**:82-85.

Kerlinger, F.N. (1986). *Foundations of behavioral research,* 2nd ed., New York, Holt, Rinehart, & Winston, Inc.

Kunnel, M.T., O'Brien, C., Hazard Munro, B., and Medoff-Cooper, B. (1988). Comparisons of rectal, femoral, axillary and skin to mattress temperatures in stable neonates, *Nursing Research,* **37**:162-164.

McNemar, Q. (1969). *Psychological statistics,* New York, John Wiley & Sons, Inc.

Shelley, S.I. (1984). *Research methods in nursing and health,* Boston, Little, Brown & Co.

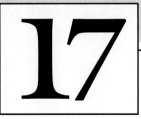

Inferential Data Analysis

Margaret Grey

LEARNING OBJECTIVES

After reading this chapter the student should be able to do the following:

◇ Identify the purpose of inferential statistics.

◇ Distinguish between a parameter and a statistic.

◇ Explain the concept of probability as it applies to the analysis of sample data.

◇ Distinguish between type I and type II error.

◇ Distinguish between parametric and nonparametric tests.

◇ List the commonly utilized statistical tests and their purposes.

◇ Critically analyze the statistics utilized in published research studies.

KEY TERMS

correlation	parametric statistics
degrees of freedom	probability
inferential statistic	sampling error
level of significance (alpha level)	scientific hypothesis
nonparametric statistic	standard error of the mean
null hypothesis	type I error
parameter	type II error

Inferential statistics are used to analyze the data collected in a research study. The reader of research studies needs to understand the purpose and application of statistics. Although it may be useful also to understand how statistical procedures are conducted, such knowledge is not critical to understanding published research findings. The purpose of this chapter is to demonstrate how researchers use inferential statistics to make conclusions about larger groups (the population of interest) from sample data. Basic concepts and terminology will be presented in the sections that follow so that the reader can begin to make sense of the statistics used in research papers. Those readers who desire a more advanced discussion should refer to the Additional Readings at the end of this chapter.

DESCRIPTIVE AND INFERENTIAL STATISTICS

In the previous chapter we discussed *descriptive statistics,* the statistics that are utilized when the researcher needs to summarize the data. In this chapter we turn our attention to the use of inferential statistics. *Inferential statistics* combine mathematical processes and logic to allow researchers to test hypotheses about a population utilizing data obtained from probability samples. Statistical inference is generally used for two purposes: to estimate the probability that statistics found in the sample accurately reflect the population **parameter** and to test hypotheses about a population. In the first purpose a *parameter* is a characteristic of a population, whereas a *statistic* is a characteristic of a sample. We use statistics to estimate population parameters. Suppose we randomly sample 100 people with chronic lung disease and use an interval scale to study their knowledge of the disease. If the mean score for these clients is 65, the mean represents the *sample statistic*. If we were able to study every client with chronic lung disease, we could also calculate an average knowledge score, and that score would be the *parameter for the population*. As you know, a researcher is rarely able to study an entire population, so inferential statistics allow the researcher to make statements about the larger population from studying the sample.

The example given alludes to two important qualifications of how a study must be conducted so that inferential statistics may be used. First, it was stated that the sample was randomly selected (see Chapter 15). Since you are already familiar with the advantages of probability sampling, it should be clear that if we wish to make statements about a population from a sample, that sample must be representative. All procedures for inferential statistics are based on the assumption that the sample was drawn with a known probability. Second, it was stated that the scale had to reach the interval level of measurement. This is because the mathematical operations involved in doing inferential statistics require this level of measurement.

HYPOTHESIS TESTING

The second, and most commonly used, purpose of inferential statistics is hypothesis testing. Statistical hypothesis testing allows researchers to make objective decisions about the outcome of their study. The use of statistical hypothesis testing allows researchers to answer such questions as "How much of this effect is a result of chance?" or "How strongly are these two variables associated with each other?"

The procedures used when making inferences are based on principles of negative inference. In other words, if a researcher studied the effect of a new educational program for clients with chronic lung disease, the researcher would actually have two hypotheses — the **scientific hypothesis** and the **null hypothesis.** The research or *scientific* hypothesis is that which the researcher believes will be the outcome of the study. In our example the scientific hypothesis would be that the educational intervention would have a marked impact on the outcome in the experimental group beyond that in the control group. The *null hypothesis,* which is the hypothesis that can actually be tested by statistical methods, would state that there is NO difference between the groups. Inferential statistics utilize the null hypothesis for testing the validity of a scientific hypothesis in sample data. The null hypothesis states that there is no actual relationship between the variables and that any observed relationship or difference is merely a function of chance fluctuations in sampling.

The concept of the null hypothesis is often confusing. Another example may help to clarify this concept. A study by Gennaro (1988), which compares levels of postpartum anxiety and depression in mothers of term and preterm infants, provides a good illustration. Dr. Gennaro was interested in determining if anxiety and depression would be higher in mothers of preterm infants than in mothers of full-term infants. She based this *scientific* hypothesis, that mothers of premature infants would have higher levels of anxiety and depression, on previous work that suggested that mothers of preterm infants may have more difficulty adapting. She administered scales measuring anxiety and depression to the two groups of mothers, and then she determined whether their scores were different. The researcher used the *null hypothesis,* that there were no differences between term and preterm mothers, to test this scientific hypothesis, and she found that mothers of preterm infants were significantly more anxious and depressed than mothers of term infants. In other words, the researcher found that the differences in the scores between the two groups were large enough as not to be caused by chance, and she could *reject* the null hypothesis.

Note that the researcher would *reject* the null hypothesis. All statistical hypothesis testing is a process of disproof or rejection. It is impossible to prove that a scientific hypothesis is true, but it is possible to show that the null hypothesis has a high probability of being incorrect. To reject the null hypothesis, then, is considered to show support for the scientific hypothesis and is the desired outcome of most studies that utilize inferential statistics (see Chapter 7).

PROBABILITY

The researcher can never prove the scientific hypothesis but can show support for it by rejecting the null hypothesis; that is, show that the null hypothesis has a high probability of being incorrect. We have now introduced the theory underlying all of the procedures to be discussed in this chapter—probability theory. **Probability** is a concept that we talk about all the time, such as the chance of rain today, but we have a difficult time defining it. The *probability* of an event is the event's long-run relative frequency in repeated trials under similar conditions (Colton, 1975). In other words, the statistician does not think of the probability of obtaining a single result from a single study but rather of the chances of obtaining the same result from an idealized study that can be carried out many times under identical conditions. It is the notion of repeated trials that allows researchers to use probability to test hypotheses.

Statistical probability is based on the concept of **sampling error.** Remember that the use of inferential statistics is based on random sampling. However, even when samples are randomly selected there is always the possibility of some errors in sampling. Therefore the characteristics of any given sample may be different from those of the entire population. Suppose a group of researchers has at their disposal a large group of clients with decubitus ulcers and they wish to study the average length of time ulcers take to heal with the usual nursing care. If the researchers studied the entire population, they might obtain an average healing time of 50 days, with a standard deviation of 10 days. Now suppose that the researchers did not have the money necessary to study all of the clients but wished instead to do several consecutive studies of these clients. For this study they first draw a sample of 25 clients, calculate the mean and standard deviation, and replace the subjects in the population before drawing the next sample. The researchers repeat this process many times so that they might end up with 50 different means. If the researchers then placed the means in a frequency distribution, it might appear as in Fig. 17-1. This frequency distribution is a sampling distribution of the means. It illustrates that the researchers might find that one sample's mean might be 50.5, the next 47.5, the next 62.5, and so on. The tendency for statistics to fluctuate from one sample to another is known as *sampling error*.

Sampling distributions are theoretical. In practice, researchers do not routinely draw consecutive samples from the same population, but usually they compute statistics and make inferences based on one sample. However, the knowledge of the properties of the sampling distribution—*if* these repeated samples are hypothetically

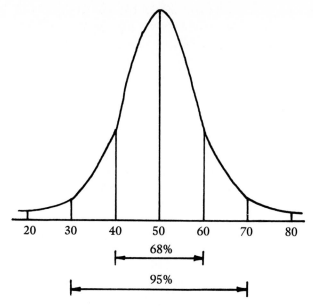

Fig. 17-1 Sampling distribution of the means.

obtained — permits the researcher to draw a conclusion based on one sample. This is possible because the sampling distribution of the means has certain known properties.

The sampling distribution of the means followed a normal curve, and the mean of the sampling distribution will be the mean of the population. As was discussed in the previous chapter, the fact that the sampling distribution of the means is normal tells us several other important things. When scores are normally distributed we know that 68% of the cases will fall between +1 SD and −1 SD or that the probability is 68 out of 100 that any one randomly drawn sample mean will lie within the range of values between ±1 SD. In the example given, if we only drew one sample, we would have a 68% chance of finding a sample mean that fell between 40 and 60. The standard deviation of a theoretical distribution of sample means is called the **standard error of the mean.** The word *error* is used because the various means that make up the distribution contain some error in their estimates of the population mean. The error is considered to be standard because it implies the magnitude of the average error, just as a standard deviation implies the average variation from one mean. The smaller the standard error, the less variable are the sample means and the more accurate are those means as estimates of the population value.

Although researchers rarely construct sampling distributions, standard error can be estimated because it bears a systematic relationship to the sample standard deviation and the size of the sample. This tells us that increasing the size of the sample will increase the accuracy of our estimates of population parameters. It should make intuitive sense that to increase the size of a sample will decrease the likelihood that one outlying score will dramatically affect the sample mean (see Chapter 16). The other reason that the sampling distribution is so important is that there are sampling distributions for all statistics. Researchers consult these distributions when making determinations about rejecting the null hypothesis.

TYPE I AND TYPE II ERRORS

The researcher's decision regarding accepting or rejecting the null hypothesis is based on a consideration of how probable it is that the observed differences are a result of chance alone. Since data on the entire population are not available, the researcher can never flatly assert that the null hypothesis is or is not true. Thus statistical inference is always based on incomplete information about a population, and it is possible for errors to occur when making this decision. There are two types of error in statistical inference: **type I error** and **type II error.**

Let us return to the example of Gennaro's (1988) study of mothers of term and preterm infants. Remember that the null hypothesis of the study was that mothers of term and preterm infants would not differ in levels of anxiety and depression. There were 41 mothers in each group at the beginning of the study. Remember that there were significant differences between the mothers in both anxiety and depression scores. If the differences that were found were truly a function of chance (for example, because these mothers were unusual in some way) and if the number studied was too small, a type I error would occur. *Type I error* is the researcher's rejection of the null hypothesis when it is actually true. If on the other hand the researcher had found that the term and preterm mothers did not differ in anxiety and depression, but the researcher had studied only a few mothers, a type II error might occur. A *type II error* is the researcher's acceptance of a null hypothesis that is actually false. The relationship of the two types is shown in Fig. 17-2.

Level of significance

The researcher does not know when an error in statistical decision making has occurred. It is possible to know only that the null hypothesis is indeed true or false if data from the total population are available. However, the researcher can control the risk of making type I errors by setting the **level of significance** before the study begins. The *level of significance* is the probability of making a type I error, or the probability of rejecting a true null hypothesis. The minimum level of significance acceptable for nursing research is 0.05. If the researcher sets *alpha,* or the level of significance, at 0.05, the researcher is willing to accept the fact that if the study were done 100 times, the decision to reject the null hypothesis would be wrong 5 times out of those 100 trials. If, as is sometimes done, the researcher wants to have a smaller risk of rejecting a true null hypothesis, the level of significance may be set at 0.01. In this case the researcher is willing to be wrong only once in 100 trials. The decision as to how strictly the alpha level should be set depends on how important it is to not make an error. For example,

Conclusion of test of significance	REALITY	
	Null hypothesis is true	Null hypotheses is not true
Not statistically significant	Correct conclusion	Type II error
Statistically significant	Type I error	Correct conclusion

Fig. 17-2 Outcome of statistical decision making.

if the results of a study are to be used to determine whether a great deal of money should be spent in an area of nursing care, the researcher may decide that the accuracy of the results is so important that an alpha level of 0.01 is chosen. In most studies, however, alpha is set at 0.05.

Perhaps you are thinking that researchers should always use the lowest alpha level possible, because it makes sense that researchers would like to keep the risk of both types of errors at a minimum. Unfortunately, decreasing the risk of making a type I error increases the risk of making a type II error. What this means is that the stricter the researcher is in preventing the rejection of a true null hypothesis, the more likely is the possibility that a false null hypothesis will be accepted. Therefore the researcher always has to accept more of a risk of one type of error when setting the alpha level.

Practical versus statistical significance

The reader should realize that there is a difference between statistical significance and practical significance. When a researcher tests a hypothesis and finds that it is statistically significant, this means that the finding is unlikely to have happened by chance. In other words, if the level of significance has been set at 0.05, the odds are 19 to 1 that the conclusion the researcher makes on the basis of the statistical test performed on sample data is correct. The researcher would reach the wrong conclusion only 5 times out of 100. Suppose a researcher is interested in the effect of loud rock music on the behavior of laboratory mice. The researcher could design an experiment to study this question and find that loud music makes the mice act strangely. A statistical test suggests that this finding is not due to chance. However, such a finding may or may not have practical significance; therefore the finding has statistical significance. Although some would argue that this study might have relevance to understanding the behavior of teenagers, some would also argue that the study has no practical value. Thus the findings of a study may have statistical significance, but they may have not practical value or significance. Although researchers should consider the practicality of a problem in the early stages of a research project (see Chapter 4), a distinction between the statistical and practical significance of the findings should also be made when discussing the results of a study.

TESTS OF STATISTICAL SIGNIFICANCE

Tests of significance may be *parametric* or *nonparametric*. Most of the studies in nursing research literature utilize parametric tests, which have the following three attributes: (1) they involve the estimation of at least one parameter, (2) they require measurement on at least an interval scale, and (3) they involve certain assumptions about the variables being studied. These assumptions usually include that the variable is normally distributed in the overall population. In contrast to parametric tests, nonparametric tests of significance are not based on the estimation of population parameters, so they involve less restrictive assumptions about the underlying distribution. Nonparametric tests are usually applied when the variables have been measured on a nominal or ordinal scale.

There has been some debate about the relative merits of the two types of statistical tests. The moderate position taken by most researchers and statisticians is that nonparametric statistics are best utilized when the data cannot be assumed to be at the interval level of measurement or when the sample is small and the normality of the underlying distribution cannot be inferred. However, if these assumptions can be made, most researchers prefer to use **parametric statistics** because they are more powerful and more flexible than *nonparametric statistics*.

There are many different statistical tests of significance that researchers utilize to test hypotheses. The procedure and the rationale for their use are similar from test to test. Once the researcher has chosen a significance level and collected the data, the data are utilized to compute the appropriate test statistic. For each test there is a related theoretical distribution that shows the probable and improbable values for that statistic. On the basis of the statistical result and the values in the distribution, the researcher either accepts or rejects the null hypothesis and then reports both the statistical result and its probability. Thus a researcher may perform a statistical test called a t test, obtain a value of 8.98, and report that it is statistically significant at the $p < 0.05$ level. This means that the researcher had 5 chances out of 100 to be wrong in concluding that this result could not have been obtained by chance. In addition, the likelihood of finding a statistic that is high enough to be statistically significant is increased as the sample size increases. This likelihood is indicated by the **degrees of freedom** that are often reported with the statistic and the probability value. Degrees of freedom is usually abbreviated as *df*.

Table 17-1 shows the most commonly used inferential statistics. The test that is utilized depends on the level of the measurement of the variables in question and the type of hypothesis being studied. Basically, these statistics test two types of hypotheses: (1) that there is a difference between groups or (2) that there is a relationship between two variables.

Table 17-1 **Tests of Difference or Association**

| Level of measurement | One sample | Two samples | | More than two samples | Correlation indexes |
		Related	Independent		
Nonparametric					
Nominal	Chi-square		Chi-square Fisher exact probabil- ity test	Chi-square	Phi coeffi- cient
Ordinal	Kolmogorov- Smirnov	Sign test Wilcoxon matched- pairs, signed rank test	Chi-square Median test Mann- Whitney U	Chi-square	Spearman rank cor- relations Kendall rank correla- tions
Parametric					
Interval or ratio	With before- after mea- sures: Correlated *t* test Repeated mea- sures Analysis of vari- ance	With matched pairs: Correlated *t* test	Independent *t* test Analysis of variance	Analysis of vari- ance	Pearson product moment correla- tion Multiple correla- tion Factor anal- ysis

Test of difference

Suppose a researcher has done an experimental study utilizing an after-only design (see Chapter 9). What the researcher hopes to determine is that the two groups are different after the introduction of the experimental treatment. If the two groups are randomly assigned and the level of measurement is at the interval level, the researcher would utilize the Student *t* test to analyze the data. If the *t* statistic were found to be high enough as to not have occurred by chance, the researcher would reject the null hypothesis and conclude that the two groups were indeed more different than would have been expected on the basis of chance. In other words, the researcher would conclude that the experimental treatment produced the desired effect. The study by Brooten, Kumar, Brown, Butts, Finkler, Bakewell-Sachs, Gibbons, and Delivoria-

Papadopoulos (1986) (Appendix A) illustrates the use of the t statistic. In this case the researchers were interested in determining whether their random assignment procedures had produced groups that were equivalent on variables of importance. They used the t statistic to show that the differences between the means of the two groups were not statistically significant.

The t statistic is commonly used in nursing research, especially when the researcher wishes to test whether two group means are more different than would be expected on the basis of chance. To use this test the variables must have been measured at the interval or ratio level, and the two groups must be independent. If the groups are related, such as in a test-retest situation, and the researcher wants to know if the subjects' scores have changed significantly, a paired or correlated t test would be used.

Sometimes a researcher either has more than two groups or wants to examine the difference between "before" and "after" scores of two groups. This would be the case in a true experiment or a Solomon four-group design. Then the researcher utilizes a test called the *analysis of variance.* Like the t test, the *analysis of variance,* abbreviated ANOVA, searches for differences in the means of scores of variables measured at the interval level.

Researchers can also evaluate differences between groups when the data do not reach the interval level. If the level of measurement is nominal, the chi-square (χ^2) test is used. Chi-square is a nonparametric statistic that determines whether the frequency found in each category is different from what would be expected by chance. As with the t test, if the calculated chi-square is high enough, the researcher would conclude that the frequencies found would not be expected on the basis of chance alone, and the null hypothesis would be rejected. The chi-square test can also be used with ordinal level data and with more than two groups. It is a commonly utilized test in nursing research.

When the data are at the ordinal level, researchers have several other nonparametric tests at their disposal. These include the sign test and the Wilcoxon matched-pairs, signed ranks test for related groups, and the median test and the Mann-Whitney U test for the independent groups. Explanation of these tests is beyond the scope of this discussion, but those readers who desire further information are referred to the Additional Readings at the end of this chapter.

A study by Tulman (1986) of mothers' patterns of handling newborns delivered by cesarean section and vaginally illustrates the used of each of these statistical techniques. The researcher was interested in the differences in initial handling between the two types of mothers. Since the two groups could not be randomly assigned, the researcher had to determine if the two groups were similar on other variables of importance before determining if the handling patterns were different. For data measured at the interval level, such as age, parity, and age of youngest child, the t statistic was used. For comparison of demographic variables, which are measured at the nominal or ordinal level, such as sex of infant, prior infant experience, race, handedness, and method of feeding, the chi-square test was used. Finally, to test whether the sequence of use of body parts was different between the two groups, ANOVA was used. The results suggested that there were no differences in infant handling between mothers experiencing vaginal and cesarean deliveries.

Tests of relationships

Researchers are often interested in exploring the relationships between two or more variables. Such studies utilize statistics that determine the **correlation,** or the degree of association, between two or more variables. Tests of the relationships between variables are sometimes considered to be descriptive statistics when they are utilized to describe the magnitude and direction of a relationship of two variables in a sample and the researcher does not wish to make statements about the larger population. Such statistics can also be inferential when they are utilized to test hypotheses about the correlations that exist in the target population.

Null hypothesis tests of the relationships between variables assume that there is no relationship between the variables. Thus, when a researcher rejects this type of null hypothesis, the conclusion is that the variables are in fact related. Suppose a researcher is interested in the relationship between the age of clients and the length of time it takes them to recover from surgery. As with other statistics discussed, the researcher would design a study to collect the appropriate data and then analyze the data utilizing measures of association. In the example, age and length of time until recovery can be considered to be interval level measurements. The researcher would use a test called the *Pearson r,* or the Pearson product moment correlation coefficient. Once the Pearson r is calculated, the researcher consults the distribution for this test to determine whether the value obtained is likely to have occurred by chance. Again, the research reports both the value of the correlation and its probability of occurring by chance.

The interpretation of correlation coefficients is often problematic for students learning statistics. Correlation coefficients can range in value from $+1.0$ to -1.0 and can also be zero. A zero coefficient means that there is no relationship between the variables. A perfect positive correlation is indicated by a $+1.0$ coefficient, and a perfect negative correlation by a -1.0 coefficient. We can illustrate the meaning of these coefficients by utilizing the example from the previous paragraph. If there were no relationship between the age of the client and the length of time the client required to recover from surgery, the researcher would find a correlation of zero. However, if the correlation were $+1.0$, this would mean that the older the client, the longer it took him to recover. A negative coefficient would imply that the younger the client, the longer it would take him to recover. Of course, relationships are rarely perfect. The magnitude of the relationship is indicated by how close the correlation comes to the absolute value of 1. Thus a correlation of -0.76 is just as strong as a correlation of $+0.76$, but the direction of the relationship is opposite. In addition, a correlation of 0.76 is stronger than a correlation of 0.32. When a researcher tests hypotheses about the relationships between two variables, the test considers whether the magnitude of the correlation is large enough to not have occurred by chance. This is the meaning of the probability value or the p value reported with correlation coefficients. As with other statistical tests of significance, the larger the sample, the greater the likelihood of finding a significant correlation. Therefore researchers also report the degrees of freedom associated with the test performed.

Refer to the paper by Baillie, Norbeck, and Barnes (1988) (Appendix B) on the effects of stress, social support, and psychological distress on family caregivers of the elderly. The purpose of this study was to examine the relationships between perceived stress of caregiving, satisfaction with social support, and psychological distress in family caregivers of impaired elderly clients. Table 3 from that study (reprinted on p. 446) contains the correlation coefficients that describe the relationships between each of the variables. For example, note that variable 7, perceived stress of caregiving, is significantly associated with variable 2, mental condition of the elderly client, with a correlation coefficient of 0.41. This number is a relatively strong correlation, and it indicates that approximately 16% (0.41 × 0.41) of the variability in perceived stress of caregiving is due to the mental condition of the elderly client.

Nominal and ordinal data can also be tested for relationships utilizing nonparametric statistics. The chi-square test can be used to study the relationships between variables measured at the nominal level, and the phi coefficient (ϕ) expresses the relationship found. Spearman rank order correlations and Kendall's tau express the correlation between variables measured at the ordinal level. All of these correlation coefficients may range in value from $+1.0$ to -1.0.

Advanced statistics

Sometimes researchers are interested in studying more complex problems that examine more than two variables at a time. Most of these are variations on two of the tests that we have discussed — ANOVA and multiple regression.

The analysis of variance is a powerful statistical test that can be utilized in a large number of situations. It can be expanded to encompass multiple data collection points, as with time series studies, where it is called time series analysis of variance. It can also be used when a researcher believes that the results of the study will depend on some antecedent variable. This procedure is called the analysis of covariance, often abbreviated ANCOVA. The *analysis of covariance test* is used when ANOVA would be used, but the researcher needs to control for another important variable that may influence the dependent variable. For example, suppose a researcher is interested in the effect of a teaching program on surgical recovery rate, but the researcher knows that the recovery rates will vary depending on the clients' ages. The researcher could limit the study to just one age group, or the researcher could control for age in the analysis utilizing ANCOVA. If a positive result were obtained, the result would indicate that regardless of the client's age, the experimental program was effective in reducing recovery time.

Nursing problems are rarely so simple that they can be explained by only two variables. When researchers are interested in understanding more about a problem than just the relationships between two variables involved, they may use a procedure called *multiple regression*. Multiple regression is the expansion of correlation to include more than two variables, and it is utilized when the researcher wants to determine what variables contribute to the explanation of the dependent variable. For example, a researcher may be interested in determining what factors help women decide to breast-feed their infants. A number of variables, such as the mother's age, previous experience with breast-feeding, number of other children, and knowledge of the advantages of breast-feeding, might be measured and then analyzed to see if they, separately and together, predict the likelihood of breast-feeding. Such a study would require the use of multiple regression. The results of a study might help nurses to know that a younger mother who had only one child might be more likely to benefit from a teaching program about breast-feeding than an older mother with several other children.

Baillie, Norbeck, and Barnes (1988), who studied factors associated with psychological distress in caregivers of the impaired elderly, were not simply interested in single relationships among the variables (Appendix B). They were interested in furthering the understanding of the stress-buffering model of social support. In order to do so, they needed to use more advanced statistics. Since the purpose of the study was to determine relationships, the authors used multiple regression techniques to study their hypotheses about the relationships between stress, social support, and psychological distress. Refer to Table 4 from this study in Appendix B. This table shows the results of the multiple regression analysis for psychological distress and depression in the caregivers. The column titled "Beta" reflects the amount of relationship between the variables when the other variables are included. Note that the relationship between support and psychological distress is negative. This result means that the more support the caregivers perceived, the lower their psychological distress. The second column, R^2, shows the amount of variance in distress accounted for by the variables, a total of 31.6%. The remaining columns report the statistical test results used to determine the relative importance of each of the variables in the regression. This table is a commonly used and accepted way to show the results of a multiple regression analysis.

There are many other statistical tests of significance. Consult one of the statistics resources listed in the Additional Readings at the end of the chapter if further information is desired or if a test not discussed is included in a study of interest to you.

CRITIQUING INFERENTIAL STATISTICAL RESULTS

Many students find that critiquing inferential statistics is difficult or even impossible if they have not taken a course in statistics. Although there is some merit to this feeling, there are aspects of the statistical analysis that should be possible to critique without the benefit of years of statistics course work. Important questions to consider when critiquing the use of inferential statistics are listed in the box on p. 324.

The first place to begin critiquing the statistical analysis of a research report is with the hypotheses. The hypotheses should indicate to you what type of statistics will be utilized. If the hypothesis indicates that a relationship will be found, you should expect to find indexes of correlation. If the study is experimental or quasiexperimental, the hypotheses would indicate that the author is looking for differences between the

Critiquing Criteria

1. Does the hypothesis indicate that the researcher is interested in testing for differences between groups or in testing for relationships?
2. What is the level of measurement chosen for the important variables?
3. Does the level of measurement permit the use of parametric statistics?
4. Is the size of the sample large enough to permit the use of parametric statistics?
5. Has the researcher provided enough information to decide whether the appropriate statistics were utilized?
6. Are the statistics utilized appropriate to the problem, the hypotheses, the method, and the sample?
7. Are the results for each of the hypotheses presented?
8. Do the tables and the text agree?
9. Are the results understandable?
10. Is a distinction made between practical significance and statistical significance? How?
11. What is the level of significance set for the study? Is it applied throughout the paper?

groups studied, and you would expect to find statistical tests of differences between means.

Then as you read the methods section of the paper, consider what level of measurement the author has utilized to measure the important variables. If the level of measurement is interval or ratio, the statistics will most likely be parametric statistics. On the other hand, if the variables are measured at the nominal or ordinal level, then the statistics utilized should be nonparametric. Also consider the size of the sample, and remember that samples have to be large enough to permit the assumption of normality. If the sample is quite small, for example, 5 to 10 subjects, the researcher may have violated the assumptions necessary for inferential statistics to be utilized. Thus the important question is whether the researcher has provided enough justification to utilize the statistics presented.

Finally, consider the results as they are presented. There should be enough data presented for each hypothesis studied to determine if the researcher actually examined each hypothesis. The tables should accurately reflect the procedure performed and be in harmony with the text. For example, the text should not indicate that a test reached statistical significance, while the tables indicate that the probability value of the test was above 0.05. If the researcher has utilized analyses that are not discussed in this text, you may want to refer to a statistics text to decide if the analysis was appropriate to the hypothesis and the level of measurement.

There are two other aspects of the data analysis section that the reader should critique. The paper should not read as if it were a statistical textbook. The results of the study in the text of the paper should be clear enough to the average reader so that the reader can determine what was done and what the results were. In addition, the author should attempt to make a distinction between practical and statistical significance. Some results may be statistically significant, but their practical importance may be doubtful. If this is so, the author should note it. Alternatively, you may find yourself reading a research report that is elegantly presented, but you come away with a "so what?" feeling. Such a feeling may indicate that the practical significance of the study and its findings have not been adequately explained in the report.

Note that the critical analysis of a research paper's statistical analysis is not done in a vacuum. It is possible to judge the adequacy of the analysis only in relationship to the other important aspects of the paper: the problem, the hypotheses, the design, the data collection methods, and the sample. Without consideration of these aspects of the research process, the statistics themselves have very little meaning. Statistics can lie; thus it is most important that the researcher use the appropriate statistic for the problem. For example, a researcher may sometimes use a nonparametric statistic when it appears that a parametric statistic is appropriate. Since parametric statistics are more powerful than nonparametric, the result of the parametric analysis may have not been what the researcher expected. However, the nonparametric result might be in the expected direction, so the researcher reports only that result.

Example of the use and critique of inferential statistics

Earlier in this chapter we referred to a study of postpartal anxiety and depression in mothers of term and preterm infants (Gennaro, 1988). The purpose of the study was to examine differences in anxiety and depression in mothers of term and preterm infants in the first postpartum week and over the next 6 weeks. This statement of purpose indicates that the author is interested in looking at differences between groups. Therefore the reader should expect that the analysis will consist of t tests or ANOVA.

The major variables were measured with standardized instruments at the interval level so that parametric statistical tests could be used. There were 41 mothers in each of the two groups at the beginning of the study, an adequate sample. However, the research can have less confidence in her findings over the 6-week follow-up period, because the sample size at the end of the study was 16 mothers of preterm infants and 10 mothers of term infants.

The researcher used the t and chi-square tests to determine if differences existed between the groups of mothers of term infants and mothers of preterm infants on demographic variables. In addition, she determined whether dropouts from the study were different on any of the variables from those who stayed in the study. These were appropriate tests, and no differences were found.

The hypotheses were tested by ANOVA. This test is appropriate to the problem, because the researcher was interested in the differences between the mothers. Results for each of the implicit hypotheses are presented, and they suggest that mothers of preterm infants are more anxious and depressed than mothers of term infants in the first postpartal week, but these differences do not persist over time. Tables agree with the text, and the results are understandable to the reader. The discussion points out that the numbers in the analysis over time are small and that these results should be interpreted with caution. Clear implications for practice are made supporting the practical significance of the study. The statistical level of significance was set at 0.05 and is consistent throughout the paper.

SUMMARY

The purpose of this chapter was to introduce the student to the use of inferential statistics as a tool to test hypotheses about populations from sample data. The emphasis was on the appropriate use of statistical tests of hypotheses in nursing research studies.

To understand how probability is utilized by researchers when they make decisions about the acceptance or rejection of a hypothesis, the theoretical distribution called the sampling distribution of the means was discussed. Because the sampling distribution of the means follows a normal curve, researchers are able to estimate the probability that a certain sample will have the same properties as the total population of interest. Sampling distributions provide the basis for all inferential statistics.

Inferential statistics allow researchers to estimate population parameters and to test hypotheses. Since little nursing research focuses on estimation of parameters as an objective for the study, the chapter concentrated on the testing of hypotheses. The use of these statistics allows researchers to make objective decisions about the outcome of the study. Such decisions are based on the rejection or acceptance of the null hypothesis, which states there is no relationship between the variables. If the null hypothesis is accepted, this result indicates that the findings are likely to have occurred by chance. If the null hypothesis is rejected, the researcher accepts the scientific hypothesis of a relationship being present between the variables and that this relationship is unlikely to have been found by chance.

Statistical hypothesis testing is subject to two types of error: type I and type II. Type I error occurs when the researcher rejects a null hypothesis that is actually true. Type II error occurs when the researcher accepts a null hypothesis that is actually false. The researcher controls the risk of making a type I error by setting the alpha level, or level of significance. Unfortunately, reducing the risk of a type I error by reducing the level of significance increases the risk of making a type II error.

The results of statistical tests are reported to be significant or nonsignificant. Statistically significant results are those whose probability of occurring is less than 0.05 or 0.01, depending on the level of significance set by the researcher.

Finally, a number of commonly used parametric and nonparametric statistical tests were discussed. These tests included those that test for differences between means, such as the t test and ANOVA, and those that test for differences in proportions, such as the chi-square test. Tests that examine data for the presence of relationships include the Pearson *r*, the sign test, the Wilcoxon matched-pairs, signed ranks test, and several others. The reader who also introduced to several advanced statistical procedures such as the anaysis of covariance and multiple regression.

These principles of statistical inference were then applied to the critical analysis of published research papers. The most important aspect of critiquing statistical analyses is the relationship of the statistics employed to the problem, design, and method used in the study. Clues to the appropriate statistical test to be utilized by the researcher should stem from the researcher's hypotheses. The reader should also determine if all of the hypotheses have been presented in the paper.

References

Baillie, V., Norbeck, J.S., and Barnes, L.E.A. (1988). Stress, social support, and psychological distress of family caregivers of the elderly, *Nursing Research,* **37**:217-222.

Brooten, D., Kumar, S., Brown, L.P., Butts, P., Finkler, S.A., Bakewell-Sachs, S., Gibbons, A., and Delivoria-Papadopoulos, M. (1986). A randomized clinical trial of early hospital discharge and home follow-up of very-low-birth-weight infants, *New England Journal of Medicine,* **315**:934-939.

Colton, T. (1975). *Statistics in medicine,* Boston, Little, Brown & Co.

Fox, D.J. (1982). *Fundamentals of research in nursing,* Norwalk, Conn., Appleton-Century-Crofts.

Gennaro, S. (1988). Postpartal anxiety and depression in mothers of term and preterm infants, *Nursing Research,* **37**:82-85.

Munro, B.H., Visitainer, M.A., and Page, E.B. (1986). *Statistical methods for health care research,* Philadelphia, J.B. Lippincott.

Tulman, L.J. (1986). Initial handling of newborn infants by vaginally and Cesarean-delivered mothers, *Nursing Research,* **35**:296-299.

Additional Readings

Bennett, S., and Bowers, D. (1976). *An introduction to multivariate techniques for the social and behavioral sciences,* New York, John Wiley & Sons, Inc.

Blalock, H.M. (1972). *Causal inferences in nonexperimental research,* New York, W.W. Norton.

Blalock, H.M. (1979). *Social statistics,* New York, McGraw-Hill Book Co.

Kerlinger, F.N., and Pedhazur, E.J. (1986). *Foundations of behavioral research,* 2nd ed., New York, Holt, Rinehart & Winston, Inc.

Knapp, R. (1984). *Basic statistics for nurses,* Norwalk, Conn., Appleton-Century-Crofts.

Pedhazur, E.J. (1982). *Multiple regression in behavioral research,* 2nd ed., New York, Holt, Rinehart & Winston, Inc.

18

Computers in Research

Christine Tassone Kovner

LEARNING OBJECTIVES

After studying this chapter the student should be able to do the following:

◇ Describe in general terms how a computer works.

◇ Compare and contrast the uses of mainframe computers and microcomputers in nursing research.

◇ Describe how a computer can be used in the various steps of the research process.

◇ Identify the steps of the research process that a computer cannot be used for and explain why.

KEY TERMS

data base	random access memory (RAM)
hardware	read only memory (ROM)
memory	software
modem	terminal
program	time-sharing

Computer use has vastly facilitated many steps in the research process. For example, statistical tests that were infrequently performed 10 years ago because of the lengthy calculations involved are now commonly performed. It would be unusual for anyone today to analyze data from a research study without at least using a calculator, and in virtually all published quantitative research a computer has been used. This chapter will discuss how the computer aids in carrying out the research process. This chapter includes an overview of computers and specifically identifies those steps in the research process that can be enhanced by using a computer.

OVERVIEW OF COMPUTERS

Computers are electronic devices that store and manipulate pieces of data. In simple terms, a computer is a series of electronic *on* and *off* switches.

Generally when people talk about computers, they are talking about the **hardware.** *Computer hardware* is the electronic equipment and includes the following four main components:

1. An input device, such as a keyboard
2. An output device, such as a monitor or a printer
3. A central processing unit (CPU)
4. The memory (RAM/ROM)

The input device is much like a typewriter, and the user simply types the information that goes into the CPU. After the instructions are entered, they are stored in the computer's **memory.** Memory can be visualized as a series of boxes and each box has room for one message, either *on* or *off*. Memory is usually available in two types—RAM and ROM. *RAM,* or **random access memory,** means that the user can read it, change it, or write over it. *ROM,* or **read only memory,** as its name implies, means that the computer can read it, but it cannot be changed. ROM is used for the computer's operating system and it tells the CPU what it should be doing. From the memory the instructions go to the CPU for processing. After the information has been processed, it is sent to one or more output devices. Historically data were entered on paper cards with holes punched in them to represent the letters or numbers. Now data are entered via keyboard or on a magnetic tape directly to the CPU. Magnetic tape is similar to the tape used in audio tape recorders.

Computers can also store information. These instructions or data are stored in the memory, on floppy disks, on magnetic tape, or on cards. Information that is stored in the memory is lost when the computer is turned off. To avoid losing data, information can be stored on 5¼-inch floppy disks that are similar to soft phonograph records, on 3½-inch firm disks, on compact disks, or on magnetic tape. These media can be kept for long periods of time and physically transported from one computer to another. In addition, hard disks are available to store large amounts of data and are generally not transportable. Information that is stored on cards can also be transported, but this is rarely used anymore because the cards are very bulky. Instructions that are put on disks or tapes to program the computer to do something, such as word processing or statistics, are called **software.**

TYPES OF COMPUTERS

The three types of computers are mainframes, minicomputers, and microcomputers. Since most researchers use mainframes or microcomputers, only those will be discussed. A mainframe is a large computer that is capable of great speed and that can be used by many people at the same time. When several people are working on one mainframe at the same time, this is called **time-sharing.** The mainframe is wired to many **terminals.** A *terminal* is an input device consisting of a keyboard and a monitor. Each person using a terminal works independently, but the people are all sharing the same mainframe. Mainframes are generally quite expensive and are owned by universities and large businesses. On the other hand, microcomputers, or personal computers (PCs), are smaller and much slower than mainframes. Usually they are used by only one person at a time, are owned by individuals or small businesses, and are relatively inexpensive. Sometimes a high-capacity microcomputer is shared by many people in a network.

Use of either a mainframe or a microcomputer requires knowledge of the computer's operating system. The operating system directs the computer to perform the desired tasks and is the language that the computer understands. For mainframes it is also necessary to know one of the editing systems; that is, the set of instructions used to direct the computer. The editing system is a series of short commands that will move letters and numbers around on the screen. For example, if the computer is directed to get a data file, "get file" might be typed in; however, if "het file" were typed by mistake, the spelling would need to be corrected from "het" to "get." The editing system is used to make the spelling correction. Both operating systems and editing systems vary from computer to computer. Each time the user works with a new mainframe, the operating and editing systems for that computer must be learned.

Microcomputers also have operating and editing systems. The most common disk operating systems are Microsoft Disk Operating System (MS-DOS), OS/2, UNIX, and Control Program for Microcomputers (CP/M). The editing systems on microcomputers serve the same purposes as those on the mainframes, and the user must know the computer's operating system before using it. If computer programs written by someone else are being used, it may not be necessary to learn the editing system.

Remote terminals

To use a mainframe the user communicates to the mainframe from a remote terminal. In most large universities and businesses these terminals are "hard wired"; that is, the terminals are hooked up directly by wires much like telephone cables to the computer. It is also possible to connect to a mainframe computer by telephone lines. One can purchase a terminal and a **modem** (the device needed to communicate from terminal to mainframe), and then by calling the mainframe's telephone number, the user can connect to it. In this way computer files can be accessed from any telephone in the world, including your own home telephone.

Microcomputers can also be used as terminals to communicate with a mainframe. Commercially available software tells the microcomputer to act as if it were a terminal. Access to the mainframe by telephone lines and modem is then possible. The obvious advantage of using a remote terminal is the ability to use the mainframe from remote locations, thereby no longer making it necessary to go to a computer center to use a mainframe. It is easy to enter the data, process them, and see the results from where you and your terminal are located. It is even possible to print those data wherever you are if you have a printer. The major disadvantage of using a modem and telephone connection is that use of a telephone line costs money. Occasionally data that are transmitted over telephone lines have errors, although there are computer programs to ensure that this does not happen.

SOFTWARE

A complicated set of directions for the computer to execute is called a **program.** Programs are called software and are written in a computer language. The computer language takes the directions and turns them into *on* and *off* switches that the CPU can manipulate. Both microcomputers and mainframes can accept sets of directions written in a computer language. Commonly used languages are FORTRAN, PASCAL, COBOL, BASIC, and LOGO. Not every computer can understand and use or compile all of these languages. It is necessary to know what languages your computer can understand.

Some software can be used by many different people. This software is sold by the person who wrote it or a company representing that person. Examples include programs that do word processing, handle statistics, set up **data bases,** and contain games. Thousands of these programs are available. Programs written for use on a mainframe cannot automatically run on a microcomputer, because their operating systems differ. For example, an Apple computer's software will not work on an IBM PC. Many of the large manufacturers prepare versions of their software for a variety of computers. The word processing program Wordstar is available for the IBM PC and

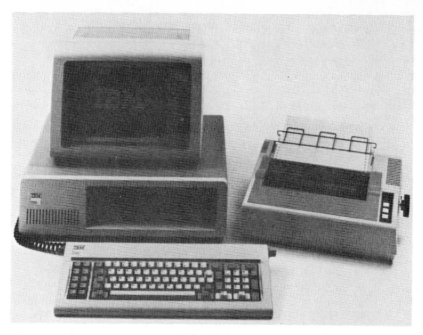

Fig. 18-1   IBM Personal Computer with keyboard, monochrome display, and 80 CPS matrix printer.

other computers (Fig. 18-1). From the user's point of view, the program operates the same way on any microcomputer. From the computer's point of view, the directions it receives to process information are different and written in a language the computer can understand. Therefore, if you are able to use Wordstar on any computer, you will also be able to use it on the IBM PC. However, it will always be necessary to learn the basics of the different operating systems for each computer so you will know how to turn the machine on and ask it for the desired program.

AN EXAMPLE OF DATA PROCESSING IN NURSING RESEARCH

Table 18-1 briefly summarizes the steps a researcher must utilize to process data on a mainframe and on a microcomputer. When using a terminal to process statistical data on a mainframe such as the Cyber CDC, the researcher must "write" a program. A software program such as the Statistical Package for the Social Sciences (SPSSX Users Guide, 1988), which uses an editing system called Xedit, is an example of a packaged computer program. SPSS commands are similar to a series of FORTRAN programs and can be compared to baking a cake with a mix rather than from scratch. Once the program is "written" (commands have to be given in the appropriate order), the researcher processes the program using the network operating system. If the researcher wants to process the same statistical data on

Table 18-1 Comparison of Mainframe Computers and Microcomputers for Data Processing	
Mainframe computer (Cyber CDC)	**Microcomputer (IBM PC)**
Network operating system: initial startup response is the character "/"; this affirms that the computer is operational	Disk operating system: response given by the computer is "A>"
Editing system: Xedit; response is "?" or "??"	Editing system: Edlin
Software: SPSSX, a statistics program	Software: SPSSX PC+, a statistics program
Languages: FORTRAN, PASCAL, COBOL	Languages: BASIC, and with special software can also run FORTRAN or PASCAL

a IBM PC or a compatible PC, he or she can use SPSSPC+ (Norusis, 1988). Processing data with SPSSX on a mainframe is significantly faster than processing similar information on a microcomputer. Versions of SPSSX are available for many mainframes; however, the network operating system and line editors vary from computer to computer. Software for microcomputers usually has to be installed for the mainframe computer.

USING THE COMPUTER IN THE RESEARCH PROCESS

Many students new to the research process think that the computer is utilized only for the statistical analysis of data collected for a research study. However, this is not true. Researchers use computers to help accomplish many of the steps in the research process. This section reviews the phases of the research process in which computers can be helpful.

Problem identification (see Chapter 4)

The computer can be used to identify problems that can be studied. As computers are being increasingly used in clinical settings, data can be accessed from these computers to identify trends in client problems, nursing care, and delivery of nursing services. For example, the computer at a large medical center can be programmed to note all cases of infections. This can be done from laboratory records or client records. With this information the nurse researcher can observe trends over time and decide if this problem is important enough to pursue. Another example of computer use in problem identification is in a rural hospital that might program its computer to note the incidence of decubiti. Again, the nurse researcher could monitor the incidence and decide if this were a problem to study. It should be noted that the computer is only an adjunct; real problem development occurs when the nurse thinks about clients, nurses, and care provided. In addition, reading literature about nursing research studies can set the problem identification process in motion.

Literature review (see Chapter 5)

A major step in the development of a research project is the literature review. It is imperative that one knows what other work has been done on a subject of interest before designing a research project. The computer is a valuable tool for reviewing the literature. The process can be conducted from home by use of a microcomputer or at most major university libraries.

The literature is listed in a *data base*. A data base is a compilation of information about something and is organized in a systematic way. Information from the data base can be presented in different ways; for example, by date, alphabetically, or by subject. Data bases exist that index everything from advertisements to health care articles to zoological literature. The most commonly used bibliographic health care data base is MEDLINE; it is produced by the United States National Library of Medicine. All articles indexed in the *Index Medicus, Index to Dental Literature,* and *International Nursing Index* since 1966 to the present are computerized in MEDLINE. MEDLINE indexes more than 3000 journals and has been including abstracts for more than 40% of the citations since 1975. More than 250,000 records are added each year.

To gain entry into this computer file, one needs to either have an account number with a commercial organization such as Dialog* or use the services of a library that has access to the files. The data bases are organized by key word codes. MEDLINE uses Medical Subject Headings developed by the National Library of Medicine. The specifics of the procedure vary, depending on the computer being used, but are basically as follows: From home, once the user has turned on the computer, the computer dials the phone number of the commercial service. An individual charge account is then entered and the actual search procedure begins. MEDLINE's procedure is quite complicated but, in essence, the data base program requests from the user a series of key words. After the key words are entered, the MEDLINE computer will transmit, via telephone wire, the list of articles associated with the key words. They will appear on the screen or they may be printed to produce a permanent copy.

If the literature search is done at a library, the procedure is similar, with either the researcher or a librarian doing the actual communicating with MEDLINE's computer. Depending on the library, the information either is printed immediately or is available at a later date. Costs for a computer search vary widely. The costs for MEDLINE include a combination of telephone charges and user time with MEDLINE. If you have an account with a commercial firm, you are usually billed monthly. Libraries generally charge on a per job basis. A typical search listing 40 articles would cost about $35. In addition, MEDLINE has completed searches for

---

* Dialog, 3460 Hillview Ave., Palo Alto, CA 94304.

commonly requested topics. These are much less expensive and can be ordered by mail directly from MEDLINE. Specific information can be found from any major library or in the *Internatioanl Nursing Index.*

The Cumulative Index to Nursing & Allied Health Literature is available on 5¼-inch floppy disks. These disks are organized by year and can be purchased for personal or institutional use.* MEDLINE is available on compact disk that requires a special disk drive. The advantage of both these formats is a one-time charge with updating charges, rather than a fee for each search.

Accuracy of literature research

The major question that arises when using a computer search concerns the accuracy of the information. Has the researcher missed any important articles? In an effort to explore this area Fox and Ventura (1984) found that a computer search of articles about nurse practitioners did not identify a high proportion of critical studies identified from other sources. This suggests that traditional methods of reviewing literature should be used in addition to computer searches.

Additional uses in the literature search

Additional uses of the computer for literature review include abstracting services and individual reference list development. In some fields there are commercially available abstracting services that produce references on a monthly basis using key words described by the researcher. These references are then sent to the researcher on a disk that can be accessed at will. At present this service is not available for nursing articles, but it is expected in the near future.

The researcher can also create and store personal reference lists and abstracts. Many software programs exist that can help the researcher organize references by key words, dates, author, or any system preferred. When the researcher then wants a list of all articles with a reference to "pain," for example, only that list needs to be called up from the data base.

Theoretical rationale development (see Chapter 6), *formulating the hypothesis* (see Chapter 7), *and selecting the design* (see Chapters 8 to 12)

At this time computers cannot perform high-level thinking skills. Therefore computers are not helpful in these steps of the research process.

Data collection (see Chapter 13)

Data collection can be aided by the computer in several ways. First, it is possible that the data that the researcher is interested in already exist as part of records collected for other reasons. One example is the National Health Survey, an ongoing national study about the use of health care services. Computer tapes of the surveys exist, and these tapes can be either rented and put on a mainframe or accessed from the federal government through a modem over the telephone line. Another example are the data

---

* 1509 Wilson Terrace, P.O. Box 871, Glendale, CA 91209.

that hospitals keep about the length of stay that is reported to various insurers and government agencies. These data can be accessed directly from the hospital.

Second, the computer can be used as a word processor to generate form letters and mailing labels that could be used in a mailed survey. The computer can be programmed so that each recipient receives a "personal" letter rather than a "Dear Colleague" letter. Survey research experts say that the response rate is higher when potential respondents receive a personalized letter.

Third, questionnaires can be prepared to use computer-readable answer sheets, like the ones we have all used to take standardized tests. These sheets are then "read" by the computer, and the data are held in a file until they are analyzed. Ultra Quest* is a microcomputer program that is used for survey research. The software is used to write questionnaires and provide descriptive results.

Operationalization and variable measurement (see Chapters 13 and 14)

Operationalizing and measuring variables can be greatly enhanced by the use of the computer. Although definitions derive from theory, the researcher must choose a reliable and valid tool for measuring the variable. Many of the variables used in nursing studies are complex constructs such as pain, anxiety, or the quality of nursing care. Researchers try to measure these constructs using scales consistent with the theoretical rationale applied in the study. The computerized version of *Mental Measurement Yearbook* contains descriptive information and reviews of instruments to measure psychological variables (Directory of Online Data Bases, 1988). This is available on the BRS information system.† However, it is sometimes necessary for the researcher to develop a new scale. In either case the reliability and validity of the tool must be ensured. This is usually done by the various statistical tests discussed in Chapter 13 that can all be done quite rapidly with a computer. Thus the reliability and validity of instruments used in research studies should be available to the reader.

The following is an example. When Hinshaw and Atwood's (1982) revision of the Risser Patient Satisfaction instrument, a scale to measure the client's satisfaction with nursing care, is used, it is necessary to know both the reliability and the validity of the scale. A common reliability test of internal consistency is the Cronbach alpha. An example of some data and the printout describing the reliability taken from the SPSS/Pct are shown in Fig. 18-2.

For a study with 100 subjects calculating the alpha with a calculator would take several hours, but a mainframe computer can do it in less than a second.

Sample selection (see Chapter 15)

The selection of the sample is one of the most important aspects of the research process. As described in Chapter 15, if a volunteer sample is used, the results can be generalized only to that volunteer group. Researchers try to choose samples that will reflect the population of interest in the study. The computer can assist in several ways. There are

---

* Brainstorm, 17200 Old Rim Court, El Paso, TX 79936.
† BRS Information Technologies, 1200 Route 7, Latham, NY 12110.

RELIABILITY ANALYSIS — SCALE (TOTAL)

ITEM-TOTAL STATISTICS

	SCALE MEAN IF ITEM DELETED	SCALE VARIANCE IF ITEM DELETED	CORRECTED ITEM-TOTAL CORRELATION	SQUARED MULTIPLE CORRELATION	ALPHA IF ITEM DELETED
QUES1	19.9636	23.1537	.7513	.5995	.9132
QUES2	19.8303	23.5334	.6955	.6663	.9152
QUES3	19.8303	23.7219	.6630	.6191	.9162
QUES4	20.0576	23.2642	.7249	.6149	.9141
QUES5	20.0061	23.2644	.7172	.6916	.9143
QUES6	19.9758	23.1848	.7438	.7032	.9135
QUES7	19.9606	23.0957	.6338	.4839	.9174
QUES8	19.9758	23.5374	.6665	.4770	.9160
QUES9	19.9788	23.8324	.6027	.4388	.9181
QUES10	20.0545	23.6323	.4865	.2657	.9237
QUES11	19.8273	24.0400	.5927	.4831	.9184
QUES12	19.9303	23.4875	.6818	.5940	.9155
QUES13	19.9970	23.5106	.5739	.4855	.9195
QUES14	19.9152	23.4882	.6329	.5057	.9171

RELIABILITY ANALYSIS — SCALE (TOTAL)

RELIABILITY COEFFICIENTS   14 ITEMS

ALPHA = .9221   STANDARDIZED ITEM ALPHA = .9247

Fig. 18-2   An example of reliability using SPSS/PC+.

computer programs that will identify the number of people necessary in the sample to achieve a stated level of significance for specific statistical tests. In addition, the computer can generate random numbers, so if the researcher wants a random sample of clients admitted to the hospital during a certain time period, random numbers can be chosen to identify chart numbers to be included in the study.

If the researcher were using a stratified sample and were interested in including the study subjects who met certain criteria (for example, clients who live in a specific part of the city), the computer could be used to choose those clients whose addresses have a specified ZIP code. The computer can be programmed to choose subjects along any parameters that the researcher sets. However, it should be kept in mind that the final sample is only as good as the original population list; that is, if the plan is to choose clients who live in ZIP code 10012, and the researcher uses as a population list those clients who go to one hospital, all those clients who live in ZIP code 10012 but who go to other hospitals will not be in the final sample. However, if the researcher uses a broader list of clients for the population list, the sample chosen will be more reflective of the population being studied.

Organizing the data for analysis and analyzing the data (see Chapters 16 and 17)

Historically the computer has been used primarily to manipulate numbers, and this continues to be the function it best serves. When organizing the data the computer can be used to sort the data, perhaps by generating lists of all those subjects with a particular diagnosis. When the data need to be analyzed, the computer is an invaluable aid. Both applications require the computer to manipulate numbers.

Analyzing data is the real forte of the computer. It should always be remembered that the computer is only as good as the information put in, so if the data are inaccurate, the analysis will be inadequate. In computer lingo, this is known as the *GIGO* axiom — *Garbage In, Garbage Out*. For example, if the data are best explained by use of multiple regression and the researcher used a *t* test, the results will be incorrectly interpreted. It is the researcher's responsibility to analyze the data appropriately. Whether the tests requested are appropriate or not, the computer will quickly perform the statistical calculation and print the result. The researcher, not the computer, must decide if the result makes sense.

To perform the most commonly required statistical programs, most researchers use commercially available software packages that are already prepared. Of course the energetic computer user could write a program to do any statistical test required. Mainframes at most major universities have one or more general statistics programs. Two examples are SPSS and Biomedical Computer Programs (BMD). These programs are continually updated by the manufacturers to make them easier to use, more accurate, and inclusive of new statistical tests. The program used usually depends on what is available to the researcher and the familiarity of the faculty with the various programs. The pros and cons of each system are not a subject for this book. The researcher should have a record of which program (including the version, such as SPSS version 8.3) was used, should questions about data analysis occur at a later date.

Fig. 18-3 shows an example of data generated by use of an SPSSX Release 2.2 +. This example shows the complexity of the output generated by a multiple regression procedure.

Statistical packages used on microcomputers are much slower than those on mainframes because of the limited hardware of microcomputers. These packages also tend to be much less comprehensive than those on mainframes and include fewer statistical tests. SPSSPC + and SAS are now available for use on microcomputers, but

30-MAR-88   SPSS-X RELEASE 2.2+ FOR VAX/VMS
13:36:38
                                                    DEC VAX-8600   VMS Y4.6

**** MULTIPLE REGRESSION

Equation Number 1   Dependent Variable   LOS 'LENGTH OF STAY'

——Variables in the Equation —

Variable	B	SE B	95% Confdnce	Intrvl B	Beta	SE B
COMP	7.444781	4.455301	−1.390249	16.279811	.163155	.097
SEX	1.280677	3.911057	−6.475096	9.036450	.031544	.096
AGE	−.058532	.239430	−.533331	.416267	−.023958	.098
MARIG	−1.685969	3.697093	−9.017443	5.645506	−.046479	.101
MENTAL	7.680106	3.293071	1.149821	14.210390	.221300	.094
(Constant)	16.010893	20.394536	−24.432239	56.454025		

———————— in ————————

Variable	Sig T
COMP	.0977
SEX	.7440
AGE	.8074
MARIG	.6493
MENTAL	.0216
(Constant)	.4342

End Block Number 2   All requested variables entered.

Fig. 18-3   An example of multiple regression data generated by SPSS-X.

the package is not identical to that used on the mainframes and includes fewer statistics. An example of data produced by SPSS/PC+ on an IBM PC is shown in Fig. 18-4.

Analyzing the results (see Chapter 19)

Perhaps the most difficult part of the research process is interpreting the results. If the hypothesis is not supported, does that mean that the hypothesis is not an accurate description of events in the world, or does it mean that flaws in the design affected the results? If the hypothesis is supported, is it because the hypothesis does reflect the way events occur in the world or that the support fell in the support category on the basis of the 5% error? The answers to these and other questions raised in Chapter 19 are judgments. The computer cannot make judgments, and so the task of interpreting the result is left to the researcher and others who may read the final research report.

RELIABILITY   ANALYSIS   —   SCALE   (TOTAL)

CORRELATION MATRIX

	QUES6	QUES7	QUES8	QUES9	QUES10
QUES6	1.0000				
QUES7	.6046	1.0000			
QUES8	.5265	.4533	1.0000		
QUES9	.4496	.4182	.4969	1.0000	
QUES10	.3907	.3078	.3439	.3760	1.0000
QUES11	.3802	.3422	.4176	.4008	.3216
QUES12	.4386	.4572	.4981	.4570	.3792
QUES13	.3834	.2700	.4041	.3470	.3090
QUES14	.4612	.3754	.4053	.4340	.3456

RELIABILITY   ANALYSIS   —   SCALE   (TOTAL)

CORRELATION MATRIX

	QUES11	QUES12	QUES13	QUES14
QUES11	1.0000			
QUES12	.6472	1.0000		
QUES13	.4916	.5905	1.0000	
QUES14	.5332	.5475	.5985	1.0000

Fig. 18-4   An example of a correlation matrix produced by SPSS/PC+.

Communication of the findings

The communication step in the research process is one of the most important. If results are not communicated to other researchers and practitioners, the nursing profession cannot advance. Results cannot and will not be used in practice. The computer, especially the microcomputer, is an aid for this step in the research process, because in addition to processing numbers, it can also process words. Using a commercially prepared software package, the researcher types on a key board and words appear on the monitor screen. If the researcher does not like the appearance of what is written on the screen, the words are simple to change. When the researcher is happy with the final version, the report can be saved on a disk and then a printer can be used to make copies for colleagues or for submission to a journal for eventual publication. Some journals, such as *Computers in Nursing,* will accept articles directly from the disk rather than on paper. This saves both printing time and mailing costs. A copy of the article can also be transmitted over the telephone line to the disk or screen of someone else's computer for virtually instant viewing.

GUIDELINES FOR ANALYZING THE USE OF COMPUTERS IN PUBLISHED RESEARCH STUDIES

Almost all researchers use computers. The task for the critiquer of research reports is to decide if a computer has been used and whether it was used judiciously.

In some papers, the researcher may say, "Data were analyzed using SPSS" or "A MEDLINE search revealed. . . ." Such statements would be presumptive evidence that the researcher utilized a computer when doing the research. If no such statement appears, the reader can make an intelligent assumption that computers were used if the sample is large (for example, greater than 20) or if inferential statistics are presented. Unless it is explicitly stated the reader will not be able to determine if the researcher has utilized the computer for other steps of the research process.

There are no unique aspects to critiquing the written research reports that have utilized computers. The guides for critiquing the sections of a research report that can be aided by the use of a computer are presented throughout this book and should be consulted. The quality of the finished work should not be affected, either positively or negatively, by the use of a computer. The computer merely serves to facilitate the researcher's work.

SUMMARY

The purpose of this chapter was to discuss the use of the computer in the research process. Computers are composed of hardware and software. A computer's hardware includes an input device, output devices, central processing unit, and memory. Computers are available in the following three sizes: mainframes, minicomputers, and microcomputers. However, most researchers in nursing use mainframes via terminals or microcomputers. Computer software provides the hardware with instructions to carry out procedures, such as statistical analysis or word processing.

The computer is a useful tool for researchers in many aspects of the research process. Computers can be helpful in problem identification, literature review, data collection procedures, measuring variables of interest, sample selection, data analysis, and communicating research findings. Because the computer is not capable of abstract thinking, it is not helpful for developing the theoretical rationale, formulating the hypothesis, selecting the design, and interpreting the results.

When analyzing published research reports, the reader should consider the steps in the research process where computers might be used and then consider whether appropriate steps to safeguard the quality of the work have been taken.

References

Computers in Nursing, a bimonthly journal published by J.B. Lippincott, East Washington Square, Philadelphia.

Directory of online data bases (1988), Vol. 9, New York, Publishers Cuadra, Elsevier.

Fox, R.N., and Ventura, M.R. (1984). Efficiency of automated literature search mechanisms, *Nursing Research,* **33:**174-177.

Hinshaw, A.S., and Atwood, J.R. (1982). A patient satisfaction instrument: precision by replication, *Nursing Research,* **31:**170-175.

Norusis, M. (1988). *SPSS/PC+ V2.0 base manual,* Chicago, SPSS, Inc.

SPSS, Inc. (1988). SPSSX user's guide, 3rd ed., Chicago, SPSS, Inc.

19

Analysis of the Findings

Geri LoBiondo-Wood

LEARNING OBJECTIVES

After studying this chapter the student should be able to do the following:

◇ Discuss the difference between the results sections of a study and the discussion of the results.

◇ Identify the format of the results section.

◇ Determine if both statistically supported and statistically nonsupported findings are discussed.

◇ Determine whether the investigator objectively reported the results.

◇ Describe how tables and figures were used in a research report.

◇ List the criteria of a meaningful table.

◇ Identify the format and components of the discussion of the results.

◇ Determine the purpose of the discussion section.

◇ Discuss the importance of interpreting both supported and nonsupported hypotheses.

◇ Discuss the importance of including generalizations and limitations of a study in the report.

◇ Determine the purpose of including recommendations in the study report.

KEY TERMS

finding
generalizability
limitation
recommendation

The ultimate goals of nursing research are to develop nursing theory and knowledge, to substantiate and improve nursing practice, thereby widening the scientific basis of the nursing profession. Nursing research not only serves nurses but also serves those individuals, families, and groups with whom we as nurses interact in a multitude of health care settings. From the viewpoint of the research consumer, the analysis of the results, interpretations, and generalizations that a researcher generates from a study become a highly important piece of the research project. The final sections of a research report are generally entitled results and discussion, and it is here that the researcher puts the final pieces of the jigsaw puzzle together to view the total picture with a critical eye. This process is analogous to evaluation, the last step in the nursing process. The reader of a research report may view these last sections as an easier step for the investigator, but it is here that a most critical and creative process comes into use. It is in these final sections of the report, after the statistical procedures have been applied, that the researcher will interrelate the statistical or numerical findings to the theoretical framework, literature, methods, hypotheses, and problem statements.

The final sections of published research reports are generally titled results and discussion, but other topics such as limitations of findings, implications for future research, recommendations, and conclusions may be separately addressed or subsumed within these sections. The presentational format of these areas is a function of the author's and the journal's stylistic considerations. The function of these final sections is then to interrelate all aspects of the research process and to discuss, interpret, and identify the limitations and generalizations relevant to the investigation and thereby further nursing research. The goal of this chapter is to introduce the student to the purpose and content of the final sections of a research investigation where data are presented, interpreted, discussed, and generalized. An understanding of what an investigator presents in these sections will assist the research consumer to critically analyze an investigator's findings.

FINDINGS

The **findings** of a study are the results, interpretations, **recommendations,** generalizations, implications for future research, and conclusions and will be addressed by separating the presentation into two major areas. These two areas are the results and the discussion of the results. The results section will focus on the results or statistical findings of the study, and the discussion of the results section will focus on the remaining topics. For both sections the rule applies, as it does to all other sections of a report, that the content needs to be presented clearly, concisely, and logically.

Results

The results section of a research report is considered to be the data-bound section of the report. It is here that the researcher presents the quantitative data or numbers generated by the descriptive and inferential statistical tests. The results of the data analysis set the stage for the interpretations or discussion section that follows the results. The results section should then reflect the problem and hypothesis tested. The information from each hypothesis should be sequentially presented. The tests used to analyze the data should be mentioned. If the exact test that was used is not explicitly stated, then the values obtained should be noted. This is done by providing the numerical values of the statistics and stating the specific correlation and probability level, or t value (see Chapters 16 and 17). Examples of these can be found in Table 19-1. These numbers and their signs should not frighten the novice. These numbers are very important, but there is much more to the research process than the numbers. They are one piece of the whole. Chapters 16 and 17 conceptually present the meanings of the numbers found in studies for the novice consumer. Whether the consumer only superficially understands statistics or has an in-depth knowledge of statistics, it should be obvious that the results are clearly stated, and the presence or lack of statistically significant results should be noted. The Additional Readings list at the end of this chapter also provides further detail for those interested in the application of statistics.

The researcher is bound to present the data for all of the hypotheses posed, such as whether the hypotheses were accepted, rejected, supported, or not supported. If the data supported the hypotheses, it may be assumed that the hypotheses were proved, but this is not true. It does not necessarily mean that the hypotheses were proved; it only means that the hypotheses were supported and that the results suggest that the relationship as posed in the hypotheses, which were derived from the theoretical framework, was probably logical. The beginning research consumer may think that if a researcher's results were not supported statistically or only partially supported, then the study is irrelevant or possibly should not have been published, but this is also not true. If the data are not supported, the critiquer should not expect the researcher to bury the work in a file. It is as important for a critiquer of research to review and understand nonsupported studies as it is for the researcher. Information obtained from nonsupported studies can often be as useful as data obtained from supported studies. Nonsupported studies can be used to suggest **limitations** of particular aspects of a study's design and procedures. Data from nonsupported studies may suggest that current modes of practice or current theory in an area may not be supported by research and therefore need to be reexamined and researched further. Data then assist a profession to generate new knowledge, as well as prevent stagnation of knowledge.

Table 19-1 **Examples of Reported Statistical Results**

Statistical test	Means of reporting results
Pearson correlation	$r = -0.39, p < 0.01$
Analysis of variance	$F = 3.59, df = 2, 48, p < 0.05$
t test	$t = 2.65, p < 0.01$
Chi-square	$\chi^2 = 2.52, df = 1, p < 0.05$

Generally it has been noted that an investigator will interpret the results in a separate section of the report. At times the reader may find that the results section contains the results and the researcher's interpretations, which generally fall into the discussion section. Integrating the results with the discussion in a report becomes the decision of the author. Integration of both sections may be utilized when a study contains several segments that may be viewed as fairly separate subproblems of a major overall problem.

An example of this type of integration is found in a study by Ventura, Young, Feldman, Pastore, Pikala, and Yates (1985). In this study the investigators' purpose was to provide cost-related data from an intervention study in the care of patients with peripheral vascular disease (PVD). The study looked at various aspects of cost and hospitalization, such as vascular-related costs and outpatient usage. Instead of two sections titled results and discussion, the investigators integrated both of these areas and discussed these areas as subproblems of the overall problem. The encompassing title that addressed results and discussion in this study was labeled Hospitalization and Costs. Subproblems or related areas tested and discussed were titled as follows: costs—PVD, costs—vascular related, costs—nonvascular, costs—combined total, outpatient hospital usage and time allocation, and costs for intervention. The investigators thus made use of conceptually discrete portions that flowed back to the overall problem. If integration is done in this manner, it should be consistent; that is, if one hypothesis or question is integrated, then so should all. The presentation should not take on a haphazard use of integration. In the Ventura study a consistent approach was used. Overall the reader will generally find the data results in a separate section from the interpretation or discussion of the results.

The investigator should also demonstrate objectivity in the presentation of the results. Phrases like "analysis of variance showed that high psychosocial care resulted in significantly greater intent to adhere to a health care regimen" (Chang, Uman, Linn, Ware, and Kane, 1985) are the appropriate means to express a result. The investigators would be accused of lacking objectivity if they had stated the results in the following manner: "Analysis of variance showed surprisingly that high psychosocial care resulted in significantly greater intent to adhere. . . ." Opinions or reactionary statements to the data in the results section therefore are inappropriate. The box on p. 349 provides

Example of Results Section

Quantitative Studies

Initial support for hypotheses I and II was shown by zero-order correlations. Perceived stress of caregiving was positively related to psychological distress ($r = 0.46$) and depression ($r = 0.49$), and satisfaction with social support was negatively related to psychological distress ($r = -0.48$) and depression ($r = -0.52$) (Baillie, Norbeck, and Barnes, 1988, p. 220).

A two-way analysis of variance with repeated measures was used to test for an overall effect of parity and significance of interaction between stage (of labor) and parity. There was a significant main effect of parity ($F[1, 82] = 4.73, p < 0.05$) and a significant interaction of parity and stage ($F[2,164] = 4.56, p < 0.05$) for the sensory component of pain (Gaston-Johansson, Fridh, and Turner-Norvell, 1988, p. 88).

Repeated measures analysis of variance was used to compare these mean times. The mean times at the four sites differed significantly ($F = 63.29, p = 0.000$). Paired t tests were used to test for differences among the four mean times (Kunnel, O'Brien, Hazard Munro, and Medoff-Cooper, 1988, p. 164).

Qualitative Studies

During the pretransplantation stage and up to 3 months after transplantation, the process of redesigning the dream is comprised of three interpersonal and intrapersonal concepts—immersion, passage, and negotiation. Immersion occurs during the stage of waiting for a donor, passage is experienced during hospitalization, and negotiation characterizes the recovery after discharge (Mishel and Murdaugh, 1987, p. 333). (The researchers go on to describe in detail each of these phases.)

The self-sustaining process consists of four sequential core concepts or phases: cognitive discomfort, distraction, cognitive comfort, and personal competence (Hinds and Martin, 1988, p. 337). (The researchers detail each of these phases.)

---

examples of objectively stated results from both quantitative and qualitative studies. It is the investigator's responsibility to objectively respond to the results. This is accomplished in the last section titled Discussion of Results. The investigator then uses the discussion of the results section to respond to and interpret the results, with a careful reflection on all aspects of the study that preceded the results.

The reader of a research report should keep in mind that the data presented are considerably reduced. A great deal more data or numbers are generated in a study, but only the critical numbers of each test need to be presented in a report. An example of summarized descriptive data is seen when only the means and standard deviations of age, education, income, and years married are presented rather than all of the subject information listed. Including all of the data in a published report would be too

Table 19-2 **Optimal Temperatures Across Sites**

Site	Optimal temperature (SD*)
Skin-to-mattress	98.11 (0.49)
Femoral	98.25 (0.42)
Axillary	98.34 (0.43)
Rectal	98.60 (0.39)

From Kunnel, M.T., O'Brien, C., Hazard Munro, B., and Medoff-Cooper, B. (1988). *Nursing Research,* 37:162-164.
*Standard deviation.

cumbersome. Individual data may be presented when a case study design is used. The condensation of data is done both in the written text and through the use of tables and figures. The use of tables and figures can facilitate the presentation of large amounts of data generated by the study.

In the study by Kunnel, O'Brien, Hazard Munro, and Medoff-Cooper (1988) (Appendix C) the researchers developed tables to visually depict the results (Tables 19-2 and 19-3). These tables allow the researchers to provide a more thorough explanation and discussion of the results. The results section then can be viewed as a summation section. Both the results of the descriptive and inferential statistics are presented for each hypothesis posed. No data should be omitted that would preclude the critiquer from gaining a full picture of the results. If tables and figures are used, they need to be concise. Although the text is the major mode of communicating the results, the tables and figures serve a supplementary but independent role. The role of tables and figures is to report results with some detail that the investigator does not enter into the text. This does not mean that tables and figures should not be mentioned in the text. The amount of detail that the author uses in the text to describe the specific tabled data varies with the needs of the researcher. Fox (1982) notes that if the text includes everything that is found in the table, the table should not appear. Good tables are those that meet the following criteria:

1. They supplement and economize the text.
2. They have precise titles and headings.
3. They are not repetitious of the text.

An example of a table that meets these criteria can be found in the study by Brooten, Kumar, Brown, Butts, Finkler, Bakewell-Sachs, Gibbons, and Delivoria-Papadopoulos (1986) (Appendix A). The research group wanted to report the characteristics of the sample of mothers and infants in their study. There were 10 separate variables, some with more than one subclassification. To describe each one of these in the text of the article would not have economized space and would have been difficult to visualize. The table developed by the researchers (Table 19-4) not only allows the reader to quickly visualize the variables but also allows the reader to compare the early discharge group and the control group.

Table 19-3 **Repeated Measures Analysis of Variance on Time to Optimal Temperature**					
Source of variance	SS	df	MS	F	p
Between subjects	801.49	98	8.18		
Within subjects	4397.75	297	14.81		
Between measures	1725.06	3	575.22	63.29	0.000
Residual	2672.09	294	9.09		
TOTAL	5199.24	395	13.16		

From Kunnel, M.T., O'Brien, C., Hazard Munro, B., and Medoff-Cooper, B. (1988). *Nursing Research,* **37**:162-164.

The research consumer will find a well-written results section is systematic, logical, concise, and drawn from all of the analyzed data. All that is written in the results section should be geared to letting the data reflect the testing of the problems and hypotheses. The length of this section therefore depends on the scope and breadth of the analysis.

Discussion of the results

In the final section of the report the investigator interpretively discusses the results of the study. It is in this section that a skilled researcher makes the data come alive. The researcher gives the numbers in quantitative studies or the concepts in qualitative studies meaning and interpretation. The reviewer may ask where the investigator extracted the meaning that is applied in this section. If the researcher does the job properly, you will find a return to the beginning of the study. The researcher returns to the earlier points in the study where a problem statement was identified and independent and dependent variables were related on the basis of a sound theoretical framework and literature review. It is in this section that the researcher discusses both the supported and nonsupported data. In this final section the limitations or weaknesses of a study are discussed in light of the design and the sample or data collection procedures. When the data are supported with a statistical significance, the discussion and interpretation are seen as a relatively easy task. The critiquer should find a discussion of how the theoretical framework was supported. In addition, the reviewer should also see the investigator's attempt to look at the data for additional or previously unrealized relationships.

Even if the data are supported, the reviewer should not believe it to be the final word. Downs (1984) cautions that the research critiquer should not be overwhelmed by small p values, since they are not indicative of research breakthroughs. Therefore researchers and reviewers should accept statistical significance with prudence. Statistically significant findings are not the sole means of establishing the study's merit. Other considerations such as theory, sample, instrumentation, and methods should also be considered.

Table 19-4 **Characteristics of Very-Low-Birth-Weight Infants and Their Families**		
Characteristic	Early-discharge group	Control group
MOTHER		
No.	36	36
Mean age, SD (range)	24, 7 yr (16-44)	23, 6 yr (12-38)
Education level		
Less than high school	42%	30.5%
High school	28%	39.0%
More than high school	30%	30.5%
Marital status		
Married	31%	33%
Unmarried	69%	67%
Race		
Black	83%	78%
White	17%	22%
FAMILY		
Hospital insurance		
Medicaid	75%	56%
Private	25%	44%
Income		
$5,000	34%	26%
$5,001-9,999	43%	32%
$10,000-49,999	17%	26%
$50,000	6%	16%

From Brooten, D., Kumar, S., Brown, L.P., Butts, P., Finkler, S.A., Bakewell-Sachs, S., Gibbons, A., and Delivoria-Papadopoulos, M. (1986). *New England Journal of Medicine,* **35:**934-939.

When the results are not statistically supported, the researcher also returns to the theoretical framework and analyzes the earlier thinking process. Results of nonsupported hypotheses do not require the investigator to go on a fault-finding tour of each piece of the project. Such a course can then become an overdone process. All research has weaknesses. This analysis is an attempt to identify the weaknesses and to suggest what the possible problem or problems were in the study. At times the theoretical thinking is correct, but the researcher finds problems or limitations that could be attributed to the tools (see Chapters 13 and 14), the sampling methods (see Chapter 15), the design (see Chapters 8 through 12), or the analysis (see Chapters 16 and 17). Therefore, when results are not supported, the investigator attempts to go on a *fact*-finding tour rather than a *fault*-finding one. The discussion then is done not to show humility or one's technical competence but rather to enable the reviewer to judge the validity of the interpretations drawn from the data and the general worth of the study (Kerlinger, 1986).

Table 19-4 **Characteristics of Very-Low-Birth-Weight Infants and Their Families — cont'd**

Characteristic	Early-discharge group	Control group
INFANTS		
Number	39	40
Mean birth weight, SD (range)	1,187, 198 g (740-1,490)	1,148, 203 g (710-1,500)
Mean gestational age at birth, SD (range)	30, 2 wk (26-37)	30, 2 wk (26-37)
Mean days of hospitalization, SD (range)	46.5, 12.5* (20-79)	57.7, 17* (21-94)
Mean weight at discharge, SD (range)	2,072, 131 g (1,880-2,500)	2,280, 179 g (1,980-2,650)
Mean gestational age at discharge, SD (range)	36, 2 wk (34-39)	38, 2 wk (34-44)
No. of infants rehospitalized		
Within 14 days	4	5
Within 18 months	10	10
No. of infants with acute care visits	29	36
No. of acute care visits	163	186
No. of infants with failure to thrive	0	1
No. of infants reported abused	2	4
No. of infants in foster care	0	2

*The difference in the two means is statistically significant ($p < 0.05$).

It is in this last section of the report that the researcher ties together all the loose ends of the study. It is from this point that reviewers of research can begin to think about clinical relevance, the need for replication, or the germination of a new idea for a prospective researcher. Finally, the reviewer of a research project should find this last section either in separate sections or subsumed within the discussion section, and it should include **generalizations** and recommendations for future research, as well as a summary or a conclusion.

Generalizations (generalizability) are inferences that the data are representative of similar phenomena in a population beyond the study's sample. Reviewers of research are cautioned not to generalize beyond the population on which a study is based. Beware of research studies that may overgeneralize. Generalizations that draw conclusions and make inferences within a particular situation and at a particular

---

Examples of Recommendations

"The findings of this study are helpful to practicing clinicians because they give credibility to planning intervention strategies that offer tangible assistance and emotional support to the caregiver, perhaps through members of the caregiver's own network" (Baillie, Norbeck, and Barnes, 1988, p.222).

"These results indicate that temperatures measured at a variety of sites provide the clinician with reliable data. . . . The results of this research indicate that the thermometer must be in place 6 minutes on the average and 11 minutes to be sure that 90% of the infants measured have reached their optimal temperature. Therefore, it is recommended that placement time be increased to achieve a more reliable measurement." (Kunnel, O'Brien, Hazard Munro, and Medoff-Cooper; 1988, p.164).

---

point in time are appropriate. An example of such a generalization is drawn from a study conducted by Baillie, Norbeck, and Barnes (1988) found in Appendix B of this text. This investigation was designed to examine the effects of stress and social support and their interaction with psychological well-being in family caregivers of impaired elderly. The researchers, when discussing the sample in light of the results, appropriately stated (p. 450).

> The ability to generalize the findings is limited by the nonrandom, predominately middle-class nature of the sample. Although the measure of perceived stress and social support had high internal consistency reliability, further work with more developed measures is needed to validate these findings. Because social support was strongly related to the psychological well-being of these caregivers, additional research is needed to explore factors that contribute to satisfaction with social support.

This type of statement is important for reviewers of research. It helps to guide thinking in terms of a study's clinical relevance, and it also suggests areas for further research. One study does not provide all of the answers, nor should it. It has been said that a good study is one that raises more questions than it answers. So the research consumer should not view an investigator's review of limitations, generalizations, and implications of the findings for practice as lack of research skill. These final steps of evaluation are critical links to the refinement of practice and the generation of future research. Evaluation of research, like evaluation of the nursing process, is not the last link in the chain but a connection between findings that may serve to improve nursing theory and nursing practice.

The final area that the investigator integrates into the discussion section is the recommendations. The *recommendations* are the investigator's suggestions for the

Critiquing Criteria

1. Are all of the results of each hypothesis presented?
2. Is the information regarding the results concisely and sequentially presented?
3. Are the tests that were used to analyze the data or the numerical values presented?
4. Are the results presented objectively?
5. If tables or figures are used, do they meet the following standards:
   a. They supplement and economize the text.
   b. They have precise titles and headings.
   c. They are not repetitious of the text.
6. Are the results interpreted in light of the hypotheses and theoretical framework and all of the other sections that preceded the results?
7. If the data are supported, does the investigator provide a discussion of how the theoretical framework was supported?
8. If the data are not supported, does the investigator attempt to identify the weaknesses and suggest what the possible problems were in the study?
9. Does the investigator discuss the study's clinical relevance?
10. Are any generalizations made?
11. Are the generalizations within the scope of the findings or beyond the findings?
12. Are any recommendations for future research stated or implied?

study's application to practice, theory, and further research. This requires the investigator to reflect on the question of what contribution to nursing does this study make? For examples of recommendations see the box above. This evaluation places the study into the realm of what is known and what needs to be known before being utilized. Fawcett (1982) noted, "It is through future exploration of the dissemination and utilization of research in nursing practice that the science of nursing will become an entity with which to be reckoned."

CRITIQUING THE RESULTS AND DISCUSSION

Criteria for critiquing the results and the discussion of the results sections are found in the box above.

The results and the discussion of the results are the researcher's opportunity to examine the logic of the hypotheses posed, the theoretical framework, the methods, and the analysis. This final section requires as much logic, conciseness, and specificity as was employed in the preceding steps of the research process. The consumer should be able to identify statements of the type of analysis that was utilized and whether or not the data statistically supported the hypotheses. These statements should be straightforward and not reflect bias (see Table 19-2). Auxiliary data or serendipitous findings may also be presented. In such auxiliary findings are presented, they should be as dispassionately presented as were the hypothesis data. The statistical tests used should also be noted. The numerical value of the obtained data should also be presented (see Table 19-1). The presentation of the tests, the numerical values found, and the statements of support or nonsupport should be clear, concise, and systematically reported. For illustrative purposes the researcher should present extensive findings in tables for the reader's consumption.

The discussion section should interpret the data, the gaps, the limitations of the study, and the conclusions, as well as give recommendations for further research. Drawing these aspects into the study should give the consumer a sense of the relationship of the findings to the theoretical framework. Statements reflecting the underlying theory are necessary, whether or not the hypotheses were supported.

If the findings were not supported, the consumer should, as the researcher did, attempt to identify, without fault-finding, possible methodological problems. Finally, a concise presentation of the study's generalizability and the implications of the findings for practice and research should be evident. The last presentation can help the research consumer to begin to rethink clinical practice, provoke discussion in clinical settings (see Chapters 20 and 21), and find similar studies that may support or refute the phenomena being studied to more fully understand the problem.

SUMMARY

It is obvious that the analysis of the findings is the final step of a research investigation. It is in this section that the consumer will find the results printed in a straightforward manner. All results should be reported whether or not they support the hypothesis. Tables and figures may be used to illustrate and condense data for presentation. Once the results are reported, the researcher interprets the results. In this presentation, usually titled Discussion, the consumer should be able to identify the key topics being discussed. The key topics, which include an interpretation of the results, are the limitations, generalizations, implications, and recommendations for future research.

The section on interpretation of the results is where the researcher draws together the theoretical framework and makes interpretations based on the findings and theory. Again, both statistically supported and nonsupported results should be interpreted. If the results are not supported, the researcher should discuss the results reflecting on the theory, as well as possible problems with the methods, procedures, design, and analysis.

In this final process, research should present limitations or weaknesses of the study. This presentation is important, because it affects the study's generalizability. The generalizations or inferences about similar findings in other samples are also presented in light of the findings. The research consumer should be alert for sweeping claims or overgeneralizations that a researcher may state. An overextension of the data can alert one to possible researcher bias.

Finally, the recommendations provide the consumer with suggestions regarding the study's application to practice, theory, and future research. These recommendations furnish the critiquer with a final perspective of the researcher on the utility of the investigation.

References

Baillie, V., Norbeck, J.S., and Barnes, L.E. (1988). Stress, social support, and psychological distress of family caregivers of the elderly, *Nursing Research,* **37**:217-222.

Brooten, D., Kumar, S., Brown, L.P., Butts, P., Finkler, S.A., Bakewell-Sachs, S., Gibbons, A., and Delivoria-Papadopoulos, M. (1986). A randomized clinical trial of early hospital discharge and home follow-up of very-low-birth-weight infants, *The New England Journal of Medicine,* **35**:934-939.

Chang, B.L., Uman, G.C., Linn, L.S., Ware, J.P., and Kane, R.L. (1985). Adherence to health care regimens among elderly women, *Nursing Research,* **34**:27-31.

Downs, F.S. (1984). *A sourcebook of nursing research,* 3rd ed., Philadelphia, F.A. Davis Co.

Fawcett, J. (1982). Utilization of nursing research findings, *Image,* **14**:57-59.

Fox, D.J. (1982). *Fundamentals of research in nursing,* 4th ed., Norwalk, Conn., Appleton-Century-Crofts.

Gaston-Johansson, F., Fridh, G., and Turner-Norvell, K. (1988). Progression of labor pain in primiparas and multiparas, *Nursing Research,* **37**:86-90.

Hinds, P.S., and Martin, J. (1988). Hopefulness and the self-sustaining process in adolescents with cancer, *Nursing Research,* **37**:336-339.

Kerlinger, F.N. (1986). *Foundations of behavioral research,* 2nd ed., New York, Holt, Rinehart & Winston, Inc.

Kunnel, M.T., O'Brien, C., Hazard Munro, B., and Medoff-Cooper, B. (1988). Comparisons of rectal, femoral, axillary, and skin-to-mattress temperatures in stable neonates, *Nursing Research,* **37**:162-164.

Mishel M.H., and Murdaugh, C.L. (1987). Family adjustment to heart transplantation: redesigning the dream, *Nursing Research,* **36**:332-338.

Ventura, M.R., Young, D.E., Feldman, M.J., Pastore, P., Pikula, S., and Yates, M.A. (1985). Cost savings as an indicator of successful nursing intervention, *Nursing Research,* **34**:50-53.

Additional Readings

Knapp, R.G. (1985). *Basic statistics for nurses,* 2nd ed., New York, John Wiley & Sons, Inc.

Pedhazer, E.J. (1982). *Multiple regression in behavioral research,* 2nd ed., New York, Holt, Rinehart, & Winston, Inc.

Voliker, B.J. (1984). *Multivariate statistics for nursing research,* New York, Grune & Stratton, Inc.

Waltz, C., and Bausell, R.B. (1981). *Nursing research: design, statistics, and computer analysis,* Philadelphia, F.A. Davis Co.

Woods, N.F., and Catanzaro, M. (1988). *Nursing research: theory & practice,* St. Louis, C.V. Mosby Co.

20

Utilizing Nursing Research

Rona F. Levin

LEARNING OBJECTIVES

After reading this chapter the student should be able to do the following:

◇ Identify the factors that contribute to the gap between the dissemination and the use of nursing research findings.

◇ Describe the mechanisms that facilitate the utilization of research finds in nursing practice.

◇ Apply the criteria for research utilization to the evaluation of findings for implementation in practice.

◇ Compare and contrast nursing research and the evaluation of practice innovations.

KEY TERMS

construct replication
replication
research base
scientific merit

Previous chapters have explored the significance of research to the practice of nursing, described the research process, and provided guidelines for the critical evaluation of research reports. Throughout this book the emphasis has been placed on your role as a consumer of nursing research. The reason for this emphasis is that the goal of research and theory development in nursing is to develop knowledge that will guide professional practice (Donaldson and Crowley, 1978). As a profession, nursing is ultimately responsible for the provision of safe and effective health care to society. Thus the ultimate purpose of research and theory development in nursing is to provide a "validated body of knowledge on which to base [this] practice" (Fawcett, 1984, p. 62).

This chapter will focus on the implementation of the role of the nursing research consumer. It begins by highlighting the present gap between research and practice, the factors that contribute to that gap, and suggestions for bridging, if not closing, the gap. The section on *utilization criteria* explores how to go about integrating research findings into practice. In other words, now that you have acquired some knowledge of the research process, what do you do with it? Unless professional practitioners of nursing use research in their practice, the goal of research and theory development in nursing will not be reached.

THE NURSE RESEARCHERS VERSUS THE NURSING RESEARCH CONSUMER

The role of the nurse researcher is not the same as the role of the nursing research consumer. According to Phillips (1986), each role requires a different set of skills. The nurse researcher requires knowledge of and skill in "theory construction, research designs and methodologies, instrumentation techniques, and statistical manipulation to conduct actual research in the field setting" (p. 8). In comparison, the nursing research consumer needs to be an expert practitioner who can use theory in the delivery of nursing care and evaluate the applicability of research findings to practice. Table 20-1 compares the specific skills to fulfill each of these roles.

Table 20-1 **Comparison of the Skills of the Nurse Researcher and the Nursing Research Consumer**

Skills of the nurse researcher	Skills of the nursing research consumer
1. The ability to generate researchable questions from clinical practice	1. The ability to use the nursing process from assessment through evaluation and to deliver expert nursing care to individual clients, to family systems, and to communities
2. The ability to operationalize theoretical concepts or conceptualize empirical events	2. The ability to use theoretical, research, and practice-based knowledge in nursing care
3. The ability to use the research process	3. The ability to use continual experience in the practice of nursing along with other educational experiences for constant professional growth and updating
4. The ability to use the philosophical principles of scientific inquiry	
5. The ability to use and develop research designs and methodology	4. The ability to evaluate the relevance and utility of research innovations based on the realities of clinical practice
6. The ability to use measurement models and to develop measurement systems	5. The ability to transfer critically and appropriately gathered information in a contrived research environment to the real world of nursing practice
7. The ability to use statistical analysis techniques	6. The ability to evaluate the effects of innovation on the client's status
8. The ability to make interpretations of collected data that are related to the theoretical base of the inquiry	7. The ability to evaluate the changes in the client's condition resulting from innovation separately from changes in the client's condition resulting from the application of other theoretically based nursing interventions and from other changes in the client's health status
9. The ability to communicate the findings of the research endeavor in a manner suitable to the potential consumer audience	8. The ability to feed back evaluative comments in the research arena

Reprinted with permission from Phillips, L.R.F. (1986, p. 9). *A clinician's guide to the critique and utilization of nursing research,* Norwalk, Conn., Appleton-Century-Crofts.

THE GAP BETWEEN RESEARCH AND PRACTICE

Unfortunately a tremendous gap exists between the dissemination and the use of research findings in nursing practice. Studies conducted by Ketefian (1975a) and Kirchhoff (1982) highlight this problem.

For example, Ketefian wanted to find out if nurses were using research findings in client care settings. She identified oral temperature determination as a common, frequent practice that had been studied and replicated. *Replication* is the repetition of a study in different settings with different samples, taken from the same or different populations. The findings of these studies had been widely disseminated for at least 5 years before her investigation.

The **research base** or group of studies on oral temperature determination indicated that the usual practice of placing a thermometer sublingually for 2 to 4 minutes did not reflect an accurate body temperature. More specifically, Nichols and Verhonick found that the optimum placement time was 9 minutes (cited in Ketefian, 1975a).

Ketefian (1975a) surveyed 87 registered nurses in New York and Massachusetts from a variety of employment settings regarding their practices of temperature determination. She found that only one nurse gave the correct placement time for an oral thermometer. Furthermore, although most respondents indicated that they thought the rectal mode was more accurate, they continued to use the oral mode in practice.

Another example of the gap that exists between the reporting of such findings and their use in practice is the results of Kirchhoff's (1982) study. She surveyed a nationwide sample of critical care nurses to "assess the impact of the published studies on the practices of restricting ice water and the measurement of rectal temperature" in cardiac patients (p. 196). Although reported research findings did not validate that these coronary precautions were necessary, they were still widely practiced. In addition, nurses' awareness of the published research was not related to changes in their practice.

Thus, as Horsley, Crane, and Bingle (1978) have pointed out, little evidence exists to indicate that research findings are being incorporated into practice. Nursing must come to terms with this issue to be accepted as a professional discipline that bases its practice on a valid body of knowledge.

Contributing factors

What are the reasons for the gap between research and practice? They can be broadly classified under the categories of educational preparation, communication, organizational resources, and resistance to change.

Educational preparation

The inclusion of research-related content in undergraduate nursing curricula is usually reserved for baccalaureate programs. It is well known, however, that most practicing nurses are graduates of diploma or associate degree programs. Thus most nurses who are expected to implement research findings in their practice do not have the educational preparation that is required to do this. Moreover, the focus of many research courses at the baccalaureate level is on the process of conducting research and on the critical evaluation of research reports. Rarely has the area of utilization been dealt with in an adequate fashion (Kirchhoff, 1983). Thus most professional nurses do not enter beginning practice with knowledge and skill needed for using research findings in practice.

Communication

Another factor that contributes to the gap between the dissemination and the use of research findings is the way in which studies are communicated to the profession. For the most part, research reports appear in research journals, publications that most practicing nurses do not read. Even if practitioners do read the published reports, they find them difficult to interpret. In a survey conducted by Miller and Messinger (1978) 75% of 499 nurses from the New York area reported having difficulty in reading research reports. The manner of presentation, which includes the use of research jargon, is aimed at an audience who has an advanced knowledge of research design and statistics.

Furthermore, nurses who are involved either in direct patient care or in the management of that care usually do not attend conferences where research findings are disseminated. Either they do not know of their existence, have not been encouraged to attend, do not see the relevance of these conferences to their practice, or are unable to take time off for attendance at conferences. As a consequence, those nurses who are in the best position to use the research findings disseminated at these conferences do not know of their existence.

Organizational resources

The organizational factors that can either facilitate or hinder research utilization in a service setting include the research climate, the availability of consultation, and the financial support.

The research climate. To be able to question current practices within our profession, an atmosphere of intellectual curiosity and freedom of thought must prevail in the workplace as well as in our educational institutions. Unfortunately, as Ketefian (1975b, p. 26) has stated, "there is a deeply ingrained adherence to tradition, authoritative sources, the 'procedure manual,' 'the way we were taught,' that makes it difficult to make room for the new." Coupled with the nonresearch attitudes that may exist within nursing services are the attitudes of physicians and administrators regarding nursing's place within the organization. For the most part the latter group still believes nursing's primary role is to carry out the physician's orders. Most physicians and hospital administrators are not even aware that nursing has its own body of knowledge that is different from medical knowledge. Even fewer are cognizant of the fact that some nurses are prepared educationally at the doctoral level to conduct their own research related to nursing phenomena, or that nurses are capable of collaborating on interdisciplinary research projects as peers.

The availability of consultation. Traditionally, doctorally prepared nurses who possess the skills needed to carry out research-related activities have been employed in academic settings. Concurrently, the nurses who are involved in the delivery of care and who are most familiar with the kinds of clinical problems that need to be addressed are employed in service settings. Unfortunately there has been little communication between these two groups. Ketefian (1975b, p. 14) suggested that the functions of developing and applying knowledge "cannot be adequately performed either by the practitioner or the researcher-scholar as that role is presently conceived, and that we probably need to conceive of new researcher roles or, in any case, a breed that has one foot in the world of research and the other in the world of practice." Phillips (1986) advocated increasing dialogue between nurse researchers and nurse clinicians.

However, many nurses, concerned about the lack of communication between researchers and practitioners, have begun to reach out to each other and realize each other's worth. A few schools of nursing and clinical agencies have begun to work together in both formal and informal relationships. The establishment of joint appointments in research between education and service is an example of a formal mechanism that provides an available research consultant to both groups. An example of an informal mechanism is the establishment of a consultative relationship between a staff nurse and her former teacher for the purpose of engaging in a research study or utilization project.

Financial support. In today's health care system with the advent of diagnostic-related groups (DRGs) and the push toward cost containment, financial resources are limited. Thus, even if the research climate in a given organization is favorable and consultation is readily available, the researcher still has to contend with the limited amount of funds available for both the conduct and utilization of nursing research.

Financial resources consist of the time that the nurse is released from the usual nursing responsibilities as well as the direct outlay of funds. In a recent survey conducted by Levin, Fitzgibbon, Belevich, and McDonald (1983) to assess the research climate in a large suburban medical center, the great majority of nurses responded that lack of time was the greatest barrier to their involvement in research activities.

Resistance to change

Most people are comfortable with the status quo. They are used to established routines and traditional ways of approaching problems. Every individual or group has a system of internalized values, beliefs, or attitudes that guides behavior. A proposed change that is perceived as threatening to this system is likely to result in resistance. Other factors that contribute to resistance to change include the following (Mauksch and Miller, 1981):

1. Lack of a felt need
2. Lack of knowledge about the change program
3. Threat to security
4. Behavior of the change agent

For example, when the introduction of a practice innovation is the change that is planned, the nursing staff may perceive it as a threat to their security because of a real inadequacy; that is, they are not familiar with the new practice and may question their ability to implement it. When the sources of resistance are known, they can be dealt with in a constructive manner.

However, not all opposition to change is defined as resistance. When change is opposed for logical reasons based on valid data, it is considered rational behavior (Mauksch and Miller, 1981). For example, a policy established at hospital X requires nurses to discard intravenous bags that have been removed from their outer wrappings and not used within 24 hours. Nurse Y has become attuned to cost-effective practices, sees this policy as very expensive, and wonders if it is supported by research findings. She reviews the literature and calls the company that manufactures the intravenous bags to obtain information related to the growth of organisms in unwrapped bags. Her search indicates that the outer wrap is not sterile to begin with, and studies have shown that bacterial growth does not occur any more often in unwrapped bags than it does in wrapped bags. Thus she opposes the new policy on logical grounds and is supported by facts.

It is also important to distinguish between resistance and interference. *Interference* is defined as those forces that hamper progress toward the change objective without being directly concerned with it (Lippett, Watson, and Westley, 1958, Chapter 4). It usually stems from a lack of resources needed to implement the change. These resources consist of time, energy, money, and qualified personnel. Let us imagine that you and your colleagues have read several studies that you believe to have relevance to your practice. You have obtained an informal consultation with a former teacher to evaluate these studies and validate your thinking. You wish to develop a proposal for implementation and evaluation of the research findings in your client care area. Because the members of your group have not attempted such a project before, you are not sure how to proceed and need additional consultation. Your former teacher, although interested in helping you, does not consider it possible to devote the necessary time and energy to the project without receiving financial reimbursement from your agency. Your group approaches the director of nursing, who has shown enthusiasm in your ideas, to ask for the necessary funds. She informs you that the nursing budget has already been submitted and approved for this year, and it did not include the services of a nursing research consultant. She goes on to say that she will try to include such an item in next year's budget, and so the project will have to be postponed. This is an example of an interfering force.

Closing the gap

Although the factors that contribute to the gap between the production and the use of knowledge may appear to be overwhelming, several mechanisms for narrowing the gap can be suggested. Some of these have been attempted on a limited basis. These mechanisms will be discussed in relation to the contributing factors outlined earlier.

Educational preparation

Professional nurses should be prepared to be intelligent research consumers. This includes the ability to critically evaluate reported studies and to determine which findings may be applicable to practice. One course in research methods taught in isolation from the rest of the curriculum fails to do this. As Levin (1983, p. 258) has pointed out previously, "Students do not come to perceive research as real or as related to their role as clinical practitioners."

One approach that may foster critical thinking about practice is to integrate research concepts throughout the curriculum. Instead of teaching fundamental nursing skills from the perspective of tradition and authority, research findings that support the demonstrated technique can be cited (Levin, 1983). For example, placing a client in a prone position with femurs internally rotated for the administration of a dorsogluteal injection has been taught for years as a valid practice to reduce discomfort. In theory, this position was supposed to result in a relaxed muscle that would reduce the discomfort of an injection. However, only recently was this hypothesis supported by research findings (Kruszewski, Lang, and Johnson, 1979).

Granted that the educator has the responsibility of integrating such concepts into a curriculum, it behooves you, as a nursing student or practitioner, to question and challenge the principles and procedures that you are taught either in school or on the job. As a professional nurse you are responsible and accountable for seeking validation for your practice and for guiding the practice of those nurses who are not prepared at the professional level and who may not have been exposed to the perspective and methods of scientific inquiry.

Consider the following example, based on an actual incident. A staff nurse working on a surgical unit had taken a course on the uses of acupuncture and acupressure. She decided to try using an acupressure technique with some clients for the alleviation of postoperative pain. Her experience suggested that the technique might be an effective pain reduction innovation. It so happened that a nurse researcher employed by the hospital and an undergraduate student interested in participating in a research project as part of her clinical practicum were assigned to this unit. Because of the staff nurse's interest in acupressure, it was decided that the student would conduct a literature review to determine what prior research had been done in this area. The search revealed that no studies on the effectiveness of acupressure for pain relief had been published. Furthermore the only literature found on the topic consisted of "how to" manuals. In reading these manuals it was discovered that the administration of a great deal of pressure on various body areas was advocated for pain relief. However, this treatment was not suggested for postoperative pain. It became obvious that the administration of unusual pressure to a client postoperatively could result in deleterious effects. The staff nurse was therefore requested to discontinue her "experimentation." The point of this anecdote is to share with you the potential danger of using a treatment or technique that has not been validated through research and to encourage you to think critically about nursing practice.

Communication

The issue of communicating research findings to nurses who are involved in direct client care has begun to be addressed by some members of our profession. One direction that needs to be taken is to publish research-based articles in journals that are read by most practicing nurses. In such a spirit, the *American Journal of Nursing* recently added a regular column, "For the Research Record," that publishes summaries of completed and ongoing studies. Although some researchers are attemping to publish the results of their studies in a form that the practicing nurse would find easier to read and understand, a review of the *American Journal of Nursing* for the period June 1983 through June 1984 revealed only one research-based, full-length article (Taylor, West, Simon, Skelton, and Rowlingson, 1983).

The content and format of articles that appear in journals are based on what the publisher believes will appeal to the readers. If professional nurses began writing to the journals that they read and requesting more research-based content, the appearance of such articles would increase. By the same token, more nurses at all levels of practice could encourage our profession's research journals (for example, *Nursing Research* and *Research in Nursing and Health*) to publish articles that are written in terms more understandable to the practicing nurse.

Another approach to closing the communication gap might be for you to request staff development programs on the research process, the evaluation of research studies, and research utilization. Many in-service education departments in clinical agencies survey the nursing staff to plan their educational activities. If a nurse who is able to teach this content is not available within the agency, it may be possible to contact a nearby school of nursing to arrange continuing education courses, or to request a faculty member to present classes for the nursing staff at the agency.

Finally, many nursing research conferences in the past few years have focused on the presentation of studies that are of a clinical nature and have direct applicability to practice. Some examples are the following: the comparison of different techniques for treating decubitus ulcers, the use of various relaxation techniques for decreasing pain, and the development and validation of nursing diagnoses. Attendance at these conferences would enhance a practitioner's awareness of potential practice innovations and increase her ability to understand and evaluate research findings. It is the responsibility of every professional nurse to keep up to date with the expanding body of knowledge of the discipline.

Because participation at these conferences can be costly, many nursing service departments have an educational fund that can be used to defray the cost of attending such programs. However, to receive reimbursement for expenses (for example, registration fees, transportation, and lodging), a formal request must be submitted. Ask your head nurse, supervisor, or in-service educator how to go about this. You may be asked to justify the relevance of these programs to your position at the agency. It is hoped that the information contained in this chapter will assist you in emphasizing the importance of your role as a research consumer.

Organizational resources

The research climate. Clearly, the key to making the conduct and utilization of research an integral part of nursing practice is the administrator of a nursing service (Fawcett, 1980). Without this individual's support any attempt at establishing a research utilization program cannot succeed. Therefore it is essential that a nurse ask relevant questions about the nursing service administrator's attitude toward nursing research in general, and utilization in particular, when interviewing for a position within an organization. Ascertaining the level of education of the head of a nursing department as well as that of the nurses in middle management can be helpful. If you know that the director of nursing has a doctorate, you are almost assured that she or he is at least aware of the significance of nursing research to practice. On the other hand, if she or he has a bachelor's degree in another field, such as in health education or business, such an awareness may be lacking. It is also important to find out whether or not these nurses have been involved in research activities, either in their educational programs or in the practice setting, and their attitudes toward innovation and positive change.

Obtaining this kind of information may be a difficult task for you, especially if you are applying for your first job. The answers to these questions, however, will tell you something about the general attitude toward nursing within the institution as well as the specific attitude toward nursing research and its application in practice. The following are some nonthreatening questions that can elicit these answers:

1. Can you share a copy of the job description for a staff nurse with me? Are there any additional expectations?
2. Do staff nurses get involved with research? How?
3. What are the criteria for promotion?
4. What kinds of committees does the nursing department have? Is there a research committee? How could I participate?

The manner in which these kinds of questions are answered as well as the answers themselves indicate the prevailing attitude toward nursing research within the department. If you perceive a negative attitude, you have the option of withdrawing your application for employment.

Given the existence of a positive attitude toward research within a nursing department, an ideal mechanism for facilitating the utilization of research in practice would be the employment of a nurse researcher by the service agency. Such a position can take several forms: (1) a full-time position, (2) a part-time position, (3) a consultant position, or (4) a joint appointment with a school of nursing. Over the past few years an increasing number of agencies have been able to develop such positions within nursing departments. Although most clinical nurse researchers (CNRs) recently surveyed (59% of 34) reported that facilitating the research of others was a major responsibility of their role, they did not identify application of research to practice as a role function (Hagle, Kirchhoff, Knafl, and Bevis, 1986). It is reasonable to assume, however, that any nurse on the staff of these agencies could request and be given help from the CNR in developing a research utilization project.

Although the number is increasing, most service agencies do not employ CNRs in any capacity. There are, however, several ways you can assist your nursing colleagues to become aware of and integrate research into their practice. A relatively simple way to begin is to form a journal club. Such a group can meet periodically to review research articles that have potential applicability to practice. Members can rotate the responsibility for finding and critiquing these studies and for presenting them to the group. The discovery of a new technique or practice approach in one article may generate enough interest in the group for pursuit of a more thorough literature search on that topic, which can form the research base for a potential utilization project.

A more formal approach is the establishment of a nursing research committee within a department of nursing service. Among the purposes of such committees are the following: (1) creating an awareness of the need for using research findings in practice, (2) identifying clinical practice problems that require investigations, (3) providing educational programs related to research utilization to nursing staff, and (4) planning, implementing, and evaluating utilization projects. Of course, to carry out these purposes committee members must possess some knowledge of research and be able to obtain the resources they do not already possess.

   The availability of consultation. If nurses who have the necessary educational preparation and research skill are not available within the organization, faculty members from nearby schools of nursing can be asked to join the committee. Such an arrangement not only provides needed expertise for the research committee but can provide faculty members with a clinical setting and ideas for the conduct of their own research. It can also foster collaborative research efforts between service and education.

   Janken, Dufault, and Yeaw (1988) described another collaborative approach to disseminating practice-relevant research findings in a service setting. Faculty from five affiliated schools of nursing joined with members of a hospital nursing service to create a climate that fostered the incorporation of research values and activities as part of the nurse's role. Unit-based roundtable research discussions were held periodically. They were facilitated by faculty members and attended by both nursing students and staff. The discussions focused on research related to common nursing problems experienced by the clients on the units. Although there was a good deal of resistance to the project at first, the discussions did eventually increase appreciation for nursing research and its relevance to practice. One example of the impact these discussions had on practice is as follows (p. 190): "After learning that moist dressings as a treatment for decubitus ulcers were ineffective unless they were in place for an extended time period, the nurses argued persuasively in favor of switching to a more expensive product, but one that adhered to the skin."

   Intradisciplinary (within nursing) collaboration is one way of facilitating the use of research in practice. *Interdisciplinary* (between professions) collaboration is another alternative. Many innovations may be interdependent in nature and therefore would require the joint efforts of medicine and nursing. The use of a clean, as opposed to a sterile, technique for tracheostomy suctioning is one example. Another is the early discharge of a specified group of clients from the acute care setting.

   Interdisciplinary collaboration begins with a collegial relationship between different health care providers. It means having respect for the perspective and knowledge that each one brings to the client care or research situation. Because other health care providers, such as physicians, may not be aware of nursing's increasing knowledge and capabilities relative to research or its unique contribution to client care, it may be necessary to convey this in informal conversation about specific client problems or situations before broaching the idea for a collaborative research project. For example, I was part of an interdisciplinary hospital Professional Standards Review Committee a number of years ago. The committee's task was to review the records of surgical clients to determine the adequacy of postoperative pain management. The focus of the physicians and pharmacists was on the proper use of analgesics. However, as a nurse, I was able to present the potential benefits of other techniques of pain management that had previously not been considered by this group and to gain the committee's support for including items regarding these interventions (for example, positioning, touching, and relaxing) as part of the audit. When a subsequent nursing research project on the use of relaxation techniques for postoperative pain was initiated, full cooperation of these health professionals was apparent.

Implicit in interdisciplinary collaboration is the notion of equal status. That means that nurses function as coinvestigators on a study or utilization project, not just as research assistants or data collectors. To be a coinvestigator means being involved in determining the purpose and method of a research project as well as coauthoring any publications that result from it.

As nurses become more articulate about the uniqueness of their profession and more knowledgeable about the research process and implementation of research in practice, and as physicians and other members of the health care team begin to realize the unique and valuable contribution that nurses make in health care, interdisciplinary collaboration in research utilization will increase.

Financial support. Collaborative approaches to research utilization not only provide the skill and expertise needed for the development, implementation, and evaluation of such projects, but may also decrease the investment of time and energy required by any one individual. Furthermore, expenses such as consultation fees and the purchase of computer time for data analysis can be defrayed. Faculty from a nearby school of nursing may be willing to forgo a consultation fee in exchange for authorship on a publication about the project. In addition, faculty may be able to draw on other resources that are more available in an academic setting than in a service setting. The use of computer services for statistical analysis of data, for example, may be available to faculty members for a minimal charge or at no cost.

Resistance to change

When the potential for change is evaluated, the first step is to assess the existence of interfering forces and try to eliminate them. As you will recall, these forces have to do with an absence of needed resources, such as time, energy, money, and skill. Measures that can decrease interfering forces have been described earlier.

The next step is to assess the actual or potential sources of resistance to change, described previously (see p. 364). When the sources of resistance are known, they can usually be dealt with in a constructive manner. For example, if nurses do not know what to expect from the introduction of a practice innovation, their fear of the unknown may become a resistive force. One way of preventing this is to explicitly communicate what the utilization project entails, why it is being carried out, how the nurses will or will not be involved, and when it will take place. Such information should be provided before the project is a fait accompli so that there is time to deal with the concerns of those nurses whose support is essential to a successful project outcome.

So far we have looked at forces that can hinder the process of change. There are also forces that can facilitate the process of change, called *driving* forces. Driving forces can be both initial and emergent facilitators of the change process. Initial facilitators include the following: (1) a dissatisfaction with the present situation, (2) a realization that the situation can be improved, and (3) feelings of external pressure, such as role expectations or competitiveness. Emergent facilitators include the following: (1) the need to complete a task or project that has begun, (2) the need to meet expectations, both external and internal, and (3) an increase in insight or a developed need on the part of the individual or group involved in the change (Lippett, Watson, and Westley, 1958, Chapter 4).

Horsley, Crane, Crabtree, and Wood (1983) have emphasized the importance of fostering an awareness of the need for change among those who will be involved in the process. They state, "Both administrative and practicing nurses must perceive some need for the change if it is to succeed" (p. 4). Participation in decision making by all persons whom the change will affect can enhance interest and motivation. The use of a suggestion box, regularly scheduled meetings where new ideas are encouraged between staff nurses and those in middle management, and participation by representatives from all levels of practice in decision-making groups are all ways to increase an awareness of the need for change.

After the development of a need for a practice change is realized and relationships among involved individuals are established, planning for the change can occur. Change takes time; a great deal of frustration can result from expecting it to occur too rapidly. However, in the long run a careful, deliberative approach to the change process will increase the chances of a successful outcome.

UTILIZATION CRITERIA

Given a climate that encourages and supports the conduct and use of nursing research, how do you decide which areas of clinical research are ready for incorporation into practice? Before 1979 little assistance in this area was available in the nursing literature. As a result of a federally funded project in the mid-1970s, "Conduct and Utilization of Research in Nursing," criteria to guide utilization efforts were established. They fall into the following three major categories (Haller, Reynolds, and Horsely, 1979):
1. Evaluating the knowledge base
2. Assessing relevance to practice
3. Determining the potential for clinical evaluation

Despite the existence of these criteria as a guide, it is not realistic to expect that you will be able to accomplish the task of research utilization on your own. However, it is essential that you understand the process and that you participate actively in it as a knowledgeable consumer. Consultation and collaboration are a necessary component of the process.

Evaluating the knowledge base

The identification of studies that can provide a valid research base for application to practice involve the following three criteria (Haller, Reynolds, and Horsely, 1979; Fawcett, 1982):
1. Replication
2. Scientific merit
3. Risk

Replication

As you may recall, *replication* is the repetition of a study in different settings with different samples, taken from the same or different populations. The replication study may be conducted by the same or different investigators. The purpose of replication is to increase the generalizability of findings (Fawcett, 1982) and to decrease the chances of committing a type I error (Haller, Reynolds, and Horsely, 1979). This error occurs when a researcher concludes falsely that a treatment or intervention has a significant effect, but in reality, this effect has occurred by chance alone.

It has been noted that replication is not commonplace in nursing research (Fawcett, 1982). When direct replication of a study has not been attempted, it is important to find instances of *construct replication*. "Construct replication is achieved when a second investigator begins with a similar problem statement but formulates original methods of measurement and design to verify the first author's findings" (Haller, Reynolds, and Horsely, 1979, p. 47).

The following two studies demonstrate construct replication. In the first study Flaherty and Fitzpatrick (1978) tested the effects of a relaxation exercise on clients' postoperative comfort level when they were getting out of bed for the first time. A sample of 42 male and female clients who underwent elective surgery, such as cholecystectomy, herniorrhaphy, or hemorrhoidectomy, was divided into experimental and control groups. The experimental group was taught a relaxation exercise the night before surgery and was reminded to use it when getting out of bed 6 to 8 hours after surgery. Comfort level was measured by a scale on which clients indicated both the degree of sensation they were experiencing and how much distress this sensation was causing them. In addition, the investigators collected data on the amount of analgesics each group required during the first 24 postoperative hours. The results of this study showed that the experimental group experienced significantly less discomfort and required fewer analgesics than the control group.

Wells (1982), building on the work of Flaherty and Fitzpatrick, used a sample of 12 clients undergoing cholecystectomy to study a similar problem: however, she looked at clients' discomfort levels during the first 3 postoperative days, not during their first ambulation. A relaxation technique that differed somewhat from the one used by Flaherty and Fitzpatrick was taught to the experimental group on the night before surgery. Wells used the same scale to measure postoperative discomfort, but her method of determining analgesic usage differed. The results did not support a difference between experimental and control groups in their use of analgesics or in sensation scores. However, in agreement with the former study, Wells found self-reported distress to be significantly different between the groups. Taken together, these studies indicate that the use of a relaxation technique has potential for the reduction of postoperative discomfort.

Ideally, the research base should consist of a synthesis of the knowledge gained from several studies whose findings are consistent. In reality this is not always possible. It is suggested that at least two valid investigations of a similar problem be identified before an innovation is considered for application to practice (Horsley, Crane, and Bingle, 1983).

Scientific merit

Once a research base has been identified, the **scientific merit** of each study that constitutes this base must be considered. Chapter 21 provides the criteria for critiquing research reports. The findings and conclusions of a study must always be evaluated in terms of the theoretical framework and design. When the goal is utilization the population from which study samples were drawn is particularly important. Are they appropriate for the clinical problem? Has at least one study used a clinical population for hypothesis testing (Haller, Reynolds, and Horsely, 1979)? The results of laboratory experiments using a "normal" population cannot be generalized to a clinical setting. For example, a recent study by Geden, Beck, Hauge, and Pohlman (1984) investigated the effects of five different pain-coping strategies on the self-reported sensation of labor contractions. The sample for this research consisted of 100 nulliparous female college undergraduates. The subjects were exposed to a laboratory stimulus that simulated labor contractions. Although one of the strategies (sensory transformation) was found to have a significant effect on self-reported pain, these results cannot be generalized to a population of women who are experiencing the actual process of labor. Replication of this study in a clinical population would be necessary before these findings could be considered for use in practice.

During the process of evaluating the scientific merit of the research base, you may come across studies that have contradictory findings. As Haller, Reynolds, and Horsely (1979, p. 48) pointed out, "Attempts are made to resolve contradictory findings either through identification of methodological weakness or through a theoretical explanation for the discrepancy. It is also recognized that in a series of replications of the same study, a nonsignificant difference may be expected to occur a certain number of times on the basis of chance alone."

Risk

The third criterion that should be applied when evaluating research for its applicability to practice is the degree of risk involved in the new intervention. Teaching clients how to use a relaxation technique to decrease postoperative discomfort or leaving an oral thermometer in place a few more minutes are innovations that entail very little if any risk. On the other hand, the elimination of coronary precautions such as avoiding the rectal mode of temperature determination does involve a certain degree of risk. When an innovation has risks associated with it, a "stronger, more established" knowledge base is required than when no risk is evident (Fawcett, 1982, p. 57); that is, if there is any risk to a client, it is imperative that several studies with a high degree of scientific merit that have been replicated with clinical populations form the knowledge base and support the benefits of the practice. You must always question whether the potential benefits of a new practice outweigh the risks.

According to Stetler and Marram (1976), if an evaluation of the scientific merit of studies leads you to conclude that findings are invalid, no further action is warranted. However, given a sound research base that supports the efficacy of a clinical innovation, an assessment of its relevance to practice follows.

ASSESSING RELEVANCE TO PRACTICE

The following are questions to be addressed in assessing an innovation's relevance to practice (Fawcett, 1982, p. 58):

> Does the study focus on a significant clinical practice problem?
> Do nurses have clinical control of the study variables?
> Is it feasible to implement the nursing action (if any such action was part of the study)?
> What is the cost of implementing the nursing action?

The first question involves a determination of the clinical merit of the research base. Simply put, you want to know if a problem of practical significance to nurses will be solved by instituting a new intervention. Fawcett (1982) cautions us to guard against the premature application of study findings. Even if findings appear to be ready for clinical use, they may lack a clear theoretical structure. When knowledge consists of a collection of atheoretical facts, it usually cannot be generalized to situations or settings outside of those where it was obtained. Therefore the clinical merit and the scientific merit of a research base must be balanced.

The second question addresses the degree of clinical control nurses have over the implementation and the evaluation of the new practice. Implementation involves the degree of independence nursing has in manipulating the independent variable. For instance, the introduction of a relaxation exercise to clients preoperatively for their use after surgery is clearly within the purview of nursing. However, the innovation sometimes requires an interdependent activity that can achieve clinical control only through collaborative efforts with other disciplines. Haller, Reynolds, and Horsely (1979) provide the example of nonsterile intermittent urinary catheterization as an innovation that requires medical cooperation.

Clinical control in the measurement of outcomes, the dependent variable(s), is also of concern. What kind of instruments have been used in the research base to measure the dependent variables? Are these readily available and applicable in practice? What new skills might be needed to use the research tools (Haller, Reynolds, and Horsely, 1979)? If you are introducing a new protocol based on research findings for oral hygiene with clients who are receiving chemotherapy, you would want to evaluate its effectiveness. One client outcome that may be indicative of the protocol's effectiveness is a decrease in the growth of organisms in the mouth at specific intervals. To measure this you would need to gain the cooperation of physicians in ordering periodic cultures.

Sometimes it is not possible to use the same tools that have been used in studies. In such cases a clinical approximation needs to be made. As an example, instead of using spirometry to measure respiratory status as an indication of the efficacy of a preoperative teaching protocol, one hospital "chose to substitute tape measurement of chest expansion and auscultation" (Haller, Reynolds, and Horsely, 1979, p. 49).

The third factor needed to be considered when assessing the relevance of an innovation to practice is *feasibility*. Are the resources, such as time, personnel, equipment, and skill, available in your practice setting (Haller, Reynolds, and Horsely, 1979)? Recall the research cited earlier that studied the effectiveness of relaxation techniques for postoperative discomfort. Although the implementation of a simple relaxation exercise during preoperative teaching sessions would not involve a great deal of time or additional personnel, it would require other resources. If an audio recording of the technique were used as a teaching tool, there would be a need for equipment, such as tape recorders and earphones. In addition, skill in using and teaching the relaxation technique would be needed by the involved nurses. Learning this skill can be accomplished in a relatively short period of time, but an organized program of instruction conducted by a knowledgeable individual would be required. To attend the classes nurses would most likely need to be given released time from their client care responsibilities.

Finally, the *cost-effectiveness* of a new practice needs to be estimated. This includes the costs of both implementation and evaluation. The research base may include variables that are related directly to cost, such as days in hospital or prevention of complications. However, it is more likely for the research base to contain variables that possess an indirect relationship to cost, such as client or staff satisfaction. In the latter case it may be necessary for you to "make a case for" the potential of an innovation to decrease actual costs before administrators are willing to invest the financial resources needed for research utilization. In the final analysis you must consider whether or not a new innovation is worth the time, energy, and cost involved in its application to practice (Stetler and Marram, 1976).

Clinical evaluation

Once a research base for a practice innovation has been identified and its relevance to clinical practice has been established, the next step is to determine the potential for clinical evaluation of the new innovation. It is important to realize that the research variables, measurement techniques, and experimental procedures may not always be amenable to direct translation into practice. Thus you need to consider how these will be transformed for purposes of implementation and evaluation.

Because utilization of research findings usually involves a transformation of the independent variable in some way, it is essential that its effects in practice or outcomes be evaluated. For example, tight controls over the administration of an experimental treatment are needed to increase the internal validity of research design. Such controls would probably include limiting the number of nurse research assistants who perform the treatment; using data collectors who are blind to the subjects' experimental condition, such as a treatment group versus a control group; and attempting to keep the setting or situation where the treatment is administered the same for all subjects. It cannot be assumed that the translation of experimental procedures into practice will achieve the same outcomes as demonstrated in controlled studies. Thus careful planning of how the experimental treatment will be incorporated into practice is essential. At the very least, those nurses who will be involved in using a practice innovation need to be taught a standardized approach for implementation.

How will client or staff outcomes be measured? Are the measurement tools used in the research studies appropriate for clinical use? Have all the variables of interest to nursing been assessed in the studies? Have variables that nursing does not have control over been included as outcome measures? Haller, Reynolds, and Horsely (1979, p. 50) explicate these problems with the following example:

> The original work on nonsterile intermittent catheterization was done by physicians. Some of the dependent variables, such as cystoscopy results, were not felt to be appropriate as nursing outcomes. On the other hand, some of the variables of keen interest to nursing were not accounted for in the research base; these included patient satisfaction, patient mobility, and degree of interaction. Therefore, an evaluation procedure was devised that included variables from the research base and also drew on introspection about clinical practice.

Sometimes the dependent variable or outcome measure is appropriate for clinical evaluation, but the research instrument is not easily incorporated into a practice situation. Many studies have used lengthy questionnaires to assess such variables as self-concept, client satisfaction, locus of control, and anxiety. The State-Trait Anxiety Inventory (STAI) (Spielberger, Gorsuch, and Lushene, 1970), for instance, has been shown to be a valid and reliable instrument and has been used in many recent studies to measure situational or characteristic anxiety. It is a 40-item questionnaire that takes approximately 15 minutes to complete. If anxiety was an outcome measure that you were interested in assessing, you might have to find a more convenient way of measuring it in your setting.

Recently I was faced with just such a situation. Staff nurses in a general hospital were looking for a simple tool to assess clients' anxiety levels. Graphic rating scales were developed (see Fig. 20-1) and compared with the STAI. Both instruments were administered to a sample of 30 nurses who were enrolled in graduate research courses at a nearby university. With the Pearson product moment coefficient of correlation (r), the following results were obtained: (1) scores of state anxiety correlated 0.80 and (2) scores of trait anxiety correlated 0.70. Given the relatively high positive relationship between the scores, the graphic rating scales were deemed to be useful for measuring anxiety in clinical practice (Levin and Crosley, 1986).

The process of evaluating a new innovation can be costly. Therefore it is imperative that a budget be drafted and approved before any efforts at implementation begin. Items such as released time for nurses to learn the new technique as well as for nurse educators or clinical specialists to teach it, the development of an evaluation protocol, purchase or development of measurement tools, direction of the project, and data collection and analysis must all be considered. As mentioned earlier, because the cost of introducing and evaluating a nursing practice innovation can be high, justification of these expenditures must be documented in the form of potential savings for the institution and the consumer.

If the service agency cannot afford to support a utilization project on its own, alternatives are available. Outside funding may be one way of obtaining the needed financial resources. As an example, the U.S. Department of Health and Human Services (DHHS), through the Division of Nursing of the Public Health Service (PHS), offers a competitive grants program for nursing research utilization projects. However, to compete for these grants the principal investigator must possess the

HOW DO YOU USUALLY FEEL?

0	1	2	3	4
Calm	Slightly anxious	Moderately anxious	Very anxious	Extremely anxious

HOW DO YOU FEEL RIGHT NOW?

0	1	2	3	4
Calm	Slightly anxious	Moderately anxious	Very anxious	Extremely anxious

Fig. 20-1 Graphic anxiety scale.

appropriate credentials, for example, doctoral preparation, previous research, and publications. Few service agencies employ such an individual; most doctorally prepared nurses with research expertise are affiliated with academic institutions.Therefore collaborative efforts between service and education, as discussed previously, may facilitate the implementation and evaluation of research findings in practice.

RESEARCH VERSUS CLINICAL EVALUATION

There are differences between conducting a research study and evaluating the use of research findings in practice. Although clinical evaluation requires a systematic process that involves standardization of treatments (independent variable), measurement of outcomes (dependent variables), and analysis of data, it does not usually require the tight methodological controls of research studies (Haller, Reynolds, and Horsely, 1979). In addition, the purposes of the projects differ. The New York State Nurses Association Council on Nursing Research, in an effort to clarify the differences between evaluation and research, identified the following criteria to use when judging whether a project is a nursing research study (NYSNA Council on Nursing Research, 1983, p. 43):

1. Rigorous scientific method is employed throughout the process from the statement of hypotheses or research question through the conclusion.
2. The purpose of the study is the discovery of new knowledge.
3. The knowledge sought falls within the body of knowledge needed for nursing.

The purpose of a clinical evaluation project is to assess the worth or effectiveness of an innovation in a specific setting. The selection of clients does not usually include probability sampling techniques. Hypothesis testing by means of inferential statistics is not employed. The design of an evaluation is usually preexperimental, such as a comparison of preimplementation and postimplementation data by frequencies, percentages, ranges, rates, and means (Haller, Reynolds, and Horsely, 1979). Thus the results of a clinical evaluation can guide the decision about whether or not to incorporate a nursing practice innovation in a specific setting with a particular group of clients, but cannot be generalized to the entire client population or to other settings.

For too long a gap has existed between research and practice. Nursing has been so engrossed in elevating its status in the health care arena that at times it has perhaps lost sight of its primary goal: the development of knowledge to guide professional practice, not the development of knowledge for its own sake. Nurse researchers and practitioners have sometimes forgotten the need to communicate with one another if this goal is to be achieved. It is up to the new generation of professional nurses, both researchers and practitioners, to work together to improve the care we provide to society. This can be accomplished only by using valid findings in practice. In your role as a knowledgeable consumer of nursing research, you have an important part to play in this effort.

SUMMARY

The members of a professional discipline use research findings as a basis for practice. In this chapter factors related to the gap between the dissemination and the use of nursing research findings in practice were discussed. These included the educational preparation of nurses, the way that research is communicated to the profession, the lack of organizational resources, and the resistance to change. Suggestions for closing the gap were provided. Criteria that can be used to evaluate research findings and assess their applicability to clinical practice were presented. The factors involved in determining the potential for clinical evaluation of a practice innovation were outlined. Finally, the differences between a research study and a clinical evaluation were highlighted.

References

Donaldson, S., and Crowley, D. (1978). The discipline of nursing, *Nursing Outlook,* **26:** 113-120.

Fawcett J. (1980). A declaration of nursing independence: the relation of theory and research to nursing practice, *Journal of Nursing Administration,* **10:**36-39.

Fawcett, J. (1982). Utilization of nursing research findings, *Image,* **14:**57-59.

Fawcett, J. (1984). Another look at utilization of nursing research, *Image,* **16:**59-62.

Flaherty, G., and Fitzpatrick, J. (1978). Relaxation technique to increase comfort level of postoperative patients: a preliminary study, *Nursing Research,* **27:**352-355.

Geden, E., Beck, N., Hauge, G., and Pohlman, S. (1984). Self-report and psycho physiological effects of five pain-coping strategies, *Nursing Research,* **33:**260-265.

Hagle, M.E., Kirchhoff, K.T., Knafl, K.A., and Bevis, M.E. (1986). The clinical nurse researcher: new perspectives, *Journal of Professional Nursing,* **2:**282-288.

Haller, K., Reynolds, M., and Horsley, J. (1979). Developing research-based innovation protocols: process, criteria, and issues, *Research in Nursing and Health,* **2:**45.

Horsley, J., Crane, J., and Bingle, J. (1978). Research utilization as an organizational process, *Journal of Nursing Administration,* **8:**4-6.

Horsley, J., Crane, J., Crabtree, M., and Wood D. (1983). *Using research to improve nursing practice: a guide,* New York, Grune & Stratton, Inc.

Janken, J.K., Dufault, M.A., and Yeaw, E.M.S. (1988). Research round tables: increasing student/staff nurse awareness of the relevancy of research to practice, *Journal of Professional Nursing,* **4:**186-191.

Ketefian, S. (1975a). Application of selected nursing research findings into nursing practice, *Nursing Research,* **24**:89-92.

Ketefian, S. (1975b). Problems in the dissemination and utilization of scientific knowledge: how can the gap be bridged? In *Translation of theory into nursing practice and education,* New York, New York University Press.

Kirchhoff, K. (1982). A diffusion survey of coronary precautions, *Nursing Research,* **31**: 196-201.

Kirchhoff, K. (1983). Using research in practice: should staff nurses be expected to use research? *Western Journal of Nursing Research,* **5**:245-247.

Kruszewski, A., Lang, S., and Johnson, J. (1979). Effect of positioning on discomfort from intramuscular injections in the dorsogluteal site, *Nursing Research,* **28**:103-105.

Levin, R. (1983). Research for the undergraduate: too much, too soon? *Nursing Outlook,* **31**:258-259.

Levin, R., and Crosley, J. (1986). Evaluation of focused data collection for the generation of nursing diagnoses. *Journal of Nursing Staff Development,* **1**:56-64.

Levin, R., Fitzgibbon, A., Belevich, R., and McDonald, A. (1983). *Assessment of nursing research climate,* Unpublished manuscript.

Lippett, R., Watson, J., and Westley, B. (1958). *The dynamics of planned change,* New York, Harcourt, Brace, Jovanovich, Inc.

Mauksch, I., and Miller M. (1981). *Implementing change in nursing,* St. Louis, The C.V. Mosby Co.

Miller, J.R., and Messinger, S.R. (1978). Obstacles to applying nursing research findings, *American Journal of Nursing,* **78**:632-634.

NYSNA Council on Nursing Research (1983). What constitutes nursing research? *Journal of New York States Nurses' Association,* **14**:42-45.

Phillips, L.R.F. (1986). *A clinician's guide to the critique and utilization of nursing research,* Norwalk, Conn., Appleton-Century-Crofts.

Spielberger, C., Gorsuch, R., and Lushene, R. (1970). *STAI manual,* Palo Alto, Calif., Consulting Psychologists Press.

Stetler, C.B., and Marram, G. (1976). Evaluating research findings for applicability in practice, *Nursing Outlook,* **24**:559-563.

Taylor, A., West, B., Simon, B., Skelton, J., and Rowlingson, J. (1983). How effective is TENS for acute pain? *American Journal of Nursing,* **83**:1171-1174.

Wells, N. (1982). The effect of relaxation on postoperative muscle tension and pain, *Nursing Research,* **31**:236-238.

21

Evaluating the Research Report

Judith A. Heermann
Betty J. Craft

LEARNING OBJECTIVES

After reading this chapter the student should be able to:

◇ Identify the influence of stylistic considerations on the presentation of a research report.

◇ Identify the purpose of the critiquing process.

◇ List the steps of the critiquing process.

◇ Describe the criteria of each step of the critiquing process.

◇ Evaluate the strengths and weaknesses of a research report.

◇ Discuss the implications of the findings of a research report for nursing practice.

◇ Construct a critique of a research report.

> **KEY TERMS**
>
> replication
> research base
> scientific merit

To determine the merit of a research report each component of a research study is examined. Criteria designed to assist the consumer in judging the relative value of a research report can be found in previous chapters. An abbreviated set of questions (Table 21-1) encapsulating the more detailed criteria is used in this chapter as the framework for two sample research critiques. These critiques are included to exemplify the process of evaluating reported research for potential application to practice and thus extending the **research base** for nursing. Readers are encouraged to refer to the earlier chapters for the detailed presentation of the critiquing criteria and explanations of the research process. The criteria and examples in this chapter apply to quantitative studies. For critiquing qualitative studies see the guidelines presented in Chapter 11.

STYLISTIC CONSIDERATIONS

Before beginning to critique research studies the evaluator should realize several important aspects related to the world of publishing. First, different journals have different publication goals. The market that a group of journals appeals to varies, and so the focus of the content and style of articles accepted for publication also varies. For example, *Nursing Research* is a journal that publishes articles on the conduct or results of research in nursing. The *Journal of Obstetric, Gynecologic, and Neonatal Nursing* also publishes research articles, but it in addition includes articles related to the knowledge, experience, trends, and policies in obstetrical, gynecological, and neonatal nursing. The emphasis in this latter journal is broader in that it contains topical as well as research articles. Consequently the style and content of the manuscript will vary according to the type of journal to which it is being submitted.

Second, the author of a research article prepares the manuscript using both personal judgment and specific guidelines. *Personal judgment* refers to the researcher's expertise developed in the course of designing, executing, and analyzing the study. As a result of this expertise, the researcher is in the position to make judgments about the content that is thought to be the most important to communicate to the profession. The decision is a function of the following:

◇ The level of the study: experimental or nonexperimental
◇ The focus of the study: basic, applied, or clinical
◇ The audience to which the results will be most appropriately communicated

Table 21-1 **Major Content Sections of a Research Report and Related Critiquing Guidelines**

Section	Questions to guide evaluation
Problem statement and purpose (see Chapter 4)	1. What is the problem and/or purpose of the research study? 2. Does the problem and/or purpose statement express a relationship between two or more variables or at least between an independent and a dependent variable? If so, what is/are the relationship(s)? 3. Does the problem statement and/or purpose specify the nature of the population being studied? What is it? 4. What significance of the problem has been identified, if any?
Review of literature and definitions (see Chapters 5 and 6)	1. What concepts are included in the review? Particularly note those concepts that are the independent and dependent variables. 2. Does the literature review make explicit the relationships among the variables or place the variables within a theoretical/conceptual framework? What are the relationships? 3. What gaps in knowledge about the problem are identified, and how does this study intend to fill those gaps? 4. Are the references cited by the author mostly primary or mostly secondary sources? Give an example of each. 5. What are the conceptual and operational definitions of the independent and dependent variables?
Hypotheses and/or research question(s) (see Chapter 7)	1. What hypothesis(es) and/or research questions are stated in the study? 2. What are the independent and dependent variables in the statement of each hypothesis? 3. What is the direction of the relationship in each hypothesis, if indicated? 4. In what form is each hypothesis stated, i.e., statistical (null) or research? 5. If research questions are stated, are they used in addition to hypotheses or to guide an exploratory study?
Sample (see Chapter 15)	1. How was the sample selected? 2. What type of sampling method is used in the study? 3. To what population may the findings be generalized? 4. Is the sample representative of the population as identified in the problem or purpose statement? 5. Is the sample size appropriate?

Continued.

Table 21-1 Major Content Sections of a Research Report and Related Critiquing Guidelines—cont'd

Section	Questions to guide evaluation
Research design (see Chapters 8 to 12)	1. What type of design is used in the study? 2. What is the rationale for the design classification? 3. Does the design seem to flow from the proposed problem statement, theoretical framework, literature review, and hypothesis?
Internal validity	1. Review each of the threats to internal validity in relation to the study. 2. Does the design have controls at an acceptable level for the threats to internal validity?
External validity	1. What are the limits to generalizability in terms of external validity?
Research approach (see Chapters 13 and 14) Methods	1. What type(s) of data collection method(s) is/are used in the study? 2. Are the data collection procedures similar for all subjects? 3. What indications are given that informed consent of the subjects has been ensured?

Instruments	1. Physiological measurement
	  a. Is a rationale given for why a particular instrument/method was selected? If so, what is it?
	  b. What provision is made for maintaining the accuracy of the instrument and its use, if any?
	2. Observational methods
	  a. Who did the observing?
	  b. How were the observers trained to minimize bias?
	  c. Was there an observational guide?
	  d. Were the observers required to make inferences about what they saw?
	  e. Is there any reason to believe that the presence of the observers affected the behavior of the subjects?
	3. Interviews
	  a. Who were the interviewers and how were they trained?
	  b. Is there evidence of any interviewer bias? If so, what is it?
	4. Questionnaires
	  a. What is the type and/or format of the questionnaire (e.g., Likert, open-ended)?
	5. Available data and records
	  a. Are the records that were utilized appropriate to the problem being studied?
	  b. Are these data being used to describe the sample or for hypothesis testing?

Table 21-1 **Major Content Sections of a Research Report and Related Critiquing Guidelines — cont'd**

Section	Questions to guide evaluation
Reliability and validity (see Chapter 14)	1. What type of reliability is reported for each instrument? 2. What level of reliability is reported and is it acceptable? 3. What type of validity is reported for each instrument? 4. Does the validity of each instrument seem adequate and why?

Analysis of data (see Chapters 16 and 17)	1. What level of measurement is used to measure each of the major variables?
	2. What descriptive and/or inferential statistics are reported?
	3. Were these descriptive and/or inferential statistics appropriate to the level of measurement for each variable?
	4. Are the inferential statistics used appropriate to the intent of the hypothesis(es)?
	5. What is the level of significance set for the study?
	6. If tables or figures are used, do they meet the following standards?
	  a. They supplement and economize the text.
	  b. They have precise titles and headings.
	  c. They are not repetitious of the text.

Conclusions, implications, and recommendations (see Chapter 19)	1. If hypothesis testing was done, was/were the hypothesis(es) supported or not supported? 2. Are the results interpreted in the context of the problem/purpose, hypothesis, and theoretical framework? 3. What does the investigator identify as possible weaknesses and/or problems in the study? 4. What clinical relevance does the investigator identify, if any? 5. What generalizations are made? 6. Are the generalizations within the scope of the findings or beyond the findings? 7. What recommendations for future research are stated or implied?
Application to clinical practice (see Chapter 20)	1. Does the study appear valid? That is, do its strengths outweigh its weaknesses? 2. Are there other studies with similar findings? 3. What risks/benefits are involved for clients? 4. Is direct application feasible in terms of time, effort, money, and legal/ethical risks? 5. Should these results be applied to clinical practice? 6. Would it be possible to replicate this study in another clinical practice setting?

Guidelines are provided by each journal for preparing research manuscripts for publication. The following major headings are essential sections in the research report:

◇ Introduction
◇ Methodology
◇ Results
◇ Discussion

Depending on stylistic considerations related to author's preferences and the publishing journal's requirements, specific content will be included in each section of the research report. Stylistic variations as factors influencing the presentation of the research study are distinct from the focus of evaluating the reported research for **scientific merit.** Constructive evaluation is based on objective, unbiased, and impartial appraisal of the study's strengths and limitations. This is one step that precedes consideration of the relative worth of the findings for clinical application. Such judgments are the hallmark of promoting a sound base for quality nursing practice.

Critique of a Research Study: Sample No. 1

The following study, "Progressive Relaxation Training in Cardiac Rehabilitation: Effect on Psychologic Variables," by Patricia Bohachick, Ph.D., R.N., published in *Nursing Research* (1984), is critiqued. The article is presented in its entirety followed by the critique on p. 395.

Progressive Relaxation Training in Cardiac Rehabilitation: Effect on Psychologic Variables

The purpose of this study was to investigate the effects of progressive relaxation training as a stress management technique for cardiac patients who were participants in a cardiac exercise program. After pretesting, 18 patients received 3 weeks of relaxation training in addition to their exercise therapy; a control group of 19 patients was not taught the technique. Pretesting used two instruments to measure stress levels—the Spielberger State-Anxiety Scale and selected dimensions of the Symptom Checklist-90-Revised. At the completion of the relaxation training program, both groups of patients were retested on stress-level measures.

An analysis of covariance was used to test for the effects of the relaxation training program. The findings were: (1) posttreatment mean anxiety scores for the treatment group were significantly lower ($p < .05$) than that of the control group; and (2) the posttest scores for the treatment group were significantly lower for the dimensions of ($p < .01$) somatization and interpersonal sensitivity and ($p < .05$) anxiety and depression than that of the control group. No systematic changes were induced in either the obsessive-compulsive or hostility dimension scores by the relaxation program.

Accepted for publication December 7, 1982. Patricia Bohachick, Ph.D., R.N., is an associate professor in the graduate program for Medical-Surgical Nursing at the University of Pittsburgh.

The principle of enhancing the physical fitness of the cardiac patient has received increased attention in the last decade. The psychologic effects of a training program on the cardiac patient are of equal importance. Investigators report that patients who have suffered myocardial infarction tend to be more depressed and anxious than the general population. Following participation in an exercise training program, these patients showed less depression and anxiety (Hellerstein and Horsten, 1966). Another technique that shows promise as a useful treatment for psychological distress is progressive relaxation training. Since cardiac patients are apt to experience psychologic distress, provision of various modes for managing this distress is important to insure full rehabilitative efforts.

Review of the Literature

Evidence That Cardiac Patients Are Prone to Psychologic Distress: Various psychologic responses have been observed in patients with angina pectoris and myocardial infarction. Evidence from a number of studies suggests that these psychologic characteristics may represent emotional sequelae of coronary heart disease. Rime and Bonami (1973), in a study of matched samples (30 cases and 30 controls), found significantly higher scores on the anxiety, obsessive-compulsive, and social introversion scales of the Minnesota Multiphasic Personality Inventory (MMPI) among patients with coronary heart disease than patients with orthopedic problems. Thiel, Parker, and Bruce (1973), in studying 50 patients with myocardial infarction, reported that these men score higher on anxiety and depression scales and display more somatization than age-matched healthy controls. Wardwell and Bahnson (1973) also observed significantly greater somatization in myocardial infarction patients than healthy community and hospitalized control groups.

Several studies suggest that emotional distress may be a precursor of coronary heart disease. Bengtsson, Hallstrom, and Tibblin (1973) found patients with angina pectoris or myocardial infarction were more likely to report a history of sustained stress, including anxiety and interpersonal conflicts, than healthy subjects. Eastwood and Trevelyan (1971) studied 124 subjects with complaints of chronic anxiety and depression and a control group without these complaints. Electrocardiographic abnormalities indicative of coronary disease were more frequently found in the anxious-depressed group than in the control group. Since 90% of the subjects with abnormal electrocardiograms were previously unaware of the abnormality, the possibility of anxiety and depression as reaction to a cardiac diagnosis seemed unlikely. Medalie, Snyder, Groen, Neufeld, Goldbout, and Riss (1973) observed high scores on anxiety scales to be associated with the later development of angina pectoris. Friedman, Ury, Klatsky, and Siegelaub (1974) reported high scores indicative of somatization to be associated with later development of myocardial infarction. In a longitudinal study of patients with coronary heart disease, Bruhn, Paredes, Adsett, and Wolf (1974) discovered depression to be associated with an increased risk of reinfarction and sudden death.

Whether emotional distress represents a risk factor for the development of coronary atherosclerosis or a reaction to the diagnosis and physical problems of cardiac pathology remains debatable. However, evidence clearly indicates that cardiac patients are inclined to experience psychological distress.

Effect of Progressive Relaxation on Psychologic Distress: One promising stress-reducing technique is progressive relaxation training. Improvement in subjective and behavioral measures of tension and anxiety and measures of performance and well-being have been reported to occur as a result of relaxation training (Peters, Benson, and Porter, 1977). Investigators report a significant decrease in anxiety in response to relaxation training as measured by Husek and Alexander's Anxiety Differential (Borkovec, Grayson, and Cooper, 1978), the Zukerman Multiple Affect Adjective Checklist, the Spielberger State Anxiety

Scale, and empirical measures of state anxiety, such as heart rate and systolic blood pressure (Stoudenmire, 1975).

Paul (1969) compared progressive relaxation with hypnotic relaxation and with self-relaxation in which subjects were asked to relax to the best of their ability. In general, progressive relaxation and hypnotic relaxation produced decreases in reports of anxiety and indices of physiologic arousal that were significantly different from self-relaxation, and progressive relaxation resulted in significantly greater effects than hypnotic relaxation. Since progressive relaxation may have a beneficial effect on psychologic distress, relaxation training may be a useful modality for promoting cardiac rehabilitation.

Hypothesis

The posttest mean of selected psychologic variables for the experimental group will be lower than that of the control group.

Method

Sample: Volunteers for the study were recruited from a cardiac exercise program that uses exercise as a therapeutic modality for promoting cardiac rehabilitation. Data on background, variables, and pretreatment psychologic measures were collected on all study subjects. After pretreatment testing and in addition to their exercise therapy, 18 patients received 3 weeks of progressive relaxation training using the technique presented by Goldfried and Davison (1976). Basically, progressive relaxation training consisted of learning to systematically tense and then relax various muscle groups while at the same time learning to attend to the feelings associated with tension and relaxation. The ultimate goal was to increase the patient's ability to identify even mild tension and to effectively eliminate that tension. Control group patients ($n = 19$) were not taught the technique. Criterion measures to assess achievement of the relaxation response were taken on experimental group subjects during training. At the completion of the relaxation training program,

both groups of patients were retested on psychologic measures.

Psychologic Distress Measures: The first measure of psychologic distress was the Anxiety State Scale of the State-Trait Anxiety Inventory (Spielberger, Gorsuch, and Lushene, 1970). This scale attempts to measure anxiety, which is defined as a transitory emotional state characterized by perceived feelings of tension, nervousness, worry, and apprehension. The scale consists of 20 statements that require people to indicate how they feel at the moment of answering the questionnaire. Respondents indicate their answers on a 4-point rating scale ranging from Not At All to Very Much. The total score is the weighed sum of all 20 responses, and ranges from a minimum score of 20 (low anxiety) to a maximum score of 80 (high anxiety).

Alpha reliability coefficients for the Anxiety State Scale range from .83 to .92. Administration of the scale under stressful and nonstressful conditions provides evidence of the construct validity of the scale. Mean scores are reported to be considerably higher under stress conditions than under normal conditions (Spielberger et al., 1970).

The Symptom Checklist-90-Revised (SCL-90-R) is a self-report scale designed to measure psychologic symptoms. The earliest form of the instrument, The Discomfort Scale, was derived from symptoms taken from the Cornell Medical Index (Parloff, Kelman, and Frank, 1954). A major revision of the scale, termed The Hopkins Symptom Checklist, was introduced by Derogatis and his associates (1974). Based on clinical experiences and psychometric analyses, the scale was subsequently revised and validated to its present form. Designed for use primarily with psychiatric patients, the scale has been shown to be sensitive to the emotional state of nonpsychiatric patients as well (Edwards, Yarvis, Mueller, Zingale, and Wagman, 1978).

In its complete form, the instrument consists of 90 items that are clustered into scores in 9 underlying symptom dimensions: somatization, anxiety, depression, in-

Table 1 **Summary Definitions of the Six SCL-90-R Symptom Dimensions**

Symptom dimension	Dimension definition

I. Somatization: The *Somatization* dimension reflects distress arising from perceptions of bodily dysfunction. Complaints focused on cardiovascular, gastrointestinal, respiratory, and other systems with strong autonomic mediation are included. Headaches, pain, and discomfort of the gross musculature and additional somatic equivalents of anxiety are components of the definition. These symptoms and signs have all been demonstrated to have high prevalence in disorders demonstrated to have a functional etiology, although all may be reflections of true physical disease.

II. Depression: The symptoms of the *Depression* dimension reflect a broad range of the manifestations of clinical depression. Symptoms of dysphoric mood and affect are represented as are signs of withdrawal of life interest, lack of motivation, and loss of vital energy. In addition, feelings of hopelessness, thoughts of suicide, and other cognitive and somatic correlates of depression are included.

III. Anxiety: The *Anxiety* dimension is composed of a set of symptoms and signs that are associated clinically with high levels of manifest anxiety. General signs such as nervousness, tension, and trembling are included in definition, as are panic attacks and feelings of terror. Cognitive components involving feelings of apprehension and dread, and some of the somatic correlates of anxiety are also included as dimensional components.

IV. Interpersonal Sensitivity: The *Interpersonal Sensitivity* dimension focuses on feelings of personal inadequacy and inferiority, particularly in comparison with others. Self-deprecation, feelings of uneasiness, and marked discomfort during interpersonal interactions are characteristic manifestations of this syndrome. In addition, individuals with high scores on INT report acute self-consciousness and negative expectancies concerning the communications and interpersonal behaviors with others.

V. Obsessive-Compulsive: The *Obsessive-Compulsive* dimension reflects symptoms that are highly identified with the same name. This measure focuses on thoughts, impulses, and actions that are experienced as unremitting and irresistible by the individual but are of an ego-alien or unwanted nature. Behaviors and experiences of a more general cognitive performance attenuation are also included in this measure.

VI. Hostility: The *Hostility* dimension reflects the thoughts, feelings or actions that are characteristic of the negative affect state of anger. The selection of items includes all three modes of manifestation and reflects qualities such as aggression, irritability, rage and resentment.

(Derogatis, 1977, pp. 7-10)

terpersonal sensitivity, hostility, obsessive-compulsiveness, phobic anxiety, paranoid ideation, and psychotism. Since normative and reliability data have been established for each dimension, selected dimensions may be used with confidence. Summary definitions of the scales used in this study and the items that comprise these are presented in Table 1.

Items of the SCL-90-R are described as a list of problems and complaints that people sometimes have. The respondent is asked to indicate how much discomfort each item has caused during the past week, including the day of answering the questionnaire. Each complaint is rated on a 5-point scale of discomfort ranging from 0 (Not At All) to 4 (Extremely). The items are then clustered into scores in the underlying symptom dimensions. Scores for the subsets are computed by calculating the mean score of the questions with the subset and each has a potential range of 0 to 4.

Two forms of reliability—internal consistency and test-retest reliability—for the SCL-90-R Symptom Dimensions are reported. The consistency with which items actually represent each symptom dimension was determined from the data of 219 symptomatic volunteers. Coefficients alpha from each of the dimensions are uniformly high, ranging from .84 to .90. Test-retest reliability coefficients for the dimensions were satisfactory, ranging between a low of .78 for hostility to a high of .86 for somatization (Derogatis, 1977).

Concurrent validity of the SCL-90-R was provided by contrasting it with other established multidimensional measures of psychopathology, the MMPI, and Middlesex Hospital Questionnaire. Each symptom dimension was shown to have its highest correlation with a like symptom construct in each of these instruments (Derogatis, 1977).

Results

To insure comparability of the experimental and control group at the outset of treatment, tests for significant differences in the pretreatment psychologic distress measures of patients in the experimental and control groups were done using an independent t test. Table 2 presents the means, standard deviations and t-test results. The t scores indicated that the two groups did not differ significantly on the various pretreatment distress level scores. Any changes on the posttreatment measures could be interpreted more confidently because of the similarity of the groups.

After establishing that there were no significant differences in the pretreatment scores

of the two groups, each psychologic variable was subjected to analysis of covariance. This analysis enabled a comparison of posttreatment psychologic distress scores in both groups by statistically controlling for any differences in the pretreatment scores that were present but not significant.

The Spielberger State-Anxiety Inventory: Mean scores for this scale administered before and after the relaxation program to experimental and control groups and adjusted posttreatment mean scores are presented in Table 3. Table 4 shows the adjusted means between and within groups and the results of the F test. The F test results for the adjusted mean changes in State-Anxiety scores were statistically significant ($p < .05$).

The Symptom Checklist-90-Revised: Pretreatment mean scores for the various dimensions of the SCL-90-R were slightly higher for the experimental group than those of the control group (Table 5). Posttreatment mean scores for each dimension were lower than pretreatment scores in both groups. The results of the analysis of covariance for the SCL-90-R dimension scores are presented in Table 6. Posttreatment mean scores for the experimental group were significantly lower for the symptom dimensions of ($p < .01$) somatization and interpersonal sensitivity and ($p < .05$) anxiety and depression than that of the control group. No systematic changes were induced in either the obsessive-compulsive or hostility dimension scores by the relaxation program.

Discussion

At the initial measurement session, the experimental group reported slightly more distress as measured by the selected dimensions of the SCL-90-R and the Spielberger State-Anxiety Inventory than did the control group. While the differences in the mean scores between the two groups were not statistically significant, the scores may have reflected a true difference between experimental and control group subjects. In an effort to insure honesty in answering the self-report items, confidentiality was

Table 2 Means, Standard Deviations and *t* Tests on Pretreatment Stress Measures for the Experimental and Control Group

Variable	Experimental (N = 18)		Control (N = 19)		t Value
	Mean	SD	Mean	SD	
State anxiety	33.17	8.47	30.37	8.06	1.03
Somatization	5.67	3.91	4.84	3.91	.64
Depression	6.72	3.75	5.89	3.96	.65
Anxiety	4.33	3.36	2.95	2.82	1.36
Interpersonal sensitivity	4.11	3.07	3.95	2.53	.18
Obsessive compulsive	8.06	4.98	6.58	5.10	.89
Hostility	3.11	2.30	2.53	1.95	.84

Table 3 Pretest, Posttest, and Adjusted Posttest Means for Anxiety State Scores

Group	Pretest	Posttest	Adjusted posttest
Experimental	33.17	29.06	28.17
Control	30.37	31.58	32.42

Table 4 Summary of ANCOVAS for Anxiety State Scale

Adjusted MS between	Adjusted MS within	F (1, 34)
162.11	21.97	7.38*

*$p < .05$

assured and participants were reminded that the validity of the results depended on their answering as truthfully as possible. However, in anticipation of an intervention strategy, experimental subjects may have been more careful in recalling and/or reporting their symptoms.

The relaxation program produced a decrease in state anxiety in the trained group, which was significantly lower than that of a comparable group of untrained patients. These results are consistent with those of other investigators who report a reliable drop on the Spielberger State-Anxiety Scale in response to

Table 5 **Pretest, Posttest, and Adjusted Posttest Means for SCL-90-R Symptom Scores**

Scale		Pretest	Posttest	Adjusted posttest
Somatization	Experimental	5.67	2.67	2.46
	Control	4.84	4.52	4.72
Depression	Experimental	6.72	3.61	3.41
	Control	5.89	5.26	5.45
Anxiety	Experimental	4.33	1.78	1.42
	Control	2.95	2.74	3.08
Interpersonal sensitivity	Experimental	4.11	1.94	1.89
	Control	3.95	3.74	3.79
Obsessive-compulsive	Experimental	8.06	6.06	5.55
	Control	6.58	5.47	5.95
Hostility	Experiment	3.11	2.44	2.21
	Control	2.53	1.89	2.12

Table 6 **Summary of ANCOVAs for SCL-90-R Symptom Measures**

Scale	Adjusted means between	Adjusted means within	$F (1, 34)$
Somatization	46.73	3.93	11.88**
Depression	38.25	5.69	6.72*
Anxiety	24.15	3.04	7.94*
Interpersonal sensitivity	33.36	3.12	10.68**
Obsessive-compulsive	1.39	5.73	0.24
Hostility	0.08	2.09	0.04

*$p < .05$
**$p < .01$

relaxation procedures (Edelman, 1970, Stoudenmire, 1975).

There was strong support to indicate that the relaxation training program improved self-report psychologic distress levels of the patients in the study group. Patients trained in relaxation techniques reported significantly less anxiety, interpersonal sensitivity, depres-sion, and somatization than control group patients. These results may be contrasted with those of a study on the effects of relaxation response breaks in a working population that used comparable measures of well-being. Pe-ters, Benson, and Porter (1977) compared a group of subjects taught relaxation tech-niques with a group that received no instructions on four indices of well-being; a symptom index, illness index, performance index and sociability-satisfaction index. The symptom index, which included a list of 51 symptoms, was comparable to the somatization scale used in this study. Additionally, a number of symptoms from the symptom index and items from the performance index of Peters et al. study (1977) mirrored the depression scale used in this study. Items from the sociability-satisfaction index could be correlated with items from the interpersonal sensitivity scale used in this study. Peters et al. (1977) found a statistically significant improvement on each of the four indices of well-being for the group practicing the relaxation technique as compared to the group that received no relaxation instruction.

Significant findings did not occur for the obsessive-compulsive or hostility symptom dimensions as had been expected for the study sampling. Other researchers also report this dimension unchanged by selected stress management intervention strategies. Grimm (1971) reported that muscle tension and relaxation effected changes in the anxiety scale but not in the hostility scale of the Multiple Affect Adjective Checklist. Baker and Lynn (1979) found significantly lower anxiety and depression but no change in hostility levels in nurses who received interventions designed to assist them in dealing with stress.

The finding that the symptom dimensions of obsessive-compulsive and hostility were not relieved by relaxation training raises the question of whether these dimensions reflect symptomatology impervious to change or whether specific psychologic interventions other than relaxation training might be necessary to alleviate these symptoms. A study on the effect of hospitalization in supporting the coping mechanisms of cancer patients that showed a reduction in the obsessive-compulsive and hostility dimensions of the SCL-90-R merely as a result of hospitalization (Craig and Abeloff, 1974) would tend to make this first interpretation less likely. In support of the second interpretation, Novaco (1976) found a combination of cognitive self-control procedures and relaxation to be an effective technique in the treatment of chronic anger problems. The cognitive procedures involved cognitive restructuring of experiences to provoke anger and the use of self-statements to manage anger. Friedman and Roseman (1974) advocated behavior modification techniques as a strategy for reducing hostility and obsessive-compulsive behavior.

Conclusions

The investigation demonstrated that it is feasible to incorporate relaxation training into a cardiac exercise program; and that, compared to a control group, cardiac patients trained in relaxation techniques demonstrate significant improvement in psychologic distress measures. The findings of this study indicate that multiple dependent variables are required to sufficiently evaluate the effects of a relaxation training program. Other researchers point out that "the relaxation response appears to influence many different aspects of physical and psychic health, but not necessarily the same aspects in different individuals" (Peters et al., 1977, p. 952). Therefore, measures of a number of parameters are necessary for satisfactorily evaluating the effectiveness of relaxation training.

The significant findings of this study show a need for more extensive research regarding the use of relaxation training as a stress management technique for cardiac patients. In this study, relaxation training was introduced as a technique that must be regularly practiced for positive effects of treatment to be accrued and maintained. However, it was acknowledged that once learned, some subjects would practice the technique only during periods of increased stress. Follow-up studies are indicated to determine patterns in the use of the technique. Studies that investigate alternate indices of changes with relaxation training would be helpful. Finally, studies that include not only pretreatment and posttreatment data but also a series of follow-up long term assessments are needed to investigate the duration of the effect of relaxation training.

Progressive relaxation training is a stress-reducing technique advocated for use in clinical nursing practice (Garbin, 1979). Identi-fying methods for validating the effectiveness of this intervention is important. The positive findings of this study suggest that relaxation may be an effective nursing intervention in promoting rehabilitation of cardiac patients.

References

Baker, B.S., and Lynn, M.R. (1979). Psychiatric nursing consultation: the use of an inservice model to assist nurses in the grief process, *Journal of Psychiatric Nursing and Mental Health Services,* **17**:15-19.

Bengtsson, C., Hallstrom, R., and Tibblin, G. (1973). Social factors, stress experience and personality traits in women with ischemic heart disease, compared to a population sample of women, *Acta Medical Scandinavica,* **53**:82-92.

Borovec, T.D., Grayson, J.B., and Cooper, K.M. (1978). Treatment of general tension: subjective and physiologic effects of progressive relaxation, *Journal of Consulting and Clinical Psychology,* **46**:518-528.

Bauhn, J.G., Paredes, A., Adsett, C.A., and Wolf, S. (1974). Psychological predictors of sudden death in myocardial infarction, *Journal of Psychosomatic Research,* **18**:187-191.

Craig, T.J., and Abeloff, M.D. (1974). Psychiatric symptomatology among hospitalized cancer patients, *American Journal of Psychiatry,* **131**: 1323-1327.

Derogatis, L.R. (1977). SCL-90-R (Revised) version, *Manual I,* Baltimore, Johns Hopkins University.

Derogatis, L.R., Lipman, R.S., Rickels, K., Uhlenhulth, E.G., and Covi, L. (1974). The Hopkins symptom checklist (HSCL): a self-report symptom inventory, *Behavioral Science,* **19**:1-15.

Eastwood, M.R., and Tevelyan, H. (1971). Stress and coronary heart disease, *Journal of Psychosomatic Research,* **15**:289-292.

Edelman, R. (1970). Effects of progressive relaxation on automatic processes, *Journal of Clinical Psychology,* **26**:421-425.

Edwards, D.W., Yarvis, R.M., Mueller, D.P., Zingale, H.C., and Wagman, W.J. (1978). Test-taking and the stability of adjustment scales, *Evaluation Quarterly,* **2**:275-291.

Friedman, G., Ury, H.K., Klatsky, A.L., and Siegelaub, A.B. (1974). A psychological questionnaire predictive of myocardial infarction: results from the Kaiser Permanente epidemiologic study of myocardial infarction, *Psychosomatic Medicine,* **36**:327-349.

Friedman, M., and Rosenman, R.H. (1974). *Type A behavior and your heart,* New York, Alfred A. Knopf, Inc.

Garbin, M. (1979). Stress research in clinical settings, *Topics in Clinical Nursing,* **1**:87-95.

Goldfried, M.R., and Davison, G.C. (1976). *Clinical behavior therapy,* New York, Holt, Rinehart, and Winston, Inc.

Grimm, P.F. (1971). Anxiety change produced by self-induced muscle tension and by relaxation with respiration feedback, *Behavior Therapy,* **2**:11-17.

Hellerstein, H.K., and Horsten, T. (1966). Assessing and preparing the patient for return to a meaningful and productive life, *Journal of Rehabilitation,* **22**:46-52.

Medalie, J.H., Synder, M., Groen, J.J., Neufeld, H.N., Goldbourt, V., and Riss, E. (1973). Angina pectoris among 10,000 men: 5 year incidence and univariate analysis, *American Journal of Medicine,* **55**:583-594.

Novaco, R.W. (1979). Treatment of chronic anger through cognitive and relaxation controls, *Journal of Consulting and Clinical Psychology,* **44**:681.

Parloff, M.B., Kelman, H.C., and Frank, J.D. (1954). Comfort, effectiveness and self-awareness as criteria of improvement in psychotherapy, *American Journal of Psychiatry,* **111**: 343-351.

Paul, G.L. (1969). Physiological effects of relaxation training hypnotic suggestion, *Journal of Abnormal Psychology,* **74**:425-437.

Peters, R.K., Benson, H., and Porter, D. (1977). Daily relaxation response breaks in a working population: Part I. Effects on self-reported measures of health performance and well-being, *American Journal of Public Health,* **67**:946-952.

Rime, B., and Bonami, M. (1973). Specificite psychosomatique et affections cardiaques coronariennes: Essai de verification de la theorie de Dunbar au moven du MMPI, *Journal of Psychosomatic Research,* **17**:345-352.

Spielberger, C.D., Gorsuch, R.L., and Lushene, R.E. (1970). *STAI manual for the state-trait-anxiety inventory,* Palo Alto, Calif., Consulting Psychologists Press.

Stoudenmire, J. (1975). A comparison of muscle relaxation training and music in the reduction of state and trait anxiety, *Journal of Clinical Psychology,* **31**:490-492.

Thiel, H.G., Parker, D., and Bruce, T.A. (1973). Stress factors and the risk of myocardial infarction, *Journal of Psychosomatic Research,* **17**:43-57.

Wardwell, W.I., and Bahnson, C.B. (1973). Behavior variables and myocardial infarction in the Southeastern Connecticut heart study, *Journal of Chronic Disease,* **26**:447-461.

Williams, B., and White, P.D. (1961). Rehabilitation of the cardiac patient, *American Journal of Cardiology,* **7**:317-319.

INTRODUCTION TO CRITIQUE NO. 1

The article "Progressive Relaxation Training in Cardiac Rehabilitation: Effect on Psychologic Variables," by Bohachick (1984), is critically examined in terms of its quality and the potential usefulness of the findings for application to nursing practice.

Problem and purpose

Bohachick (1984) states the purpose of the study as "to investigate the effect of progressive relaxation training as a stress management technique for cardiac patients who were participants in a cardiac exercise program" (p. 386). In this purpose statement progressive relaxation training is the independent variable affecting the dependent variable of stress through subjects' learning of a relaxation technique. The population of interest is specified as patients with cardiac disease who were participants in a cardiac exercise program.

Bohachick (1984) notes that patients who have had a myocardial infarct tend to be more anxious and depressed than the general population. Emotional distress is identified as a possible precursor to heart disease and depression, with increased risk of reinfarct and sudden death. The significance of the problem then is suggested in the statement, "Since progressive relaxation may have a beneficial effect on psychologic distress, relaxation training may be a useful modality for promoting cardiac rehabilitation" (p. 388). The management of distress is identified as important to ensure full rehabilitative efforts.

Review of literature and definitions

The literature review incorporates information on psychologic distress in patients with cardiac disease and on the effect of progressive relaxation on psychologic distress. The association of psychologic distress with cardiac difficulty provides the framework for the notion that cardiac problems might be decreased through the improvement of one's psychologic status. It is suggested that progressive relaxation might decrease psychologic distress and thereby promote cardiac rehabilitation.

Bohachick (1984) suggests that in addition to the existing emphasis on physical fitness, attention be given to the psychologic effects of a training program on patients with cardiac disease, the gap to which she addresses her research. The literature review provides evidence for the effect of progressive relaxation in decreasing psychologic distress, and the occurrence of psychologic distress in patients with cardiac disease along with the need to demonstrate the efficacy of progressive relaxation techniques in managing psychologic distress in these patients.

The theoretical base developed by Bohachick (1984) is derived almost entirely from primary sources. An example is the research by Rime and Bonami that is cited by Bohachick (1984, p. 387) as having found significantly higher scores on selected psychologic measures among patients with coronary disease when compared with patients with orthopedic problems. The reference to Garbin (Bohachick, 1984, p. 394) seems to focus on a review of relevant research literature and therefore constitutes an example of a secondary source.

The independent and dependent variables are operationally defined. Progressive relaxation training, the independent variable, is said to be "learning to systematically tense and then relax various muscle groups while at the same time learning to attend to the feelings associated with tension and relaxation" (Bohachick, 1984, p. 388). The dependent variable, psychologic distress, is operationalized by the Anxiety State Scale of the State-Trait Anxiety Inventory and the Symptom Checklist-90-Revised (SCL-90-R). The symptom dimensions from the symptom checklist that are used include (1) somatization, (2) depression, (3) anxiety, (4) interpersonal sensitivity, (5) obsessive-compulsive behavior, and (6) hostility (p. 389).

Hypotheses and/or research questions

The only hypothesis is stated as, "The posttest mean of selected psychologic variables for the experimental group will be lower than that of the control group" (p. 388). The dependent variable is specified as psychologic variables. Whereas the independent variable is not specified in the statement of the research hypothesis, it is known by reading the article to be progressive relaxation training. The hypothesis, stated in research form, predicts that the measurement of psychologic distress for the experimental group will be lower than that of the control group as a result of the first group having received relaxation training. No research questions are included.

Sample

The sample, comprised of volunteers "recruited from a cardiac exercise program that uses exercise as a therapeutic modality" (Bohachick, 1984, p. 388), is one of convenience. The minimal description of subject characteristics (e.g., age, treatment, length of time since myocardial infarction) within this nonprobability sample limits generalization to the sample itself. The sample selected for inclusion in the research project matches that proposed in the purpose statement, "cardiac patients who were participants in a cardiac exercise program" (p. 386). The number of subjects included (18 experimental and 19 control) approaches the minimum of 20 recommended for each group.

Research design

The quasiexperimental design used by Bohachick (1984) manipulates the independent variable by providing relaxation training to the experimental group and includes a control group. But since neither random selection nor assignment of subjects to groups is used, the design is not a true experiment. The logic underlying the research design can be discerned by examining (1) the purpose statement, which proposes investigating the effects of progressive relaxation training, (2) the theoretical framework (as presented in the literature review), which supports the efficacy of relaxation training for affecting psychologic distress, and (3) the hypothesis, which predicts a decrease in the mean of the psychologic variables in the experimental group.

Internal validity

Examination of threats to internal validity reveals no indication of difficulty associated with history or maturation with this adult population over a brief span of time. The procedure by which subjects were assigned to groups and selection criteria is not described, suggesting the possibility of selection bias. Subject loss is not discussed, which makes determination of threats associated with mortality impossible. Bohachick (1984) identifies the possibility that the experimental group may have been more careful when recalling and/or reporting their symptoms. Thus the repeated use of the psychologic measures may contribute to test-retest bias. There is no specification of comparable time spent with the subjects in the control group to compensate for time spent in relaxation training with subjects in the experimental group. Thus there would appear to be a potential for change in the dependent variables associated with being in the experimental group other than the treatment, a threat associated with instrumentation. Internal validity is probably at an acceptable level, although it would appear from the available information that improvement might be possible in terms of instrumentation and sampling.

External validity

Generalizability of findings is limited because of the paucity of information about the setting and about the characteristics of subjects included in the convenience sample. The findings may be generalized only to the sample.

Research approach
Methods

Data collection is accomplished through the use of questionnaires. Experimental and control subjects completed the questionnaires before and after treatment. In addition, criterion measures to assess the achievement of relaxation responses were completed (at unspecified time[s]) on experimental subjects during the progressive relaxation training program.

Bohachick (1984) reported that subjects were assured of the confidentiality of their responses. Since all participants were volunteers, it may be assumed that they consented to participate.

Instruments

The Anxiety State Scale of the State-Trait Anxiety Inventory consists of 20 statements that subjects rate using a 4-point scale with descriptors ranging from Not at All to Very Much. The SCL-90-R includes 90 items listing problems on which subjects rate discomfort during the past week on a 5-point scale ranging from 0 (Not at All) to 4 (Extremely). Both of these are Likert-type scales.

Reliability and validity

The Anxiety State Scale is reported as the first measure of psychologic distress. Alpha reliability scores reported for this measure range from 0.83 to 0.92; these are within acceptable limits. Construct validity was established by administration of the Scale under stressful and nonstressful conditions. The mean scores obtained under stressful conditions were considerably higher. Adequacy of the established validity seems satisfactory.

The other measure of psychologic distress was the SCL-90-R. Bohachick (1984) reports that normative and reliability data have been established for each of the nine dimensions so that "selected dimensions may be used with confidence" (p. 389). Six of the nine dimensions used include somatization, depression, anxiety, interpersonal sensitivity, obsessive-compulsive behavior, and hostility. Two forms of reliability, internal consistency and test-retest, are reported. Coefficient alphas for each dimension range from 0.84 to 0.90; these constitute acceptable levels of reliability. Test-retest coefficients range from a low of 0.78 for hostility to a high of 0.86 for somatization. These reliability levels are also within acceptable limits.

Concurrent validity for the SCL-90-R is based on comparisons "with other established multidimensional measures of psychopathology, the MMPI, and Middlesex Hospital Questionnaire" (p. 390). In this comparison, "Each symptom dimension was shown to have its highest correlation with a like symptom construct in each of these instruments" (p. 390). This approach to establishing validity is appropriate and seems adequate.

Analysis of data

The two measures of psychologic stress (the dependent variable) use interval levels of measurements. The Anxiety State Scale uses a Likert scale for subject responses to the 20 items. The scores are summed with a possible range of 20 (low anxiety) to 80 (high anxiety). The SCL-90-R consists of responses to items asking for ratings of complaints of discomfort on a 5-point scale. Scores for each of the symptom dimensions are "computed by calculating the mean score of the questions within the subset" (Bohachick, 1984, p. 390). Potential scores range from 0 to 4.

Bohachick (1984) reports results of data analysis in which descriptive and inferential statistics were used. Descriptive statistics reported are means and standard deviations of pretreatment stress measures and means for posttreatment stress measures. Results of the analysis that uses inferential statistics are reported. The independent t test establishes comparability of pretreatment psychologic distress in patients included in the experimental and control groups. Analysis of covariance "enabled a comparison of posttreatment psychologic distress scores in both groups by statistically controlling for any differences in the pretreatment scores that are present but not significant" (p. 390). Analysis of covariance is used to test for significant differences between groups in the adjusted mean scores of both the State Anxiety and the SCL-90-R symptom measures.

The statistics reported are appropriate for use with interval data. The use of inferential statistics to test the differences in posttest means for psychologic stress in the experimental and control groups is appropriate to the stated intent of testing the hypothesis that the mean of the experimental group will be lower. The level of significance set for the study is 0.05.

Six tables are used to present detailed information. These tables are precisely titled and headed, and they supplement the content on data analysis that is presented in the narrative. Unnecessary repetition is avoided.

Conclusions, implications, and recommendations

The hypothesis prediction of differential changes in experimental and control subjects on psychologic variables is supported for anxiety ($p < 0.05$), somatization ($p < 0.01$), interpersonal sensitivity ($p < 0.01$), and depression ($p < 0.05$). The predicted change is not supported for the obsessive-compulsive and hostility dimensions. The findings relate to the identified purpose of investigating the effects of progressive relaxation training on stress management of patients involved in a cardiac exercise program. "There was strong support to indicate that the relaxation training program improved self-report psychologic distress levels of the patients in the study group" (Bohachick, 1984, p. 392). Results are compared with work of other researchers and address the possibility of managing emotional distress, which is theorized to be a precursor to chronic heart disease.

Bohachick (1984) identifies possible problems in the study. First, it is noted that experimental subjects might have been more careful in recalling and/or reporting their symptoms. Second, possible explanations for the lack of significant changes in the obsessive-compulsive and hostility dimensions are discussed.

Clinical relevance is specifically addressed. Bohachick (1984) states, "The investigation demonstrated that it is feasible to incorporate relaxation training into a cardiac exercise program; and that, compared to a control group, cardiac patients trained in relaxation techniques demonstrate significant improvement in psychologic distress measures" (p. 393). Generalization is qualified in the statement, "The positive findings of this study suggest that relaxation may be an effective nursing intervention in promoting rehabilitation of cardiac patients" (p. 287). The caution in the use of the terms "suggest" and "may be" keeps generalizations within the scope of the findings.

Bohachick (1984) recommends further research. One suggestion is for more extensive research on the use of relaxation training as a stress management technique for patients with cardiac disease. Specific research foci suggested are follow-up studies to determine patterns in the use of relaxation; investigation of alternative indices of change with relaxation training; and long-term follow-up study of the duration of the effect of relaxation training.

Application to clinical practice

The validity of Bohachick's (1984) research seems satisfactory. Details related to areas of concern are found in the sections on sample and on internal and external validity. Whereas issues of instrumentation and generalizability reinforce seeking support of findings from other investigations or from **replication,** the strengths of conceptualization, research design, and the potential benefit to client care make this an important contribution.

Bohachick (1984) compares and contrasts her research findings of improved psychologic distress levels with those reported by other investigators who used different populations. Munro, Creamer, Haggerty, and Cooper (1988) report use of relaxation therapy in patients after myocardial infarction. They found improved diastolic blood pressure but did not find a significant effect on psychologic and social functioning. Outcome measures used by Bohachick (1984) and Munro et al. (1988) are different. Although consistent improvement in psychologic functioning was not supported, no deleterious psychologic effect emerged in analysis of the effects of relaxation training in cardiac rehabilitation.

No risks are identified for clients with cardiac disease who learn stress management by the use of relaxation training, as reported by Bohachick (1984). The potential benefits for enhancing cardiac rehabilitation seem to support incorporation of relaxation training.

Effective utilization of relaxation training necessitates training of personnel and the investment of clients' and professionals' time to incorporate relaxation into rehabilitation programs. The efficacy of the technique and cost-effectiveness are yet to be demonstrated based on the literature reviewed. Relative benefit to the client is congruent with ethical practice. Feasibility of direct application requires examination of resources, costs, and legal constraints associated with specific clinical settings.

Despite the potential benefit and feasibility of application to clinical practice, the results are not yet ready for unequivocal use. The available empirical evidence does not provide confidence for generalized acceptance of effectiveness of relaxation training. However, it is deemed desirable to replicate Bohachick's study in another clinical practice setting to further clarify the effect of relaxation training on cardiac rehabilitation.

Critique of a Research Study: Sample No. 2

The study "Comparison of Intramuscular Injection Techniques to Reduce Site Discomfort and Lesions," by Mary Frances Keen, D.N.Sc., R.N., published in *Nursing Research* (1986), is critiqued. The article is presented first; the critique follows on p. 407.

Comparison of Intramuscular Injection Techniques to Reduce Site Discomfort and Lesions*

The Z-track intramuscular injection technique was compared with the standard injection technique for incidence and severity of discomfort and lesions at the injection site. Fifty subjects received injections of meperidine hydrochloride alone or in combination with promethazine hydrochloride every 3 to 4 hours for a total of two to eight injections. Subjects served as their own controls by receiving both techniques. They were evaluated for the presence and severity of discomfort on a 4-point Likert scale. Injection site lesions were determined by visualization and palpation. The Z-track technique significantly decreased incidence of selected descriptors of discomfort and lesions at selected time intervals, severity of discomfort at selected time intervals, and severity of lesions at all time intervals postinjection.

Intramuscular injections are a common therapeutic technique performed by nurses. However, adverse effects of frequent injections may include pain (Joubert, de Menezes, & Fernandez, 1972; Travell, 1955) and the formation of cutaneous, subcutaneous, and intramuscular lesions (Aberfield, Bienenstock, Shapiro, Namba, & Grob, 1968; DeHaan, Schellenberg, & Sobota, 1974; Hanson, 1966). The purpose of this study was to compare the effects of Z-track intramuscular injection and standard intramuscular injection techniques on the incidence and severity of discomfort and lesions in subjects receiving frequent injections. Although the Z-track technique has periodically been recommended for all intramuscular injections, the technique

has primarily been reserved for use with iron dextran preparations, which are known to be particularly irritating and permanently staining to the subcutaneous tissues.

Review of the literature

Although reports of adverse effects secondary to injection therapy in selected patients are common in the literature, the actual frequency of such occurrences is insufficiently documented. Roberts (1975) conducted a systematic study to determine the frequency of discomfort and skin reactions in a hospitalized population receiving injections as part of a prescribed medical regimen. Prolonged discomfort was defined as any pain, burning, numbness, or other uncomfortable sensation experienced by the subject longer than 15 minutes after an intramuscular injection; prolonged discomfort was noted in 20 of the 60 subjects (33%).

Roberts (1975) defined injection site lesions as any palpable or observable aberration (e.g., ecchymosis, erythema, papules, or nodules) at the injection site. Fifty-three subjects (88%) had at least one visible injection site lesion; nine of the lesions were judged to be unacceptable injection reactions (e.g., one or more nodules). Subjects with acceptable injection reactions received a mean number of 16.3 injections; those with unacceptable reactions received a mean number of 25.7 injections. Roberts' study suggests that the populaton at highest risk are patients receiving repeated injections over a period of days or weeks.

One suggested cause for the development of lesions and subsequent postinjection discomfort has been the deposition of the injected solution into the subcutaneous tissue rather than the intended musculature. Erroneous deposition of the injected solution may be due to a variety of factors, e.g., needles of insufficient length. The leakage of solution

*Copyright 1986 American Journal of Nursing Company. Reprinted from *NR,* July/August 1986, Vol. 35, No. 4. Used with permission. All rights reserved.

Mary Frances Keen, DNSc, RN, is an associate professor in the School of Nursing, University of Miami, Coral Gables, FL.

Accepted for publication December 10, 1985.

The assistance of Denise Kulick-Ciuffo, MS, RN, in data collection is acknowledged.

into the subcutaneous tissue after withdrawal of the needle due to the use of a straight injection pathway is another suggested factor. Shaffer (1929), using roentgenograms of intramuscular injections of heavy metals, e.g., bismuth, demonstrated that a straight injection pathway, such as that created by a standard intramuscular injection, permits flowback of injected solution along the injection path. Shaffer also demonstrated on roentgenogram that a broken injection pathway produced by the Z-track injection method would prevent this flowback of injected solution.

Hypotheses

I. The incidence and degree of severity of subject discomfort will be less following administration of the Z-track intramuscular injection technique than following administration of the standard intramuscular injection technique.

II. The incidence and degree of severity of injection site lesions will be less following administration of the Z-track intramuscular injection technique than following administration of the standard intramuscular injection technique.

Method

Sample: A sample of 50 subjects was chosen, based on review of the literature and consultation with a statistician. Thirty-seven subjects were male, 13 were female; 30 subjects were black, 20 were white. Ages ranged from 21 to 57 years (M age = 35.5 years ± 5.3 years). The largest part of the sample were diagnosed as acute and/or chronic pancreatitis (34%) or sickle cell anemia (28%); these two diagnoses were prevalent because the study required that subjects be receiving prescribed doses of intramuscular meperidine hydrochloride at regular intervals. All subjects were within 20% limits of normal weight for height (Metropolitan Life Insurance Company, 1959) and gave informed consent.

The convenience sample was composed of available subjects who met the study require-

ments and who had no interfering illnesses, such as generalized or localized edema or coagulation abnormalities, or preexisting injection site aberrations, such as skin rash, neurosensory loss, or unilateral changes.

Subjects were inpatients on selected medical and surgical units of a university medical center hospital. They received a minimum of two intramuscular injections of meperidine hydrochloride alone or in combination with promethazine hydrochloride every 3 to 4 hours as part of a prescribed medical regimen. Individual subjects received the same medication or combination of medications at each injection.

Measurement: Discomfort was interpreted as subjects' experience of burning, stinging, aching, being sore, or hurting when touched or moving the leg. Intensity of the sensation was rated on a 4-point Likert scale (0-3) by descriptors of none, mild, moderate, or severe. The discomfort questionnaire was administered by the nurse researcher verbally after each injection (one treatment interval postinjection) and by the research assistant each evening the subject was enrolled in the study.

Site lesions at the time of injection were interpreted as the development of resistance to needle penetration, resistance to injection of the solution, or seepage of the injected solution from the injection site following withdrawal of the needle.

Postinjection site lesions were interpreted as a finding of (a) pigmentation changes observed by comparison with the surrounding skin color (the site was measured for color using a paint chip color scale and for size using a clear metric ruler); (b) skin sloughing measured by observation for local peeling or flaking of skin; (c) swelling as determined by palpation and measurement with a clear metric ruler; and (d) induration as determined by palpation and measurement with a clear metric ruler.

If an area of discoloration, swelling, or induration was irregularly shaped, the size was recorded by using a clear piece of cellophane and a black felt-tip marking pen to duplicate the area. At the conclusion of the study, areas of discoloration, induration, or swelling were reproduced on 3×5 cards and sorted by three nurses to determine a scale of severity for point assignment. Observations of injection site lesions were recorded by the researcher at the time of injection, at the time of each subsequent injection (two treatment intervals postinjection), and by the research assistant each evening the subject was enrolled in the study.

Pilot Study: Interrater reliability was established during a pilot study using eight subjects. The subjects were examined by the nurse researcher using the measures of site lesions, given an injection, and then interviewed using the measures of discomfort. One-half hour later, the subjects were reexamined and interviewed by the research assistant. Scores were compared using the Pearson product moment correlation test. Interrater reliability for measures of discomfort was $r = .88$; interrater reliability for measures of site lesions was $r = .70$.

Procedure: Subjects were assigned to a treatment group upon entry into the study by use of a table of random numbers. Treatment Group A received the Z-track technique in the left ventrogluteal site and the standard technique in the right ventrogluteal site; Treatment Group B received the standard technique in the left ventrogluteal site and the Z-track technique in the right ventrogluteal site. By receiving both injection techniques, subjects served as their own controls, given the assumption that the right and left ventrogluteal sites were not significantly different, a criterion for entry into the study. Information as to the specific injection method being used in each site was withheld from the research assistant, the subjects, and the staff nurses caring for the subjects.

The right and left ventrogluteal sites were used exclusively during the course of the study and had not been used for at least one month prior to entry into the study. Subjects began the study with the first injection in the left ventrogluteal site, and the method of injection (standard or Z-track) remained constant for the site. The ventrogluteal site was chosen because of the absence of major nerves and blood vessels, the visibility of the site, and the infrequency with which the site is used by others.

All injections were given by the nurse researcher with a 1½-inch, 22-gauge, disposable needle with a 3cc disposable syringe. The meperidine hydrochloride was withdrawn from a single dose vial using one needle. If the subject was to also receive promethazine hydrochloride, the medication was drawn into the syringe following the meperidine hydrochloride. The ¼cc of air was drawn into the syringe, and the needle was changed to another 1½-inch, 22-gauge needle. The total volume of medication received in each injection varied from 0.75 to 3cc ($M = 1.65 \pm 0.65$cc). The most frequently occurring volume was 1cc (30%). During the study, volumes received in the right and left ventrogluteal sites remained equal but not necessarily constant. For example, at injections 1 and 2, a subject might have received 1cc in each site, but at injections 3 and 4, the subject could have received 2cc in each site.

Subjects were placed in a side-lying position with the upper leg flexed in a 20° angle (Kruszewski, Lang, & Johnson, 1979), and the ventrogluteal area was adequately exposed. The area was examined by visualization and palpation for the presence of tenderness or lesions that would prohibit further use of the site. Subjects' report of pain or extreme discomfort precluded use of the site.

The ventrogluteal site was localized using the procedure described by von Hochstetter (1956). Four injection points within the designated site were used by the investigator for purposes of site rotation. A maximum of four injections per ventrogluteal site was given due to the limited size of the area.

The skin was cleansed with two 70% isoprophyl alcohol swabs using a circular motion, starting at the center and moving outward, for a period of 15 seconds for each swab (Story, 1952). The alcohol was then allowed to dry. Needle puncture was made rapidly to a depth of 1½ inches at a near 90° angle to the skin with the needle directed slightly upward toward the crest of the ilium (von Hochstetter, 1956). The needle was aspirated for five seconds (Stokes, Beerman, & Ingraham, 1944); if clear of blood, the fluid was injected with a slow, steady pressure over a period of 10 seconds/cc (Zelman, 1961). The needle was withdrawn rapidly and light finger massage was applied with a dry 2 × 2 gauze square for 15 seconds (Zelman, 1961). The Z-track technique differed from the standard technique only in the use of lateral displacement of the cutaneous tissues prior to site cleansing and needle insertion. The lateral tension was released immediately after withdrawal of the needle.

Immediately following the injection, the subject was questioned about feelings of discomfort at the present injection site as well as the prior injection site. Each evening the subject was in the study the research assistant examined the left and right sites by visualization and palpation and questioned the subject about discomfort in both sites.

Data Analysis: Data were tabulated to determine incidence of discomfort and site lesions at four time intervals: immediately postinjection, one treatment interval postinjection (discomfort only), two treatment intervals postinjection (lesions only), and in the evening of each day. Frequencies of discomfort and lesions of specific descriptors were examined using chi square. Discomfort and lesions scores were examined using a *t* test for related measures.

Results

During the course of the study 240 injections were given. The total number of injections administered to each subject varied from two to eight; the most frequent numbers were four (40%) and six (44%). Each subject received an equal number of injections in the left and right ventrogluteal sites. The treatment interval between injections varied from 2.5 to 5 hours (M time interval = 3.5 ± 1 hour). The inter-

val between injections for each subject remained constant at the time interval ordered by the physician and requested by the subject (± .5 hours). Seventeen subjects (34%) received only meperidine hydrochloride, and 33 subjects (66%) received the combination of meperidine hydrochloride and promethazine hydrochloride.

Incidence of Discomfort: Immediately postinjection, 45 of the 50 subjects (90%) reported the presence of some form of discomfort with the standard technique, and 43 subjects (86%) reported some form of discomfort with the Z-track technique. When complaints of discomfort immediately postinjection for the total number of injections given (N = 240) were examined, the presence of discomfort was noted for 95 of the 120 standard injections (79%) and 92 of the 120 Z-track injections (77%). At one treatment interval postinjection, 33 of the 50 subjects (66%) reported discomfort in the standard site, but 10 of the 50 subjects (20%) who had received the Z-track technique reported discomfort. When the total number of discomfort questionnaires administered at one-treatment interval (n = 190) was examined, discomfort was noted in 50 of the 95 standard injections (53%) and in 28 of the 95 Z-track injections (29%).

On the evening of the first study day, 19 of the 29 subjects (66%) who had received a standard injection as their last injection reported discomfort. Of the 21 subjects who had received the Z-track as their last injection, 14 (67%) reported discomfort; of these 21 subjects, 12 (57%) reported discomfort in the standard injection site (they had received a standard injection prior to the Z-track). Of the 29 subjects who had received a Z-track injection prior to the standard injection, 12 (41%) reported discomfort in the Z-track injection site.

When the frequencies of the specific descriptors of discomfort were examined using the chi-square test, the following complaints were found to be statistically significant: (a) The Z-track injection method caused a significantly greater number of hurt-when-touched responses (at the injection site) immediately postinjection, $\chi^2 = 4.47$, $p < .05$. (b) The Standard injection method caused a significantly greater number of aches, $\chi^2 = 7.00$, $p < .05$, and hurts-when-touched responses, $\chi^2 = 6.19$, $p < .05$, at one-treatment interval postinjection. (c) The standard injection method caused a significantly greater number of aches, $\chi^2 = 5.39$, $p < .05$, and hurts, $\chi^2 = 1.50$, $p < .05$, during the first evening at the previous injection site.

Severity of Discomfort: Using a t test for related measures, combined discomfort scores for all time intervals, discomfort scores recorded immediately postinjection, and discomfort scores at one-treatment interval postinjection demonstrated no significant difference between the standard and Z-track injection techniques. However, discomfort scores in the evening of the subjects' first day in the study showed significance, supporting hypothesis I at $p < .02$, $t = 2.58$, $n = 50$.

Incidence of Lesions: At the time of injection, 35 incidences of resistance to needle penetration and to injection of solution, or seepage of solution from the injection site, were noted in a total of 120 standard injections (30%). Of the 120 Z-track injections, 13 incidences of resistance or seepage were recorded (11%).

At two-treatment intervals, when the site for reinjection was examined, the presence of a lesion was reported in 30 of the 72 observations (42%) at the site of a standard injection compared to 5 in 72 observations (7%) at the site of a Z-track injection. If the incidence of lesions is determined by number of subjects rather than by number of site observations, 22 of the 50 subjects (44%) had some type of lesion at the standard site; with use of the Z-track, only 12 of the 50 subjects (25%) had a lesion.

In the first evening of the study, lesions were reported in 20 of the 50 subjects (40%) at the standard injection site, compared with 8 of the 50 subjects (16%) at the Z-track site.

When frequencies of the specific indicators of injection site lesions were examined using chi square, the following indicators were found to be statistically significant: (a) The standard injection method was associated with significantly greater resistance to the injection of solution at the time of injection, $\chi^2 = 13.78$, $p < .05$. (b) The standard injection method caused a significantly greater number of pigmentation changes at two-treatment intervals postinjection, $\chi^2 = 16.99$, $p < .05$. (c) The standard injection method caused a significantly greater number of pigmentation changes, $\chi^2 = 11.58$, $p < .05$, and swellings, $\chi^2 = 6.66$, $p < .05$, in the evening of the first day.

Severity of Lesions: Using a t test for related measures, the combined lesion scores for all observations demonstrated significance at the $p < .001$ level ($N = 50$) in support of the Z-track method, $t = 6.70$. Objective scores recorded at the time of injection, $t = 5.30$, and at two-treatment intervals postinjection, $t = 4.74$, also showed significance supporting hypothesis II at the $p < .001$ level. Objective scores recorded in the evening of the subject's first day on the study supported the hypothesis at the $p < .01$ level, ($t = 2.90$).

T tests for related measures performed on the specific indicators of injection site lesions demonstrated that the significant indicators were pigmentation changes at two-treatment intervals postinjection, $t = 2.48$, $p < .02$, pigmentation changes in the evening of the first day, $t = 3.86$, $p < .001$, and swelling in the first evening, $t = 3.05$, $p < .001$. Pearson product moment correlations were demonstrated at $p < .001$ between: (a) pigmentation changes at two-treatment intervals postinjection and in the first evening, $r = .40$; (b) pigmentation changes and swelling in the first evening, $r = .38$; (c) swelling and induration at two-treatment intervals, $r = .28$; (d) pigmentation changes at two-treatment intervals and swelling in the first evening, $r = .22$.

Discussion

The mixed results in relation to the incidence of discomfort are interesting. Immediately postinjection the Z-track method increased the incidence of discomfort, but at one-treatment interval postinjection the discomfort was decreased. The same was true the evening of the first day for the site used previously but not for the site used more recently. These findings support a theory that the Z-track technique would not cause a decrease in the initial discomfort of injection; instead, the Z-track may affect discomfort secondary to leakage and deposition of the injected solution into the subcutaneous tissue.

This theory is further supported by findings related to the severity of discomfort. Subjective scores immediately postinjection and at one-treatment interval did not demonstrate a significant difference; however, subjective scores recorded in the evening of the first day did demonstrate that the Z-track method caused significantly less severe discomfort than did the standard method. A time interval may be necessary before injection lesions develop. Development of significant pigmentation changes and swelling at the standard site the first evening would support this explanation; expressions of discomfort thus would be assumed to coincide with lesion development.

Another possible explanation for the mixed results may be that the earlier complaints of discomfort were gathered by the nurse researcher, the same person who gave the injections. Complaints of discomfort in the evening were gathered by the research assistant. The research assistant may have been more objective in the manner of asking questions on the questionnaire, or the subjects may have been influenced by awareness of the testing situation and hesitant to report discomfort to the person giving the needed injection.

Although the potential for investigator bias may have been a major drawback of the study design, the pilot study determining interrater reliability on the measures of discomfort and lesions did not support this notion. If the observations of the research assistant only had been reported in this study, the hypotheses would continue to be supported by the severity of discomfort, $p < .02$, and lesions, $p < .01$, as well as the frequency of specific descriptors of complaints of aching and hurting, pigmentation changes, and swelling, $p < .05$.

Strengths of the design that helped minimize the effects of investigator bias were: (a) Subjects served as their own controls by receiving both injection techniques. (b) All injections were given by the nurse researcher in accordance with strict injection procedures. (c) The research assistant and the subjects were aware of the two techniques being investigated but knew nothing of the treatment method being used in each ventrogluteal site.

Clinical Implications: The results of this study illustrate that nurses can decrease the incidence and severity of injection site lesions and possible subsequent discomfort by using the Z-track injection method. Although this method has previously been reserved primarily for use with iron dextran preparations, the literature and theoretical framework suggest that the technique would be appropriate for all injections. This study points out that the method could be particularly helpful for patients who receive frequent injections over extended periods of time.

References

Aberfield, D.C., Bienenstock, H., Shapiro, M.S., Namba, I., & Grob, D. (1968). Diffuse myopathy related to meperidine addiction in a mother and child. *Archives of Neurology, 19,* 384-388.

DeHaan, R.M., Schellenberg, M.A., & Sobota, J.T. (1974). Assessing local reactions and serum enzyme changes from intramuscular injections: A preliminary evaluation. *Journal of Clinical Pharmacology, 14,* 183-191.

Hanson, D.J. (1966). Acute and chronic lesions from intramuscular injections. *Hospital Formulary Management, 1*(9), 31-34.

Joubert, L., de Menezes, J.P., & Fernandez, C.A. (1972). Measurement of variations in pain associated with intramuscular injections. *Journal of International Medical Research, 1,* 61-64.

Kruszewski, A.Z., Lang, S.H., & Johnson, J.E. (1979). Effects of positioning on discomfort. *Nursing Research, 28*(2), 103-105.

Metropolitan Life Insurance Company, (1959, November-December). New weight standards for men and women. *Statistical Bulletin, 40,* 1-4.

Roberts, R.A., (1975). *Frequency of discomfort and skin reactions from intramuscular injections.* Masters thesis, Case Western Reserve University, Cleveland.

Shaffer, L.W. (1929). The fate of intragluteal injections. *Archives of Dermatology and Syphilogy, 19,* 347-364.

Stokes, J.H., Beerman, H., & Ingraham, R., Jr. (1944). *Modern clinical syphilogy* (3rd ed., pp. 302-309). Philadelphia: W.B. Saunders Co.

Story, P. (1952). Testing of skin disinfectants. *British Medical Journal, 2,* 1128.

Travell, J. (1955). Factors affecting pain of injection. *Journal of the American Medical Association, 158,* 368-371.

von Hochstetter, A.V. (1956). Problems and technique of intragluteal injection. Part II. Influence of injection technique on the development of syringe injection injuries. *Schweizerische Medizinische Wochenschrift, 86,* 69-76.

Zelman, S. (1961). Notes on techniques of intramuscular injections. The avoidance of needless pain and morbidity. *American Journal of the Medical Sciences, 241,* 563-574.

INTRODUCTION TO CRITIQUE NO. 2

This critique examines the research reported by Keen (1986) that compares intramuscular techniques as a mechanism to reduce site discomfort and lesions. The purpose of this examination is to determine the quality of the research as evidenced in the report and its potential usefulness for nursing practice.

Problem and purpose

The identified purpose is "to compare the effects of Z-track intramuscular injection and standard intramuscular injection techniques on the incidence and severity of discomfort and lesions in subjects receiving frequent injections" (Keen, 1986, p. 401). The types of intramuscular injection techniques are the independent variables affecting the incidence and severity of discomfort and lesions, the dependent variables. The population is identified as those individuals receiving frequent injections.

Keen (1986) identifies the significance of the problem when discussing the frequency of intramuscular injections, a commonly used therapeutic technique that may result in frequent pain and cutaneous, subcutaneous, and intramuscular lesions. The Z-track technique has been recommended as the technique of choice but is not commonly used other than with iron preparations.

Review of literature and definitions

The literature review includes the following concepts: standard and Z-track injection therapy, discomfort, site lesions, and population at risk. The posited relationship among the variables suggests a cause of adverse effects that points to an intervention. The discomfort and site lesions associated with injection therapy are thought to be caused by deposition of the injected solution in subcutaneous tissue rather than into muscle. Thus the Z-track technique may prevent adverse effects by prohibiting the leakage of solution into subcutaneous tissue after the needle is withdrawn. Studies are summarized that identify populations receiving repeated injections over days or weeks as at risk for adverse effects, which supports the problem statement. In summary, the author clearly reviews literature related to the specified independent and dependent variables, states the relationship expected among them, and provides the theoretical framework for the study.

Keen (1986) identifies a gap in the literature as being the insufficient documentation of the frequency of adverse effects of injection therapy. Approximately equal numbers of primary and secondary sources are reviewed. The reference by Kruszewski, Lang, and Johnson, in which the authors report their research, constitutes a primary source (cited in Keen, 1986). The textbook by Stokes, Beerman, and Ingraham, an example of a secondary source, is used to provide information on injection technique (cited in Keen, 1986).

The dependent variables, discomfort and lesions, are measured according to intensity and severity. The incidence of discomfort is operationally defined by the subject's report "of burning, stinging, aching, being sore, or hurting when touched or moving the leg" (Keen, 1986, p. 402). The subjects indicate the severity of discomfort by rating the intensity of the sensation on a 4-point Likert scale (0 to 3) using the descriptors of none, mild, moderate, or severe.

The incidence of site lesion was defined at the time of injection as resistance to needle penetration and to the injection of solution as well as seepage of injected solution after withdrawal of the needle. The incidence of postinjection site lesions was determined by the presence of pigmentation changes, skin sloughing, swelling, and/or induration. Site lesion severity was determined by reproducing lesions on 3×5 inch cards, which were sorted by three nurses at the conclusion of the study to determine a scale of severity for point assignment. The criteria for determining severity and the range of the scale are unclear.

The independent variables, standard injection and Z-track injection technique, are clearly operationalized. The standard injection technique is operationally defined as a needle puncture "made rapidly to a depth of $1\frac{1}{2}$ inches at a near 90° angle to the skin with the needle directed slightly upward toward the crest of the ilium. . . . The needle was aspirated for five seconds. . . ; if clear of blood, the fluid was injected with a slow, steady pressure over a period of 10 seconds/cc. . . . The needle was withdrawn rapidly and light finger massage was applied with a dry 2×2 gauze square for 15 seconds . . ." (Keen, 1986, p. 404). The operational definition of the Z-track technique specifies that it "differed from the standard technique only in the use of lateral displacement of the cutaneous tissues prior to site cleansing and needle insertion. The lateral tension was released immediately after withdrawal of the needle" (Keen, 1986, p. 404).

Hypotheses and/or research questions

Keen (1986) presents two hypotheses that are stated in a concise, objective, and declarative manner. The first, "The incidence and degree of severity of subject discomfort will be less following administration of the Z-track intramuscular injection technique than following administration of the standard intramuscular injection technique" (p. 402), specifies the dependent variables as degree and severity of subject discomfort. The second, "The incidence and degree of severity of injection site lesions will be less following administration of the Z-track intramuscular injection technique than following administration of the standard intramuscular injection technique" (p. 402), specifies as the dependent variables the incidence and degree of severity of injection site lesions. The independent variables in both hypotheses are the Z-track and the standard intramuscular injection techniques.

Both hypotheses are stated in the research form. The direction is specified by the prediction of "less" incidence and severity of discomfort and site lesions after the use of Z-track than after the use of standard intramuscular injection technique. No research questions are stated in the study.

Sample

The researcher accepted available subjects from selected medical and surgical units who met the sample criteria, who had no interfering illnesses, and who agreed to participate. This comprises a convenience sample, a nonprobability technique. Since the sample is not randomly selected, caution is required in generalizing findings beyond the sample.

The population indicated in the problem statement is made up of individuals requiring frequent injections. This population is narrowed by the selection criteria. Since random selection is not used, the sample may not be representative of the population receiving frequent injections.

The researcher reports that the appropriateness of the sample size was ensured through consultation with a statistician and the literature review. The sample of 50 would be satisfactory for use with a *t* test or chi-square statistic.

Research design

A quasiexperimental design is used. The deviation from the true experimental design requirements of randomization, control group, and manipulation occurs in the use of the subjects as their own controls. The researcher provides rationale for the use of the subjects as their own controls, specifically, that individual subjective experience of discomfort and individual tissue responses to trauma will vary. Randomization is achieved with the use of a table of random numbers to assign subjects to one of two treatment groups on entry into the study. The groups' treatment is manipulated by varying the designation of which ventrogluteal site to use for Z-track and which for standard intramuscular technique.

The design is appropriate for comparing two injection techniques, which is the purpose of the study, and for testing the stated hypotheses that were developed from the theoretical framework as presented in the literature review.

Internal validity

The threats to the internal validity are scrutinized to determine if the independent variable really made a difference in the study. There are no apparent threats associated with history, maturation, or testing. Since the researcher did not report any loss of subjects, mortality did not appear to affect the results. Although self-selection of subjects and use of a convenience sample may pose validity threats, the use of subjects as their own controls seems to minimize the risk of there being an effect on differences in responses to the two injection techniques.

Instrumentation threats associated with the potential for observer bias are controlled through the protocol used for measurement of lesions. In the discussion section the investigator notes that there may have been investigator bias in the study design. From the discussion of procedures and the reported results of the pilot study, instrumentation does not seem to be a major problem.

The controls for potential threats to internal validity are at an acceptable level. Thus confidence in the findings is enhanced by the elimination of alternative explanations for any differences in lesions or comfort other than the injection technique.

External validity

Caution in generalizing related to possible sample biases is discussed under "Sample" in this critique. A description of the clinical setting and criteria for inclusion in the sample are provided by Keen (1986) so that comparable patients and settings to which findings may be generalized can be identified by nurses.

Research approach
Methods

Data collection methods include observation and interview based on use of a structured schedule/questionnaire. The author identifies the mechanism for determining presence of pain and/or lesions and specifies that the same procedures were used for all subjects. Keen (1986) reports that the subjects gave informed consent.

Instruments

Observations of skin lesions were made by the investigator and a research assistant. These observers were trained in the course of the pilot study. Possible bias may be associated with judgments made about site lesions at the time of injection. The nurse-researcher was not blind to the injection technique being used, and this posed a threat to the objectivity of judgment related to resistance at the site to penetration of the needle and injection of solution. Observation guides used for site lesions post injection included a paint chip color scale and a clear metric ruler to judge pigmentation changes, skin sloughing, swelling, and induration. Irregularly shaped lesions were duplicated with clear cellophane and black felt-tip pen to record their size. Inferences regarding the severity of the site lesions were made by three nurses. The occurrence of lesions would not have been influenced by the presence of the observers.

The interview used to measure the incidence and severity of discomfort is not described in detail. The questionnaire that guided the interview was said to operationalize discomfort as "burning, stinging, aching, being sore or hurting when touched or moving the leg" (p. 402). Interviews were completed by the nurse-researcher and the research assistant whose training was discussed in the documentation of a pilot study. Keen (1986) identifies possible interviewer bias related to (1) differences in objectivity in asking questions between the researcher, who knew which injection technique was used, and the assistant and (2) differences in subjects' responses to the researcher who administered the injections and to the research assistant. Although the possibility of interviewer bias exists, the control invoked through use of subjects as their own controls seems to minimize the influence of multiple interviewers on the finding.

Reliability and validity

Interrater reliability for each of the instruments is based on a pilot study. Interrater reliability for discomfort ($r = 0.88$) and for lesions ($r = 0.70$) is acceptable.

The validity of the instruments is not reported. Face validity is apparent to the reader because of the match between sensations assessed as indicative of discomfort. The measures used seem to be legitimate indicators of the variables measured (discomfort and site lesions), although the validity is not precisely specified.

Analysis of data

The dependent variable of discomfort was measured initially by having subjects report the presence of burning, stinging, aching, being sore, or hurting, which is a nominal level of measurement. The ratings of intensity of discomfort, based on a 4-point Likert scale (0 to 3), are treated as interval level data. The dependent variable of site lesions was measured at the time of injection to be the occurrence of resistance to needle penetration or to injection of solution and/or seepage of injected solution on withdrawal of the needle; this is a nominal level of measurement. The presence of lesions after injection was based on pigmentation changes, skin sloughing, swelling, and induration, a nominal measure. Keen (1986) reports the determination of a scale of severity and the assignment of points for the lesions; these data are treated as interval level data by the author.

Descriptive statistics used to describe the sample characteristics include frequencies, mean, standard deviation, and percentages. Frequencies and percentages are used to report the occurrence of discomfort and lesions. Mean and standard deviation are used appropriately for subjects' age, a ratio level of measurement. Frequencies and percentages may be used at any level of measurement and therefore are used appropriately.

Inferential statistics used include chi-square statistic, t test, and Pearson product moment correlation. The inferential statistical test used for incidence of discomfort and lesions is chi square, which is appropriate for nominal levels of measurement. Both the t test and Pearson product moment correlation require interval level of measurement. These tests are used for analyzing severity of lesions and discomfort measured by scales that are treated as interval. The t test and chi-square statistic are inferential statistical procedures that test for differences. Therefore they are appropriate to test the hypotheses, which are designed to detect differences in discomfort and lesions occurring with standard and Z-track injection techniques.

Keen (1986) appears to be using 0.05 or less as the alpha level for significance, although this is not specifically stated. No tables or figures are presented.

Conclusions, implications, and recommendations

The results of the hypotheses testing are mixed. Hypothesis I was not supported when immediate postinjection measures were used but was supported at one treatment interval post injection and the evening after injections. Hypothesis II was supported. The interpretation of the results is done in terms of the hypotheses, which incorporates the theory that could explain the differences in the findings between Z-track and standard injections. The author provides rationale for failure to find a decrease in the initial discomfort with the use of Z-track injections. Keen (1986) also examines the findings in relation to the methodology used.

The researcher discusses investigator bias as a possible problem associated with hesitance of subjects to report discomfort to the investigator who gave the injection. It is also suggested that the research assistant who was blind to the experimental condition may have been more objective in posing the questions on the questionnaire.

Specific clinical implications for the study are considered. Keen (1986) notes "that nurses can decrease the incidence and severity of injection site lesions and possible subsequent discomfort" and that the "study points out that the method could be particularly helpful for patients who receive frequent injections over extended periods of time" (p. 406). These generalizations are consistent with the findings of the hypothesis testing. Keen's cautious approach in terms of specific applications seems congruent with the limitations of the nonprobability sampling technique.

No suggestions for future research are stated or implied.

Application to clinical practice

The study appears valid. The strengths outweigh the limitations, and the author has addressed potential limitations such as those associated with investigator bias. Whereas no research addressing the problem is incorporated by Keen in the literature review of this article, it would be appropriate to ascertain whether or not other related studies are reported in the literature.

One risk of the use of Z-track technique is the possible increase in client discomfort at the time of injection. Keen's research also suggests potential benefit of decreased discomfort and lesions at subsequent treatment intervals or the evening after the injections. Direct application would be feasible in terms of time, effort, or money if the possible initial expenditure for instruction in the Z-track technique is recognized. Potential risk to the client is an ethical concern that limits feasibility of direct application. Until additional research yields similar results, direct application is not justified. *Replication* of the study would have the potential of validating the findings and supporting clinical application. It would be necessary to contact Keen (1986) to obtain the specific tools used to measure the variables in order to replicate the research study.

References

Bohachick, P. (1984). Progressive relaxation training in cardiac rehabilitation: effect on psychologic variables, *Nursing Research,* **33**:283-287.

Keen, M.F. (1986). Comparison of intramuscular injection techniques to reduce site discomfort and lesions, *Nursing Research,* **35**:207-210.

Munro, B.H., Creamer, A.M., Haggerty, M.R., and Cooper, F.S. (1988). Effect of relaxation therapy of post-myocardial infarction patients' rehabilitation, *Nursing Research,* **37**:231-235.

Additional Readings

American Psychological Association. (1983). *Publication manual of the American Psychological Association,* 3rd ed., Washington, D.C., The Association.

Downs, F.S., and Newman, M.A. (1984). *Source book of nursing research,* 3rd ed., Philadelphia, F.A. Davis.

Jacox, A., and Prescott, P. (1978). Determining a study's relevance for clinical practice, *American Journal of Nursing,* **78**:1882-1889.

Kerlinger, F.N. (1986). *Foundations of behavioral research,* 3rd ed., New York, Holt, Rinehart, & Winston, Inc.

Stetler, C.B., and Marram, G. (1976). Evaluating research for applicability in practice, *Nursing Outlook,* **24**:559-563.

GLOSSARY

alternate form (reliability)   Two or more alternate forms of a measure are administered to the same subjects at different times. The scores of the two tests determine the degree of relationship between the measures.

animal rights   Guidelines used to protect the rights of animals in the conduct of research.

antecedent variable   A variable that affects the dependent variable but occurs before the introduction of the independent variable.

anonymity   A research participant's protection in a study so that no one, not even the researcher, can link the subject with the information given.

applied research   Tests the practical limits of descriptive theories but does not examine the efficacy of actions taken by practitioners.

assumption   A basic principle assumed to be true without the need for scientific proof.

basic research   Theoretical or pure research that generates, tests, and expands theories that explain or predict a phenomenon.

bias   A distortion in the data analysis results.

case study   A qualitative research approach using multiple sources of data in an in-depth study of a single case or a small number of cases.

chance error   Attributable to fluctuations in subject characteristics that occur at a specific point in time and are often beyond the awareness and control of the examiner.

clinical research   Examines the effects of nursing processes on health status.

close-ended item   Questions that the respondent may answer with only one of a fixed number of choices.

cluster sampling   A probability sampling strategy that involves a successive random sampling of units. The units sampled progress from large to small.

concealment   Refers to whether the subject(s) know that they are being observed.

concept   An image or symbolic representation of an abstract idea.

conceptual definition   Conveys the general meaning of the concept. It reflects the theory used in the study of that concept.

conceptual literature   Published material that deals with theory and propositions about phenomena.

concurrent validity   The degree of correlation of two measures of the same concept that are administered at the same time.

confidentiality   Assurance that a research participant's identity cannot be linked to the information that was provided to the researcher.

constancy   Methods and procedures of data collection are the same for all subjects.

constant comparative method   The method of data analysis in grounded theory, culminating in identification of a main theme or core variable.

construct   An abstraction that is adapted for a scientific purpose.

construct replication   The use of original methods, such as sampling techniques, instruments, or research design, to study a problem that has been investigated previously.

construct validity　The extent to which an instrument is said to measure a theoretical construct or trait.

consumer　One who actively uses and applies research findings in nursing practice.

content analysis　A technique for the objective, systematic, and quantitative description of communications and documentary evidence.

content validity　The degree to which the content of the measure represents the universe of content, or the domain of a given behavior.

control　Measures used to hold uniform or constant the conditions under which an investigation occurs.

control group　The group in an experimental investigation that does not receive an intervention or treatment; the comparison group.

convenience sampling　A nonprobability sampling strategy that utilizes the most readily accessible persons or objects as subjects in a study.

correlation　The degree of association between two variables.

correlational study　A type of nonexperimental research design that examines the relationship between two or more variables.

criterion-related validity　Indicates the degree of relationship between performance on the measure and actual behavior either in the present (concurrent) or in the future (predictive).

critique　The process of objectively and critically evaluating a research report's content for scientific merit and application to practice, theory, or education.

Cronbach alpha　Test of internal consistency that simultaneously compares each item in a scale to all others.

cross-sectional study　A nonexperimental research design that looks at data at one point in time; that is, in the immediate present.

data　Information systematically collected in the course of a study; the plural of datum.

data base　A compilation of information about a topic organized in a systematic way.

data-based literature　Published material that reports results of research studies.

deductive reasoning　A logical thought process in which hypotheses are derived from theory; reasoning moves from the general to the particular.

degrees of freedom　The number of quantities that are unknown minus the number of independent equations linking these unknowns; a function of the number in the sample.

delimitation　Those characteristics that restrict the population to a homogeneous group of subjects.

dependent variable　In experimental studies the presumed effect of the independent or experimental variable on the outcome.

descriptive statistics　Statistical methods used to describe and summarize sample data.

developmental study　A type of nonexperimental research design that is concerned with not only the existing status and interrelationship of phenomena but also changes that take place as a function of time.

direct observation A method for measuring psychological and physiological behaviors for purposes of evaluating change and facilitating recovery.

directional hypothesis One that specifies the expected direction of the relationship between the independent and dependent variables.

ecological validity Generalization of results to other settings or environmental conditions.

element The most basic unit about which information is collected.

eligibility criteria Those characteristics that restrict the population to a homogeneous group of subjects.

equivalence Consistency or agreement among observers utilizing the same measurement tool or agreement among alternate forms of a tool.

error variance The extent to which the variance in test scores is attributable to error rather than a true measure of the behaviors.

ethics The use of a moral code in research.

ethnography A qualitative research approach designed to produce cultural theory.

evaluative research The utilization of scientific research methods and procedures for the purpose of making an evaluation.

ex post facto study A type of nonexperimental research design that examines the relationships among the variables after the variations have occurred.

experiment A scientific investigation where observations are made and data are collected by means of the characteristics of control, randomization, and manipulation.

experimental design A research design that has the following properties: randomization, control, and manipulation.

experimental group The group in an experimental investigation that receives an intervention or treatment.

external criticism Establishment of genuineness, validity, and credibility of a document.

external validity The degree to which findings of a study can be generalized to other populations or environments.

extraneous variable Variables that interfere with the operations of the phenomena being studied.

findings Statistical results of a study.

frequency distribution Descriptive statistical method for summarizing the occurrences of events under study.

generalizability The inferences that the data are representative of similar phenomena in a population beyond the studied sample.

grounded theory Theory that is constructed inductively from a base of observations of the world as it is lived by a selected group of people.

hardware The electronic equipment that makes a computer. Usually includes an input device, an output device, a central processing unit, and a memory.

historical research Studies designed to systematically compile data and critically present, evaluate, and interpret facts regarding former people, events, or occurrences.

history   The internal validity threat that refers to events outside of the experimental setting that may affect the dependent variable.

homogeneity   Similarity of conditions.

hypothesis   An assumptive statement about the relationship between two or more variables.

independent variable   The antecedent or the variable that has the presumed effect on the dependent variable.

inductive reasoning   A logical thought process in which generalizations are developed from specific observations; reasoning moves from the particular to the general.

inferential statistics   Procedures that combine mathematical processes and logic to test hypotheses about a population with the help of sample data.

informed consent   An ethical principle that requires a researcher to obtain the voluntary participation of subjects after informing them of potential benefits and risks.

institutional review board   A board established in agencies to review biomedical and behavioral research involving human subjects within the agency or in programs sponsored by the agency.

instrumentation   Changes in the measurement of the variables that may account for changes in the obtained measurement.

internal consistency   The extent to which items within a scale reflect or measure the same concept.

internal criticism   Establishment of the reliability or consistency of information within a document.

internal validity   The degree to which it can be inferred that the experimental treatment, rather than an uncontrolled condition, resulted in the observed effects.

interrater reliability   An index of the constituency between observers or scorers. This is usually used with the direct observation method.

interrelationship studies   The classification of a nonexperimental research design that attempts to trace relationships among variables. The four types are correlational, ex post facto, prediction, and developmental.

interval   The level of measurement that provides different levels or gradations in response. The differences or intervals between responses are assumed to be approximately equal.

interval measurement level   Level used to show rankings of events or objects on a scale with equal intervals between numbers but with an arbitrary zero (example, centigrade temperature).

intervening variable   A variable that occurs during an experimental or quasiexperimental study that affects the dependent variable.

intervention   Deals with whether or not the observer provokes actions from those who are being observed.

item-total correlation   The relationship between each of the items on a scale and the total scale.

key informant   In ethnographic research a member of the culture under study who is knowledgeable about the culture and willing to collaborate with the researcher.

Kuder-Richardson coefficient   The estimate of homogeneity utilized for instruments that use a dichotomous response pattern.

kurtosis   The relative peakness or flatness of a distribution.

level of significance (alpha level)   The risk of making a type I error, set by the researcher before the study begins.

levels of measurement   Categorization of the precision with which an event can be measured (nominal, ordinal, interval, and ratio).

limitation   Weakness of a study.

lived experience   In phenomenological research a term used to refer to the focus on living through events and circumstances (prelingual) rather than thinking about these events and circumstances (conceptualized experience).

longitudinal study   A nonexperimental research design where a researcher collects data from the same group at different points in time.

manipulation   The provision of some experimental treatment, in one or varying degrees, to some of the subjects in the study.

maturation   Developmental, biological, or psychological processes that operate within an individual as a function of time and are external to the events of the investigation.

mean   A measure of central tendency; the arithmetic average of all scores.

measure of central tendency   Descriptive statistical procedure that describes the average member of a sample (mean, median, and mode).

measure of variability   Descriptive statistical procedure that describes how much dispersion there is in sample data.

measurement   The assignment of numbers to objects or events according to rules.

median   A measure of central tendency; the middle score.

memory   The amount of working space that the computer has; an IBM PC is usually sold with 64K bytes of RAM (random access memory). Different amounts of memory are required for specific uses.

methodological research   The controlled investigation and measurement of the means of gathering and analyzing data.

modal percentage   A measure of variability; percent of cases in the mode.

modality   The number of peaks in a frequency distribution.

mode   A measure of central tendency; most frequent score or result.

modem   The device needed to communicate from a terminal to a mainframe computer.

mortality   The loss of subjects from time 1 data collection to time 2 data collection.

nominal   The level of measurement that simply assigns data into categories that are mutually exclusive.

nominal measurement level   Level used to classify objects or events into categories without any relative ranking (examples, sex, hair color).

nondirectional hypothesis   One that indicates the existence of a relationship between the variables but does not specify the anticipated direction of the relationship.

nonexperimental research   Research where an investigator observes a phenomenon without manipulating the independent variable(s).

nonparametric statistics   Statistics that are usually utilized when variables are measured at the nominal or ordinal level because they do not estimate population parameters and involve less restrictive assumptions about the underlying distribution.

nonprobability sampling   A procedure where elements are chosen by nonrandom methods.

normal curve   A curve that is symmetrical about the mean and unimodal.

null hypothesis   A statement that there is no relationship between the variables and that any relationship observed is a function of chance or fluctuations in sampling.

objective   Data that are not influenced by anyone who collects the information.

objectivity   The use of facts without distortion by personal feelings or bias.

open-ended item   Question that the respondent may answer in his or her own words.

operational definition   The measurements utilized to observe or measure a variable; delineates the procedures or operations required to measure a concept.

operationalization   The process of translating concepts into observable, measurable phenomena.

ordinal   The level of measurement that systematically categorizes data in an ordered or ranked manner. Ordinal measures do not permit a high level of differentiation among subjects.

ordinal measurement level   Level used to show rankings of events or objects; numbers are not equidistant and zero is arbitrary (class ranking).

parallel form (validity)   *See* **alternate form (validity).**

parameter   A characteristic of a population.

parametric statistics   Inferential statistics that involve the estimation of at least one parameter, require measurement at the interval level or above, and involve assumptions about the variables being studied. These assumptions usually include the fact that the variable is normally distributed.

percentile   A measure of variability; percent of cases a given score exceeds.

phenomenological research   Based on the investigation of the description of experience as it is lived.

phenomenology   A qualitative research approach that aims to describe experience as it is lived through, before it is conceptualized.

philosophical research   Based on the investigation of the truths and principles of existence, knowledge, and conduct.

population   A well-defined set that has certain specified properties.

population validity   Generalization of results to other populations.

prediction study   A type of nonexperimental research design that attempts to make a forecast or prediction derived from particular phenomena.

predictive validity   The degree of correlation between the measure of the concept and some future measure of the same concept.

primary source   First-hand account of events, such as reports of research studies written by the investigator.

probability   The probability of an event is the event's long-run relative frequency in repeated trials under similar conditions.

probability sampling   A procedure that utilizes some form of random selection when the sample units are chosen.

problem statement   An interrogative sentence or statement about the relationship between two or more variables.

process consent   In qualitative research the ongoing negotiation with subjects for their participation in a study.

product testing   Testing of medical devices.

program   A list of instructions in machine-readable language written so that a computer's hardware can carry out an operation; software.

propositions   The linkage of concepts that lays a foundation for the development of methods that test relationships.

prospective study   Nonexperimental study that begins with an exploration of assumed causes and then moves forward in time to the presumed effect.

psychometrics   The theory and development of measurement instruments.

purposive sampling   A nonprobability sampling strategy where the researcher selects subjects who are considered to be typical of the population.

qualitative measurement   The items or observed behaviors are assigned to mutually exclusive categories that are representative of the kinds of behavior exhibited by the subjects.

quantitative measurement   The assignment of items or behaviors to categories that represent the amount of a possessed characteristic.

quasiexperimental design   A study design where random assignment is not utilized but the independent variable is manipulated and certain mechanisms of control are utilized.

questionnaire   A self-administered, highly structured instrument that is a direct method for studying relationships and testing hypotheses.

quota-sampling   A nonprobability sampling strategy that identifies the strata of the population and proportionately represents the strata in the sample.

random access memory (RAM)   A computer's memory that the user can read or change.

random selection   A selection process in which each element of the population has an equal and independent chance of being included in the sample.

randomization   A sampling selection procedure in which each person or element in a population has an equal chance of being selected to either the experimental group or the control group.

range   A measure of variability; difference between the highest and lowest scores in a set of sample data.

ratio   The highest level of measurement that possesses the characteristics of categorizing, ordering, and ranking and also has an absolute or natural zero that has empirical meaning.

ratio measurement level   Level that ranks the order of events or objects and that has equal intervals and an absolute zero (examples, height, weight).

reactivity The distortion created when those who are being observed change their behavior because they know that they are being observed.

read only memory (ROM) A computer's memory that can be read but not changed.

recommendation Application of a study to practice, theory, and future research.

reliability The consistency or constancy of a measuring instrument.

replication The repetition of a study that uses different samples and is conducted in different settings.

representative sample A sample whose key characteristics closely approximate those of the population.

research The systematic, logical, and empirical inquiry into the possible relationships among particular phenomena to produce verifiable knowledge.

research base The accumulated knowledge gained from several studies that investigate a similar problem.

research hypothesis A statement about the expected relationship between the variables; also known as a scientific hypothesis.

retrospective data Data that have been manifested, such as scores on a standard examination.

retrospective study A nonexperimental research design that begins with the phenomenon of interest (dependent variable) in the present and examines its relationship to another variable (independent variable) in the past.

review of the literature An extensive, exhaustive, systematic, and critical examination of publications relevant to a research endeavor.

sample A subset of sampling units from a population.

sampling A process in which representative units of a population are selected for study in a research investigation.

sampling error The tendency for statistics to fluctuate from one sample to another.

sampling interval The standard distance between the elements chosen for the sample.

sampling unit The element or set of elements used for selecting the sample.

scale A self-report inventory that provides a set of response symbols for each item. A rating or score is assigned to each response.

scientific approach A logical, orderly, and objective means of generating and testing ideas.

scientific hypothesis The researcher's expectation about the outcome of a study; also known as the research hypothesis.

scientific merit The degree of validity of a study or group of studies.

secondary source Account of events written by someone other than the person involved; may include summaries of research, textbooks, or biographies.

selection bias The internal validity threat that arises when pretreatment differences between the experimental group and the control group are present.

semiquartile range A measure of variability; range of the middle 50% of the scores.

simple random sampling A probability sampling strategy where the population is defined, a sampling frame is listed, and a subset from which the sample will be chosen is selected; members randomly selected.

skew   Measure of the asymmetry of a set of scores.

software   Computer programs, or lists of instructions in machine language, that allow the computer to perform specified operations such as statistics or word processing; program.

split-half reliability   An index of the comparison between the scores on one half of a test with those on the other half to determine the consistency in response to items that reflect specific content.

stability   An instrument's ability to produce the same results with repeated testing.

standard deviation   A measure of variability; measure of average deviation of scores from the mean.

standard error of the mean   The standard deviation of a theoretical distribution of sample means. It indicates the average error in the estimation of the population mean.

statistical hypothesis   States that there is no relationship between the independent and dependent variables. The statistical hypothesis is also known as the null hypothesis.

statistical reliability   An index of the interval consistency of responses to all items of a single form of a measure that is administered at one time.

stratified random sampling   A probability sampling strategy where the population is divided into strata or subgroups. An appropriate number of elements from each subgroup are randomly selected based on their proportion in the population.

survey research   A type of nonexperimental research design that collects descriptions of existing phenomena for the purpose of using the data to justify or assess current conditions or to make plans for improvement of conditions.

systematic   Data collection carried out in the same manner with all subjects.

systematic error   Attributable to lasting characteristics of the subject that do not tend to fluctuate from one time to another.

systematic sampling   A probability sampling strategy that involves the selection of subjects randomly drawn from a population list at fixed intervals.

terminal   An input device for a mainframe consisting of a keyboard and a monitor.

test   A self-report inventory that provides for one response to each item that the examiner assigns a rating or score. Inferences are made from the total score about the degree to which a subject possesses whatever trait, emotion, attitude, or behavior the test is supposed to measure.

testability   Variables of a proposed study that lend themselves to observation, measurement, and analysis.

testing   The effects of taking a pretest on the scores of a posttest.

test-retest reliability   Administration of the same instrument twice to the same subjects under the same conditions within a prescribed time interval, with a comparison of the paired scores to determine the stability of the measure.

theoretical framework   A context in which to examine a problem; the theoretical rationale for the development of hypotheses.

theoretical sampling   In the grounded theory approach to research the researcher's deliberate selection of field experiences to test his/her ideas about the data.

theory   A set of interrelated constructs or concepts, definitions, and propositions that present a systematic view of phenomena by specifying relations among variables, with the purpose of explaining and predicting phenomena.

time-sharing   Several users working on one mainframe via terminals at the same time.

type I error   The rejection of a null hypothesis that is actually true.

type II error   The acceptance of a null hypothesis that is actually false.

validation sample   The sample that provides the initial data for determining the reliability and validity of a measurement tool.

validity   Determination of whether a measurement instrument actually measures what it is purported to measure.

variable   Property that takes on different values in a research study.

Z score   Used to compare measurements in standard units; examines the relative distance of the scores from the mean.

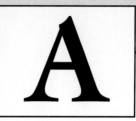

A RANDOMIZED CLINICAL TRIAL OF EARLY HOSPITAL DISCHARGE AND HOME FOLLOW-UP OF VERY-LOW-BIRTH-WEIGHT INFANTS*

Dorothy Brooten, Ph.D., Savitri Kumar, M.D.,
Linda P. Brown, Ph.D., Priscilla Butts, M.S.N.,
Steven A. Finkler, Ph.D., Susan Bakewell-Sachs, M.S.N.,
Ann Gibbons, M.S.N., and Maria Delivoria-Papadopoulos, M.D.

* Reprinted with permission from *New England Journal of Medicine*, 1986, Vol. 315, pp. 934-939.
Copyright 1986 Massachusetts Medical Society.

Abstract—To determine the safety, efficacy, and cost savings of early hospital discharge of very-low-birth-weight infants (≤ 1500 g), we randomly assigned infants to one of two groups. Infants in the control group (n = 40) were discharged according to routine nursery criteria, which included a weight of about 2200 g. Those in the early-discharge group (n = 39) were discharged before they reached this weight if they met a standard set of conditions. For families of infants in the early-discharge group, instruction, counseling, home visits, and daily on-call availability of a hospital-based nurse specialist for 18 months were provided. Infants in the early-discharge group were discharged a mean of 11 days earlier, weighed 200 g less, and were two weeks younger at discharge than control infants. The mean hospital charge for the early-discharge group was 27 percent less than that for the control group ($47,520 vs. $64,940; P < 0.01), and the mean physician's charge was 22 percent less ($5,933 vs. $7,649; P < 0.01). The mean cost of the home follow-up care in the early-discharge group was $576, yielding a net saving of $18,560 for each infant. The two groups did not differ in the numbers of rehospitalizations and acute care visits, or in measures of physical and mental growth. We conclude that early discharge of very-low-birth-weight infants, with follow-up care in the home by a nurse specialist, is safe and cost effective. (N Engl J Med 1986; 315:934-9.)

From the Division of Women's Health and Childbearing, University of Pennsylvania School of Nursing, and the Division of Neonatology, Department of Pediatrics, University of Pennsylvania School of Medicine, Philadelphia. Address reprint requests to Dr. Brooten at the Division of Women's Health and Childbearing, University of Pennsylvania School of Nursing, Nursing Education Bldg. S2, Philadelphia, PA 19104.

Supported by a grant (6742) from the Robert Wood Johnson Foundation and a grant (5-R21-NU0082) from the Division of Nursing, Health Resources Administration, U.S. Department of Health and Human Services.

More than 230,000 low-birth-weight infants are born annually in the United States, and more than 36,000 of these infants weigh less than 1500 g.[1-6] In addition, the proportion of live births made up by infants weighing less than 1500 g has changed little in the past several decades.[7,8] Although advances in neonatal intensive care have been credited with reducing mortality and morbidity in this group,[9-11] recent studies suggest that the environment of the neonatal intensive care unit—with its bright lights and high noise levels—may have a permanent adverse effect on an infant's hearing, vision, and motor coordination.[12-14] Prolonged hospitalization increases the infant's chances of contracting infections and has been associated with failure to thrive, child abuse, and parental feelings of inadequacy.[15-18] Hospital care for these infants is one of the most expensive of all types of hospitalization.[19,20] Despite initial hospital expenditures averaging up to $167,000 for very-low-birth-weight infants,[21] formalized home care services are almost completely lacking after these infants are discharged. This lack of services is particularly troubling since this group is at high risk for failure to thrive, problems associated with chronic lung disease, anemia, seizures, and developmental delays, as well as parenting problems.[22] In the first year of life, the rate of rehospitalization for very-low-birth-weight infants is four times the rate for normal-birth-weight infants (≥ 2500 g) and their postneonatal death rate is five times as high.[10] Compounding these problems, a disproportionate number of very-low-birth-weight infants are born to poor, young mothers with questionable resources to provide adequate care after discharge.[23]

Although home visits by nurses have been used in a variety of medical specialties to improve care and decrease health care costs, the efficacy of visits by perinatal nurse specialists to very-low-birth-weight infants after discharge has not been documented. This clinical trial was undertaken to examine whether it is safe and economical to discharge very-low-birth-weight infants (≤ 1500 g) early if they meet certain conditions and to subsidize home care services with any savings that result from shorter hospitalizations.

Methods

Infants with birth weights of 1500 g or less who were born at the Hospital of the University of Pennsylvania between October 1982 and December 1984 were randomly assigned to one of two groups, after their parents gave informed consent to their participation in the study. Infants in the control group were discharged according to routine nursery policy, which required that the infant be clinically well, feeding well, and weigh approximately 2200 g. Although parents received support and instruction from nursery nurses about their infant and his or her care after discharge, no routine home follow-up care by nurses was provided for this group.

Infants in the early-discharge group were discharged before they weighed 2200 g so long as they met the following criteria: (1) they were clinically well and able to feed by nipple every four hours; (2) they were able to maintain their body temperature in an open crib in room air; (3) no evidence of serious apnea or bradycardia was found in a 12-hour recording of the infant's heart rate and respiration; (4) the mother or other caretaker demonstrated satisfactory care-taking skills; and (5) the physical home environment and facilities for the care of the infant were adequate.

Infants and families in the early-discharge group received home follow-up care provided by a nurse. Since specialty practice in the care of these high-risk infants and their families formally occurs at the master's-degree level in nursing, one full-time nurse and two part-time relief nurses with master's degrees in perinatal and neonatal nursing were hired to provide follow-up care to the families. A nurse specialist contacted one or both parents soon after the infant's birth and at least once a week during the infant's hospitalization to promote the parents' interaction with the infant; to evaluate the parents' perceptions and concerns

about the infant; to teach parents to bathe, handle, and soothe the infant, to take his or her temperature, and to prevent infection; and to provide information about the infant's sleep patterns, differences in infant temperature, reportable signs and symptoms, and times for routine medical care. Weekly contact with parents helped to establish a rapport between parents and the nurse specialist and provided continuity for the parents as the infant was transferred from the intensive care unit to the intermediate care unit and then home.

Before discharge, parents were required to demonstrate satisfactorily the basic care-taking skills described above and a basic knowledge of any medications or special procedures required in the infant's care. Approximately one week before discharge, the nurse specialist made a home visit to coordinate planning for the discharge and to evaluate the adequacy of heat in the home, the safety of the environment, and the adequacy of facilities for the care of the newborn. When problems were encountered, the nurse specialist consulted with physicians, hospital social-service personnel, and others in the community.

After the infant was discharged, the nurse made home visits during the first week and at 1, 9, 12, and 18 months. The visits included a physical examination of the infant, developmental screening, confirmation of appointments for medical follow-up care, an assessment of the parents' coping ability and care-taking skills and support systems, and instruction and counseling regarding infant care and infant stimulation, if needed. The nurse was in contact with the parents by telephone at least three times a week for the first two weeks after discharge and weekly thereafter for eight weeks. The nurse specialist was on call from 8:00 a.m. to 10:00 p.m. Monday through Friday and from 8:00 a.m. to noon on weekends, to respond to parents' concerns and special problems. Medical backup for the nurse was provided by neonatologists at the hospital. Long-term medical follow-up care for infants in both groups was provided either by the hospital's high-risk follow-up clinic or by private pediatricians.

Infants with life-threatening congenital anomalies, grade 4 intraventricular hemorrhage, extensive surgical intervention, oxygen dependence for a period of more than 10 weeks, or a combination of these factors were excluded from the study.

Sample

Of 136 infants eligible for enrollment at birth, 57 were not included in the study because of death (6 infants), the complications described above as reasons for exclusion (34), family complications (7), or their parents' refusal to participate (10). The sample included 72 mothers and 79 infants; 36 mothers and 39 infants (3 sets of twins) in the early-discharge group, and 36 mothers and 40 infants (4 sets of twins) in the control group (Table 1). There were no statistically significant differences between the groups in terms of the mother's age, educational level, marital status, race, or number of children; the family structure; the availability of a telephone in the home; the type of transportation available in an emergency; the family's reported annual income; the type of health insurance; or the number of children under five years of age (a variable associated with increased infection rates among low-birth-weight infants after discharge). Although no data on living conditions were gathered on the control group, inadequate heating, food, and formula were problems during follow-up for 11 percent of the families in the early-discharge group.

There were no statistically significant differences between the groups in terms of the infants' mean birth weight, gestational age, appropriateness of size for gestational age, number of days of ventilation, or number of days spent in the intensive care nursery. Seventy infants were of appropriate size for gestational age at birth, whereas nine infants were small for gestational age (four in the early-discharge group and five in the control group). Ninety-seven percent of the infants

had complicating conditions while they were hospitalized; these included respiratory distress syndrome (30 in the early-discharge group and 35 in the control group); necrotizing enterocolitis (2 in each group); surgery (1 in each group); and jaundice requiring phototherapy (37 in the early-discharge group and 39 in the control group).

Twenty-five infants (32 percent) were discharged with apnea monitors (14 in the early-discharge group and 11 in the control group). Fifty-nine infants (75 percent) were discharged with medications such as theophylline or vitamin E to be administered at home by their parents (28 in the early-discharge group and 31 in the control group). Because of the time limits of the study, 12 infants, 6 in each group, were followed for less than 18 months.

Statistical Analysis

All data are expressed as means $\pm$ SD. The significance of differences was determined by unpaired t-tests.

Results

Infants in the early-discharge group were discharged from the hospital a mean of 11.2 days earlier, weighed 200 g less, and were approximately two weeks younger at discharge than the infants in the control group (Table 2). The difference in the average length of hospital stay between the groups was statistically significant ($P < 0.05$).

There were no statistically significant differences between the groups in terms of the number of rehospitalizations, the number of acute care visits, the incidence of failure to thrive, reported child abuse, or foster placement during the 18-month follow-up period. The two cases of reported child abuse in the early-discharge group were in families that did not comply with requirements for medical follow-up during the child's second year of life. Infants in two of the four families in the control group in which child abuse was reported were physically abused and required foster care. One infant in the early-discharge

Table 1 **Characteristics of Very-Low-Birth-Weight Infants and Their Families**

Characteristic	Early-discharge group	Control group
Mother		
Number	36	36
Mean age ± SD (range)	24 ± 7 yr	23 ± 6 yr
	(16–44)	(12–38)
Education level		
Less than high school	42%	30.5%
High school	28%	39.0%
More than high school	30%	30.5%
Marital status		
Married	31%	33%
Unmarried	69%	67%
Race		
Black	83%	78%
White	17%	22%
Family		
Hospital insurance		
Medicaid	75%	56%
Private	25%	44%
Income		
< $5,000	34%	26%
$5,001–9,999	43%	32%
$10,000–49,000	17%	26%
> $50,000	6%	16%
Infants		
Number	39	40
Mean birth weight ± SD (range)	1187 ± 198 g	1148 ± 203 g
	(740–1490)	(710–1500)
Mean gestational age at birth ± SD (range)	30 ± 2 wk	30 ± 2 wk
	(26–37)	(26–37)

group died of sudden infant death syndrome during the first year of follow-up. There were no deaths in the control group.

There were no statistically significant differences between the groups in the developmental quotient of infants as measured by the Bayley scale of infant development. Two infants, one in each group, had developmental quotients below 80. Seven infants (four in the early-discharge group and three in the control group) were at or below the fifth percentile in physical growth (weight and length) at the end of the follow-up period. Of these seven infants, one was a twin and two had been small

Table 2 **Characteristics of Very-Low-Birth-Weight Infants at Discharge and During Follow-up**

Characteristic	Early-discharge group (N = 39)	Control group (N = 40)
Mean days of hospitalization	46.5 ± 12.5*	57.7 ± 17*
± SD (range)	(20–79)	(21–94)
Mean weight at discharge	2072 ± 131 g	2280 ± 179 g
± SD (range)	(1880–2500)	(1980–2650)
Mean gestational age at discharge	36 ± 2 wk	38 ± 2 wk
± SD (range)	(34–39)	(34–44)
No. of infants rehospitalized		
Within 14 days	4	5
Within 18 months	10	10
No. of infants with acute care visits	29	36
No. of acute care visits	163	186
No. of infants with failure to thrive	0	1
No. of infants reported abused	2	4
No. of infants in foster care	0	2

* The difference in the two means is statistically significant (P < 0.05).

for gestational age at birth. These three infants were in the experimental group.

Despite the nurse's maintaining frequent telephone contact with the parents in the early-discharge group, according to the study protocol, parents initiated more than 300 telephone calls to the nurse during the follow-up period. Seventy-four percent of the calls were made within the first six months after discharge. Parents' concerns were classified into five major areas and ranked according to frequency. The five areas were newborn health problems (30 percent), concerns about routine care of the newborn (25 percent), giving information (22 percent), requesting information (13 percent), and maternal concerns (10 percent). Newborn health problems included questions regarding apnea monitoring, respiratory infections, gastrointestinal problems, fevers, hernias, medicines, skin rashes, injuries, ear infections, and nonspecific symptoms. Concerns about routine newborn care in-

cluded questions or problems with feeding, elimination, hearing, sleep, hygiene, immunization, and development. Giving information included reports by the parents of the infant's condition, providing new telephone numbers for parents, and canceling or making appointments for home visits by the nurse or for the follow-up clinic. Requests for information included questions about tests and equipment, requests for physicians' telephone numbers and referrals to community agencies and parent support groups. Maternal concerns included questions about the resumption of sexual activities, frustrations about living conditions, scheduling clinic appointments, and problems with monitor companies. The number and type of telephone calls initiated by parents did not differ according to the type of medical insurance held by the parents.

Total charges for the initial hospitalizations for the 79 infants were $4,974,710, consisting of $4,450,910 in hospital charges and

Table 3 Costs of Care for Very-Low-Birth-Weight Infants

	Early-discharge group	Control group
Charges for initial hospitalization ($)		
No. of infants	39	40
Total	1,853,297	2,597,613
Mean	47,520*	64,940*
Range	21,729–106,409	23,619–131,882
SD	19,856	31,545
Charges for physician's services ($)		
No. of infants	38†	39†
Total	225,465	298,335
Mean	5,933‡	7,649‡
Range	2,275–10,625	3,125–15,725
SD	2,164	3,169
Costs related to nurse specialist's services ($)		
No. of families	36	0
Total cost of nurse specialist's time	19,264	—
Mean cost of nurse specialist's time	535	—
Total telephone charges	966	—
Mean telephone charges	27	—
Total travel costs	500	—
Mean travel costs	14	—

* The difference between the two means is statistically significant (P < 0.01) by a one-tailed test.
† Physician's charge data were unavailable for one infant in each group.
‡ The difference between the two means is statistically significant (P < 0.01) by a one-tailed test.

$523,800 for physicians' fees (Table 3). The average hospital charge was $56,341 and the average physician's charge was $6,803 for each infant. The difference in the mean hospital charge between the early-discharge group ($47,520) and the control group ($64,940) was $17,420; this difference was statistically significant (P < 0.01). The difference in the mean physician's charge between the early-discharge group ($5,933) and the control group ($7,649) was $1,716, which was also significant (P < 0.01). The mean hospital charge for the early-discharge group was 26.8 percent less than that for the control group. The mean physician's charge was 22.4 percent less than that for the control group. The mean combined hospital and physician's charges for the early-discharge group were $19,136, or 26.4 percent less than for the control group.

The difference between the groups cannot all be counted as savings, since the costs of the nurse specialist's services must be included for the early-discharge group. The parents of the infants discharged early were not charged for the nurse's services, so no charge data exist. Therefore, the actual cost of providing this care was used for this part of the analysis. The cost of the time spent by the nurse in direct care of the infants and families was considered, as well as telephone time, time spent on home visits, travel time to and from home visits, and administrative time. Telephone charges and travel costs were included in the analysis.

The total cost of the home follow-up care for 33 infants for 18 months and 6 infants for 6 months was $20,730 (Table 3). This is a mean cost of $576 per infant and consists of the following: the cost of the time spent by the nurse specialist with families before discharge (a mean of $137 per family), the time spent by the nurse specialist with families after discharge ($398 per family), $27 for telephone calls, and $14 in travel costs for home visits. All the families in the early-discharge group lived within 45 miles (72 km) of the hospital.

Discussion

Programs of early hospital discharge for low-birth-weight infants can potentially decrease iatrogenic illness and hospital-acquired infections, enhance parent–infant interaction, and decrease hospital costs for care. With the introduction of diagnosis-related groups and prospective payment systems, such programs are an economic necessity. However, such programs are scarce in the United States, and the majority of them have dealt with healthy infants with higher birth weights and greater gestational age than the infants in our study, and most of the infants have been born to middle-class families.[24-28] Moreover, few of these programs provide the much-needed assistance in caring for the infant during the important transition period in the home, after hospital discharge.

On the basis of our findings, we conclude that early discharge of very-low-birth-weight infants according to the standards used in this study is safe, feasible, and cost effective and provides continuity of care. The hospital-based approach has several advantages: it provides continuity of care by having a nurse with specialized knowledge and skills in caring for these families and infants provide the direct care; it includes the nurse as an integral part of the hospital staff and community network, with backup available from physicians familiar with the past progress of the infant; and it makes the services of the nurse available to the families seven days a week through a telephone service. The continued home monitoring of the infant's physical status, the parents' ability to cope, their compliance with specialized medical procedures, and their use of any equipment required for high-risk infants discharged early mean that home follow-up care must be provided by nurses who have specialized in high-risk neonatal care. The need for this kind of follow-up care can only increase as smaller infants with many complex health problems survive and as the complexity of their home care increases.

Using the study methods described above, we found that infants in the early-discharge group were able to be discharged 11.2 days earlier than controls (46.5 vs. 57.7 days). These figures compare with nationally reported means of 63 and 57 days of hospitalization[10,29] for infants with birth weights under 1500 g. The early-discharge group in our study had a mean birth weight of only 1187 g.

The safety of early discharge using this approach is supported by the similar numbers of rehospitalizations and acute care visits for infants in the early-discharge and control groups, which are also comparable to nationally reported figures.[29,30] Furthermore, there were no infants with failure to thrive because of parental neglect, there was no reported physical abuse of infants, and there were no foster placements among the infants in the early-discharge group who were followed by the nurse specialist. These outcomes were achieved in a sample in which 42 percent of the mothers had less than a high-school education, 69 percent were unmarried, 75 percent were insured by Medicaid, 69 percent had a reported annual income of less than $7,500, 11 percent had no telephone, and 72 percent had to rely on the police or public transportation in an emergency.

In addition to its safety, this type of hospital-based home follow-up care for high-risk infants is feasible and cost effective. Even with the largely poor, often transient, mothers in the early-discharge group, loss of high-risk infants to medical follow-up was not a problem in this study. Because of the continuity of care provided by the nurse, her ability to handle the problems of high-risk infants and their parents' concerns, and her availability seven days a week, all but one family in the early-discharge group remained in the study until its completion. That one family moved to another part of the country. Moreover, the direct cost of the nurse specialist's services was very low, especially as compared with the charges for hospitalization and physicians' services for these infants. The mean savings in hospital and physician's charges for the early-discharge group totaled $19,136, or 26.4 percent of the average charge for the control group, minus the added cost of the nurse specialist ($576). This yielded a net savings of $18,560 per infant, or 25.6 percent of the charges for the control group.

Since data on actual charges were used for physicians' and hospital fees, whereas data on costs were used to determine the offsetting expenses related to the services provided by the nurse specialist, the costs calculated for the two groups of infants were not fully comparable. However, $576 is only 0.8 percent of the combined mean hospital and physician's fees for the control group. If the nurse services were charged at 50 percent more or even at double their direct cost, they would still constitute only 1.2 percent or 1.6 percent of that amount, respectively. Thus, even if the charge for these services were $1,152 (i.e., $576 × 2), the savings would far outweigh these charges.

These figures should be compared with the hospital and physician charges for the early-discharge group, which were 26.4 percent lower than those for the control group. The results of this study suggest the potential for substantial savings in health care costs if our approach were followed nationwide. If only half the 36,000 very-low-birth-weight infants born in the United States each year were discharged early according to the protocol we tested, the annual savings could be as much as

$334 million ($19,136 − $576 × 18,000).

It should be noted that the data on the cost of hospital and physician's care were based on actual charges, not on costs. From the perspective of private insurers and self-paying patients, that is a reasonable approach. However, it may overstate the potential savings to society if charges exceed costs — as they do in some, but not necessarily all, cases. If the hospital and physician's charges were 25 percent, 50 percent, 75 percent, or 100 percent more than the costs of delivering the services, then the potential cost savings from early discharge of half the very-low-birth-weight infants born each year would be $265 million, $219 million, $186 million, or $162 million, respectively. Thus, even estimating conservatively that half the very-low-birth-weight infants could be discharged early and assuming that charges for all items were double the actual costs, the total savings nationwide could be as much as $162 million annually.

Earlier discharge of low-birth-weight infants provides numerous potential benefits. These benefits may be offset, however, if high-risk infants are discharged early, and impose increased and highly stressful responsibilities for monitoring and care on their parents. This is particularly true if the parents lack the benefit of supportive programs and continuous contact with persons who are knowledgeable about and familiar with the problems and care of their infants since birth. A need for this type of support and continuity of care was suggested in our study by the number and types of calls the parents made to the nurse, the number of infants who required home apnea monitoring and medication, the number of families that remained in the study, and subsequently, the number of infants who continued to receive medical follow-up.

As prospective payment systems expand, it may well be financially beneficial for hospitals themselves to institute programs such as the one described here. For a hospital, the value of such a service lies in the improved, extended service it can provide to the families of high-risk infants, especially in view of the demonstrated need for such a program and its usefulness to families. Society also stands to benefit in many ways that cannot be quantified—in the support provided to families through the difficult period after discharge, and the potential reduction in child abuse and foster placement, for example, as well as in reduced health care costs.

References

1. National Center for Health Statistics. Monthly vital statistics report, 1975. Vol. 25. No. 10. Washington, D.C.: Department of Health, Education, and Welfare, 1976. (DHEW publication no. (HRA) 77-1120.)

2. *Idem.* Monthly vital statistics report, 1976. Vol. 26. No. 12. Washington, D.C.: Department of Health, Education, and Welfare, 1978. (DHEW publication no. (HRA) 78-1120.)

3. *Idem.* Monthly vital statistics report, 1977. Vol. 27. No. 11. Washington, D.C.: Department of Health, Education, and Welfare, 1979. (DHEW publication no. (HRA) 79-1120.)

4. *Idem.* Monthly vital statistics report, 1978. Vol. 29. No. 1. Washington, D.C.: Department of Health, Education, and Welfare, 1980. (DHEW publication no. (PHS) 80-1120.)

5. *Idem.* Monthly vital statistics report, 1979. Vol. 28. No. 13. Washington, D.C.: Department of Health, Education, and Welfare, 1980. (DHHS publication no. (PHS) 81-1120.)

6. *Idem.* Monthly vital statistics report, 1981. Vol. 30. No. 12. Washington, D.C.: Department of Health, Education, and Welfare, 1982. (DHHS publication no. (PHS) 82-1120.)

7. Lee K-S, Paneth N, Gartner LM, Pearlman MA, Gruss L. Neonatal mortality: an analysis of the recent improvement in the United States. Am J Public Health 1980; 70:15-21.

8. Cohen R, Stevenson D. Prenatal care for VLBW infants. Perinatol Neonatol 1983; 7:13-6.

9. Buckwald S, Zorn WA, Egan EA. Mortality and follow-up data for neonates weighing 500 to 800 g at birth. Am J Dis Child 1984; 138:779-82.

10. McCormick MC. The contribution of low birth weight to infant mortality and childhood morbidity. N Engl J Med 1985; 312:82-90.

11. Saigal S, Rosenbaum P, Stoskopf B, Milner R. Follow-up of infants 501 to 1,500 gm birth weight delivered to residents of a geographically defined region with perinatal intensive care facilities. J Pediatr 1982; 100:606-13.

12. Gottfried AW, Wallace-Lande P, Sherman-Brown S, King J, Coen C, Hodgman JE. Physical and social environment of newborn infants in special care units. Science 1981; 214:673-5.

13. Bess FH, Peek BF, Chapman JJ. Further observations on noise levels in infant incubators. Pediatrics 1979; 63:100-6.

14. Glass P, Avery GB, Subramanian KNS, Keys MP, Sostek AM, Friendly DS. Effect of bright lights in the hospital nursery on the incidence of retinopathy of prematurity. N Engl J Med 1985; 313:401-4.

15. Desmond MM, Vorderman A, Salinas M. The family and premature infant after neonatal intensive care. Texas Med 1980; 76(1):60-3.

16. Hayes J. Premature infant development: the relationship of neonatal stimulation, birth condition and home environment. Pediatr Nurs 1980; 6(Nov-Dec):33-36.

17. Jeffcoate JA, Humphrey ME, Lloyd JK. Disturbance in parent-child relationship following preterm delivery. Dev Med Child Neurol 1979; 21:344-52.

18. Larson CP. Efficacy of prenatal and postpartum home visits on child health and development. Pediatrics 1980; 66:191-7.

19. Schroeder SA, Showstack JA, Roberts HE. Frequency and clinical description of high-cost patients in 17 acute-care hospitals. N Engl J Med 1979; 300:1306-9.

20. Kaufman SL, Shepard DS. Costs of neonatal intensive care by day of stay. Inquiry 1982; 19:167-78.

21. Walker D-JB, Feldman A, Vohr BR, Oh W. Cost-benefit analysis of neonatal intensive care for infants weighing less than 1,000 grams at birth. Pediatrics 1984; 74:20-5.

22. Hurt H. Continuing care of the high-risk infant. Clin Perinatol 1984; 11:3-17.

23. National Center for Health Statistics. Factors associated with low birth-weight. Washington, D.C.: Department of Health, Education, and

Welfare. (DHEW publication no. (PHS) 80-1915.)

24. Bauer CH, Tinklepaugh W. Low birth weight babies in the hospital: a survey of recent changes in their care, with special emphasis on early discharge. Clin Pediatr 1971; 10:467-9.

25. Berg RB, Salisbury AJ. Discharging infants of low birth weight: reconsideration of current practice. Am J Dis Child 1971; 122:414-7.

26. Britton HL, Britton JR. Efficacy of early newborn discharge in a middle-class population. Am J Dis Child 1984; 138:1041-6.

27. Dillard RG, Korones SB. Lower discharge weight and shortened nursery stay for low-birth-weight infants. N Engl J Med 1973; 288:131-3.

28. Hurt H, Gealt L, Johnson M, Wurtz M, Brodsky N. Home visiting nurses are beneficial in care of intensive care nursery graduates. Pediatr Res 1985; 19 (4:Part 2):239A, abstract.

29. Hack M, DeMonterice D, Merkatz IR, Jones P, Fanaroff AA. Rehospitalization of the very-low-birth-weight infant: a continuum of perinatal and environmental morbidity. Am J Dis Child 1981; 135:263-5.

30. McCormick MC, Shapiro S, Starfield BH. Rehospitalization in the first year of life for high-risk survivors. Pediatrics 1980; 66:991-9.

B

STRESS, SOCIAL SUPPORT, AND PSYCHOLOGICAL DISTRESS OF FAMILY CAREGIVERS OF THE ELDERLY*

Virginia Baillie, Jane S. Norbeck, and Lou Ellen A. Barnes

The effects of stress and social support and their interaction with the psychological well-being of 87 family caregivers of impaired elderly were examined. Perceived stress and satisfaction with support accounted for 32% to 36% of the variance in psychological distress or depression, p < .001; however, when characteristics of the caregiver situation were included in the models, the effects of perceived stress were found to be spurious. The revised models accounted for 44% to 48% of the variance in psychological distress or depression, p < .000, and included years of caregiving and mental impairment of the elder instead of perceived stress. Although there were no buffering effects for social support, main effects accounted for 19% to 22% of the variance in psychological distress or depression. The findings indicate that caregivers who are caring for a mentally impaired elder, who have been providing care for an extended time, and who have low social support are at high risk for psychological distress or depression.

The number of elder persons will more than double in the next four decades (Doty, Liu, & Wiener, 1985). These increases, in combination with the decline in federal funds for programs for the elderly, will place further demands on families to provide the caregiving services needed by their elderly members (Stoller, 1983).

The toll of caregiving on family caregivers can be high (Clark & Rakowski, 1983). In

Accepted for publication January 22, 1988.

This study was supported by a grant from the Preventive Health Care for the Aging Program of the California Department of Health to the Public Health Nursing Division, Monterey County Health Department, Salinas, CA, for 1985–1986.

Virginia Baillie, MA, RN, CS, is a family and mental health therapist in private practice in Salinas, CA. At the time of the study she was employed by the Monterey County Health Department, Salinas, CA.

Jane S. Norbeck, DNSc, FAAN, is a professor and chairman, Department of Mental Health, Community, and Administrative Nursing, School of Nursing, University of California, San Francisco.

Lou Ellen A. Barnes, MS, RN, is a doctoral student at the School of Nursing, University of California, San Francisco.

a sample of 510 caregivers, George and Gwyther (1986) found that caregivers were significantly lower in all mental health indicators and had significantly lower social participation than age peers with no caregiving responsibilities. The groups did not differ in physical health or finances. Other studies have described burden (Poulshock & Deimling, 1984; Zarit, Reever, & Bach-Peterson, 1980), strain (Cantor, 1983), or other outcomes experienced by caregivers (Archbold, 1982; Fengler & Goodrich, 1979; Jones & Vetter, 1984).

Background of the Study

Most studies have used exploratory or descriptive designs to identify and categorize the numerous emotional, physical, social, and financial difficulties associated with caregiving. Because these studies differ in sample characteristics, antecedent and outcome variables studied, and analytical strategies, it is difficult to compare findings across studies. The atheoretical nature of most of this work and the predominant use of univariate research designs further complicates the ability to draw conclusions from these diverse findings.

Antecedent variables to caregiver burden, strain, or diminished well-being that have been studied can be clustered into the categories of (a) demographic characteristics of caregivers and of elders, (b) characteristics of the caregiving situation, (c) and variables that mediate the effects of caregiver stress.

Studies that have examined demographic characteristics of caregivers or of elders have shown mixed results. For example, Cantor (1983) found that type of relationship between caregiver and the elder (e.g., spouse, child, relative, friend) accounted for 28% of the variance in impact on the lives of caregivers, and 37% of the variance in caregiver strain. George and Gwyther (1986) also found that spouses had lower well-being than other categories of caregivers. In contrast, neither Robinson (1983) nor Zarit et al. (1980) found significant differences in strain or burden for caregivers with different relationships to the elder. These discrepancies do not appear to be explained by different mixes of relationship groups in the samples. Similar lack of agreement exists for demographic variables of caregiver's age, sex, income, and education (e.g., Gilhooly, 1984; Montgomery, Gonyea, & Hooyman, 1985; Pratt, Schmall, Wright, & Cleland, 1985).

Findings concerning characteristics of the caregiving situation and caregiver burden or satisfaction also have been equivocal. Variables such as the mental condition of the patient, the level of impairment, or the amount of care required have been supported in some studies and not in others (e.g., Worchester & Quayhagen, 1983; Zarit et al., 1980). A common finding, however, is that medical problems or physical care needs are less important factors than psychological problems or mental impairment of the elder (Poulshock & Deimling, 1984; Worchester & Quayhagen).

Of the variables that potentially mediate stress, social support has been studied most frequently. George and Gwyther (1986) reported that the group of caregivers who indicated they needed more social support were significantly lower in all four dimensions of well-being than those who reported having enough social support. In a study of 29 caregivers, Zarit et al. (1980) found that the frequency of family visits to the elder was significantly related to caregiver burden, $r = .48$, but other variables, such as the elder's cognitive impairment, duration of illness, memory problems, behavioral problems, or level of functional impairment were not. Scott, Roberto, and Hutton (1986) found that family support was positively related to coping effectiveness and reduced burden in a study of 23 caregivers of Alzheimer's patients, and Gilhooly (1984) found that satisfaction with help from relatives had the highest correlation with caregiver mental health of the 22 variables measured ($n = 37$). Social support measured as helpfulness was not a significant predictor of depression in a study of 44 caregivers by Fiore, Becker, and Coppel (1983); however, in a later study (Fiore, Becker, & Cox, 1986)

of the four operationalizations of social support, satisfaction was the only significant predictor of depression and general psychopathology among 68 caregivers. Subjects in both of these studies were spouses of patients with Alzheimer's disease. Findings from the 1986 study suggest that the lack of significance for social support in the 1983 study may reflect the validity of construct measurement.

The purpose of this study was to investigate the effects of perceived caregiver stress and social support on the psychological distress of family caregivers of the elderly, using the stress-buffering model of social support to test both main and interaction effects (House, 1981). A secondary purpose was to explore demographic variables and characteristics of the caregiving situation that might contribute additional explained variance in psychological distress in caregivers. Psychological distress was operationalized as the total score from a negative mood scale. The depression subscale was also used as a separate outcome measure because depression has been studied so frequently with this population.

Hypotheses
Consistent with theory and research in social support, three hypotheses were generated:
I. Perceived stress of caregiving will be positively related to psychological distress.
II. Satisfaction with social support will be negatively related to psychological distress.
III. Social support will have a buffering effect on the relationship between perceived caregiver stress and psychological distress.

Specific demographic characteristics or characteristics of the caregiving situation related to psychological distress were incorporated into the stress-buffering model as precursor variables on the assumption that these characteristics or conditions are causally prior to perceptions of stress or support (Cohen & Cohen, 1975).

Table 1 Relationships Between Caregivers and Elderly Person (*n* = 87)

Caregivers	Percentage	Elders	Percentage
1. Spouse	18.4		
		Husband	9.2
		Wife	9.2
2. Adult child	48.3		
		Mother	40.2
		Father	8.0
3. Other relative	25.3		
		Mother-in-law	12.6
		Grandparent	5.7
		Other	4.6
		Father-in-law	2.3
4. Friend, other	8.0		
		Friend	6.9
		Other	1.1

Method

Subjects: Subjects were recruited and tested at the initial meeting of educational groups for caregivers sponsored by a county health department. The participation rate was 95%. All participants signed a consent form indicating their voluntary participation in the study. A total of 100 individuals participated; however, only the 87 caregivers who provided care in their own home or in the elder's home without pay were included in the study. The 87 caregivers provided care to elders with care needs ranging from supportive activities (e.g., shopping, errands, managing finances, providing an environment adjusted to the elder's physical limitations, or frequently checking up on the elder) to almost constant care or supervision. The caregivers considered their caregiving activities essential to maintaining the elder in the community and often personally stressful.

The 87 family caregivers in the sample were predominately female (76%), married (71%), and white (78%). Only 2% had not completed high school; 47% had completed college or postgraduate studies. The caregivers' mean age was 52.5 years (*SD* = 13.96; range,

22–91). The elderly persons they cared for had a mean age of 77.7 years (*SD* = 8.99; range, 55–92). The caregivers had given care for an average of 3.4 years (*SD* = 3.59; range, ⅔ year–25 years). The caregiving occurred in the elder's home in 46% of the cases, and in the caregiver's home in 54% of the cases. The relationship of the caregiver to the elderly person is shown in Table 1.

A total of 170 diagnoses for the elderly persons were listed by the caregivers. Among the elderly, 97% had one or more diagnoses; 50%, two or more; 25%, three or more, 14%, four or more; and 2%, five. In contrast, 68% of the caregivers did not list diagnoses for themselves, and the total number of diagnoses was only 40. Of the caregivers, the most frequent diagnosis was hypertension, reported by one-third of those giving diagnoses. Caregivers' ratings of their elderly family member's physical, mental, and functional status are presented on Table 2.

Measures: All measures in this study were based on self-report by caregivers on written questionnaires that took 30 to 45 minutes to complete.

Table 2 Characteristics of Elders and Their Caregiving needs ($n = 87$)

Physical condition of elder

1. Healthy	37.9
2. Chronically ill	62.1

Mental condition of elder

1. Alert	47.1
2. Mentally impaired or confused	52.9

Level of functioning of elder

1. Manages all personal and health care needs independently	13.8
2. Manages personal and health care needs with some help and supervision	39.1
3. Dependent on caregiver for personal care and supervision most of the time	26.4
4. Totally dependent on caregiver for personal and health care and supervision	20.7

Mobility of elder

1. Walks without assistance	48.3
2. Walks with assistance of cane	23.0
3. Walks with assistance of walker	16.1
4. Walks with assistance of person	5.8
5. Semi-wheelchair bound	3.5
6. Totally wheelchair bound	2.3
7. Bedfast	1.2

Hours of care needed daily

1. 0-4	37.9
2. 5-12	29.9
3. 13-24	32.2

Demographic variables were measured by single-item checklists or questions. For purposes of calculating zero-order correlations and entry into multiple regressions, the nominal variables of race and marital status were dichotomized into white/nonwhite and married/not married; location of caregiving had only two levels. Thus, these nominal variables were essentially entered as dummy or blocked variables.

Characteristics of the caregiving situation were measured by single-item checklists describing the elderly person's physical condition, mental condition, mobility, level of functioning, and hours of care required, according to the response categories listed in Table 2. The duration of caregiving was measured in years or fractions of years. The validity of the caregivers' ratings of the elders' physical or mental condition was checked against the open-ended diagnoses reported for each elder.

For the variable of physical condition, the diagnoses of physical illnesses or conditions for the elders rated physically healthy were compared with those rated chronically ill. Diagnoses that reflect conditions or symptoms (e.g., arthritis, hypertension, hearing loss, or heart problems) were common to both groups; but diagnoses of actual chronic disease states appeared only in the group that had been rated chronically ill. The diagnoses that appeared exclusively in the chronically ill group ($n = 54$) included diabetes (9), emphysema or chronic obstructive pulmonary disease (6), chronic back pain (3), Parkinson's disease (2), heart attack (2), advanced liver disease (1), asthma (1), colitis (1), and ulcers (1). Additionally, 17% of the group rated chronically ill had three or more diagnoses. In contrast, only one individual or 3% of the group rated healthy had three diagnoses; no one had four or five diagnoses. The chronically ill group had an average of 1.4 physical diagnoses compared with 0.56 for the healthy group, and none of the diagnoses reported for the healthy group reflected chronic illnesses other than arthritis.

The variable of mental condition showed a similar level of confirmation of the ratings of alert versus mentally impaired or confused. Of the group rated alert, only one individual (2%) had the diagnosis of senility. Of the group rated mentally impaired or confused, 78% had diagnoses clearly consistent with mental impairment (Alzheimer's disease, senility, confusion–disorientation); 13% had diagnoses potentially consistent with cognitive impairment (brain cancer, paranoia, manic depression, chronic alcoholism); 9% had only diagnoses of physical illnesses. Thus, 91% of the cases rated mentally impaired had diagnoses consistent with cognitive impairment compared with 2% of the group rated alert.

Perceived stress of caregiving was measured by a 16-item questionnaire that was developed for this study and pretested with a pilot sample. Item content was based on both clinical experience with this population and on stressful factors identified in the family caregiving literature. It included stress arising from the elder person's behavior, communication ability, emotional or mental state, or relationship with the caregiver; time demands in caregiving; physical or task aspects of caregiving; effects on other family members; and financial considerations. Each item was rated on a 5-point Likert scale, ranging from *no stress* to *high stress*. The standardized alpha test for internal consistency reliability for the study sample was .90.

Satisfaction with social support was measured with an 8-item questionnaire developed for this study and pretested with a pilot sample. Items covered satisfaction in the areas of emotional support, acceptance in caregiver role by family members, contact with others in the social network, and tangible help from others. Items were rated on a 5-point Likert scale, ranging from *not at all satisfied* to *very satisfied*. The standardized alpha test for internal consistency reliability for the study sample was .84.

Psychological distress was measured with the Profile of Mood States (POMS) developed by McNair, Lorr, and Droppleman (1971). This 65-item adjective rating scale measures six identifiable mood states: anxiety, depression, anger, vigor, fatigue, and confusion. Factor analytic studies have established the independence of the six states. Test–retest reliability ranged from .65 to .74. Internal consistency was .90 or above for all items within each factor. Predictive and construct validity were established through various studies, including short-term psychotherapy studies, outpatient drug trials, and studies of emotion-inducing conditions. Concurrent validity was established through significant correlations with three clinically derived scores from the Hopkins Symptoms Distress Scales (Derogatis, 1977). The standardized alpha test for internal consistency reliability for the study sample was .89 on total negative mood and also .89 on the 15-item depression subscale.

Results

Preliminary Analysis: A correlation matrix of all study variables was examined to identify: (a) demographic variables or characteristics of the caregiving situation related to the substantive study variables of perceived stress of caregiving, satisfaction with social support, the total psychological distress score, or the depression subscale score and (b) possible sources of multicollinearity among study variables.

Caregiver age was related significantly to four characteristics of the caregiving situation (years of caregiving, hours of care needed, level of functioning of elder, and mobility of elder) with correlations ranging from .28 to .48. Location of caregiving was related significantly to hours of care needed, $r = .54$, in which hours of care were greater for care provided in the caregiver's home compared to the elder's home.

Relationship between caregiver and elder, using the four categories in Table 1, was examined for relationships with the study variables through analysis of variance. No significant differences were found among groups on the four substantive study variables; however, Scheffé's contrasts showed that spouse caregivers reported significantly more hours of care needed, $F (3, 83) = 7.473$, $p = .0002$, and lower level of functioning of elder, $F (3, 83) = 4.618, p = .005$, than the other three caregiver groups.

A correlation matrix of the remaining variables describing characteristics of the caregiving situation and the substantive study variables is presented in Table 3. Two variables, physical condition of the elder and mobility of the elder, were not related to the substantive study variables, although they were related to each other and to level of functioning. The variables of mental condition, level of functioning, hours of care needed, and years of caregiving were related to the study variables of perceived stress of caregiving, total psychological distress, and depression. Initial support for Hypotheses I and II was shown by these zero-order correlations. Perceived stress of caregiving was positively related to psychological distress, $r = .46$, and depression, $r = .49$, and satisfaction with social support was negatively related to psychological distress, $r = -.48$, and depression, $r = -.52$.

Multiple regression analyses were conducted to test the buffering hypothesis (III) and to study the effects of demographic and caregiving variables in conjunction with the study variables (perceived stress and support satisfaction) on the outcome variables of the total psychological distress score and the depression subscale.

First, the hypothesized relationships were tested by entering perceived stress in the models in the first step, satisfaction with support in the second step, and the interaction term to test the buffering hypothesis in the third step. Table 4 shows that perceived stress of caregiving accounted for 21% of the variance in total psychological distress and 24% of the variance in depression. Satisfaction with support accounted for an additional 10% of the variance in total psychological distress and 12% of the variance in depression. Either positive or negative signs for the regression coefficients for the relationships appeared as predicted in the hypotheses. In each regression, the interaction term of perceived stress times social support was entered in the third step; however, in neither regression did the interaction term meet criteria for entry into the models. The total explained variance for total psychological distress was 32%; for depression, 36%. Thus, the first two hypotheses were supported, but the third hypothesis was not.

Next, analyses were conducted to determine whether the addition of demographic variables or characteristics of the caregiving situation would increase the amount of variance explained. First, the demographic variables of caregiver age, sex, race (dichotomized), educational level, marital status (dichotomized), number of children in the home, elder age, and location of caregiving were included at Step 1 using forward stepwise entry. None of these variables met criteria for entry into the models.

Second, the six variables describing the characteristics of caregiving were entered in the second step. Of these, two met entry criteria for inclusion in the models: mental condition of the elder and years of caregiving. Together these caregiving variables accounted for 25% of the variance in total psychological

Table 3 Pearson Correlations, Means, and Standard Deviations of Variables in Analysis (*n* = 85)

Variables	1	2	3	4	5	6	7	8	9	10	M	SD
1. Physical condition of elder	1.00										1.6	0.5
2. Mental condition	-.17	1.00									1.5	0.5
3. Mobility of elder	.31**	.08	1.00								2.0	1.4
4. Level of functioning of elder	.06	.49***	.34***	1.00							2.5	1.0
5. Hours of care needed	.03	.39***	.19	.61***	1.00						1.9	0.8
6. Years of caregiving	.00	-.10	-.14	-.01	.11	1.00					3.4	3.6
7. Perceived stress of caregiving	.03	.41***	.14	.44***	.17	.10	1.00				33.2	14.3
8. Satisfaction with social support	-.04	-.15	.06	-.28**	.27**	.04	-.42***	1.00			18.0	6.7
9. Psychological distress	-.10	.41***	.06	.36***	.41***	.25*	.46***	-.48***	1.00		67.7	36.2
10. Depression	-.10	.43***	.06	.38***	.41***	.24*	.49***	-.52***	.94***	1.00	14.4	10.8

NOTE: *p* values are 2-tailed.
*p < .05, **p < .01, ***p < .001.

Table 4 **Regression of Main and Interaction Effects of Perceived Stress, and Satisfaction with Social Support on Total Psychological Distress and on Depression ($n = 85$)**

Source of variation	Beta	R^2	r^2 Change	F Change	p Change
Total psychological distress					
1. Perceived stress	.462	.213	.213	22.5	.000
2. Support satisfaction	−.353	.316	.103	12.3	.001
Depression					
1. Perceived stress	.494	.244	.244	26.8	.000
2. Support satisfaction	−.381	.364	.120	15.5	.000

Note: Variables were entered hierarchically with forward entry. Perceived stress was entered in Step 1, support satisfaction in Step 2, and at Step 3, the interaction term (perceived stress multiplied by support satisfaction) did not meet criteria for entry.

distress and 26% of the variance in depression. The four caregiving variables that did not enter the models were physical condition of the elder, level of functioning of the elder, hours of care needed, and mobility of the elder.

Perceived stress was entered into the models at Step 3 and satisfaction with support at Step 4. The interaction term failed to meet criteria for entry into the models at Step 5. After all variables were in the full models, the variable of perceived stress was no longer significant. Thus, the relationship of perceived stress to the outcome variables were spurious when the more direct stress variables (mental condition of the elder and years of caregiving) were in the models. The regressions were rerun without perceived stress and the final regressions met essential assumptions (Verran & Ferketich, 1987). The results are shown in Table 5: Satisfaction with support accounted for 19% of the variance in total psychological distress and 22% of the variance in depression. The total explained variance for total psycho

logical distress was 44% and for depression, 48%.

The addition of variables describing characteristics of the caregiving situation increased the overall R^2 by 13% for total psychological distress and by 12% for depression and revealed that the relationship between perceived stress and the outcome variables was spurious when these more specific stressor variables were in the models.

Because the effect of social support was substantial, additional analyses were conducted to explore qualities of the caregivers' support systems that might warrant further study. Table 6 displays the primary source of support identified by the caregivers. When broken down by marital status, the primary source of support for married and unmarried caregivers appears to differ markedly. Spouses are the primary source of support for the married caregivers, and in only one instance was a spouse also the elder person being cared for. Unmarried caregivers relied most heavily

Table 5 Regression of Demographic and Caregiving Variables, Perceived Stress, and Satisfaction with Social Support on Total Psychological Distress and on Depression ($n = 85$)

Source of variation	Beta	R^2	R^2 Change	F Change	p Change
Total psychological distress					
1. Mental condition of elder	.409	.167	.167	16.6	.000
Years of caregiving	.294	.252	.085	9.4	.003
2. Support satisfaction	− .440	.442	.189	27.5	.000
Depression					
1. Mental condition of elder	.427	.182	.182	18.5	.000
Years of caregiving	.284	.262	.080	8.9	.004
2. Support satisfaction	− .475	.483	.221	34.6	.000

Note: Variables were entered hierarchically in sets with forward stepwise entry. Eight demographic variables were included in the first set, but none met criteria for entry into the models. The next set included six characteristics of the caregiving situation, but only two met entry criteria and are shown in Step 1. The study variables were entered individually, starting with perceived stress, then support satisfaction, and finally the interaction term which did not meet criteria for entry. Perceived stress entered the models but was found to be a spurious relationship after all variables were in the models; thus, support satisfaction entered at Step 2 in the final regressions.

on friends as their primary sources of support, but they also used siblings and other relatives to a greater extent than did the married caregivers. Married caregivers' made greater use of support from health care providers and from their own children.

To further understand social support, another regression was done in which the eight demographic variables were included in Step 1 and the six conditions of caregiving were included in Step 2. Only one variable, hours of care needed daily, entered the equation, accounting for 8% of the variance in satisfaction with support. Thus, many other unmeasured factors account for caregivers' satisfaction with their support.

Discussion

The main effects of perceived stress and satisfaction with social support on psychological distress and depression (the first two hypotheses) were supported in the predicted directions in both univariate and multivariate analysis; however, when more specific indicators of caregiver demands were included in the models, the relationships between perceived stress and the outcome variables were found to be spurious. Thus, Hypothesis I was only partially supported, and the findings suggest that objective indicators of caregiver demand are more potent than a measure of perceived stress in explaining the psychological distress of caregivers.

Table 6 **Primary Sources of Support Listed by Caregivers in Percent for Total Group and for Single and Married Subgroups**

Primary source of support	Total group (*n* = 87)	Not married (*n* = 25)	Married (*n* = 62)
Spouse	44.8	0.0	62.3
Friend	25.0	59.3	11.6
Child	6.3	3.7	7.2
Health worker or counselor	6.3	3.7	7.2
Other*	5.2	3.7	5.8
Siblings	4.2	11.1	1.4
Other relatives	4.2	11.1	1.4
Neighbor	2.1	3.7	1.4
Self	2.1	3.7	1.4

* Other responses included church, support group, and unspecified.

The main effect for social support in predicting psychological distress was substantial (Hypothesis II); however, there was no evidence of a buffering effect of social support (Hypothesis III). Although some of the studies in the social support field find significant buffering effects for social support, many find only main effects. The findings from this study are consistent with the majority of studies in the social support field, except that the magnitude of the effects of social support in this study (19%-22%) is larger than usually found, perhaps because a situation-specific support measure was used instead of a general support measure. The importance of social support among caregivers in this study parallels and extends the univariate findings noted earlier (Fiore et al., 1986; George & Gwyther, 1986; Scott et al., 1986).

Only two conditions of caregiving were found to be significant predictors of psychological distress: the mental condition of the elder and the years of caregiving. Neither the physical condition of the elder nor the mobility rating of the elder was significantly related to any of the study variables, despite various chronic illnesses among 62% of the elderly and limited mobility for 30%. Even though the degree of dependence or need for supervision and the hours of care required daily had significant zero-order correlations with the outcome variables, they did not impact on the psychological distress of the caregiver when the elder's mental impairment and the number of years of caregiving were included in the models. These findings point to the importance of multivariate analysis to sort out which effects remain when variables are considered as they work together.

The fact that none of the demographic characteristics of the caregivers or elders were related to the caregiver's psychological distress is not surprising, given the highly inconsistent findings about demographic variables in other caregiver studies. Two of these variables addressed other role demands on the caregivers: the marital role and the parenting role. It is possible that the support derived from the marital role offsets marital role demands; however, the number of children living in the home would seem more likely to affect caregiver well-being. Unfortunately, the role demands from employment were not examined in this study and should be examined in future studies.

That the relationship between perceived stress and psychological distress proved to be spurious when two key characteristics of the caregiving situation (mental impairment of the elder and duration of caregiving) were included in the models raises questions about the utility of the related concepts of caregiver burden or strain as these concepts relate to the well-being of caregivers. Most of the research on caregiver burden or strain has not related these variables to mental or physical health outcomes of the caregivers. Robinson (1983) did this, but she found a significant relationship, $r = .31$, only between strain and anxiety, and not between strain and depression, hostility, or morale. Poulshock and Deimling (1984) reported zero-order correlations ranging from .18 to .30 between burden subscales and depression. The effect size of the relationships between burden or strain and psychological distress variables in these studies is extremely modest, accounting for only 3% to 10% of the variance in caregiver mental health, if significant at all. Although the concepts of burden or strain do not appear to be highly predictive of caregiver well-being, burden scores have been associated with subsequent nursing home placement (Zarit, Todd, & Zarit, 1986). But the magnitude of this effect in conjunction with other predictor variables was not reported.

In this study, the effects of social support on psychological well-being were nearly double when using characteristics of the caregiving situation as indicators of stress rather than using the measure of perceived stress. It appears that caregivers who are caring for a mentally impaired elder, who have been providing care for an extended time, and who have low social support are at high risk for psychological distress or depression. This triad of factors echoes the literature which describes the difficulties presented by the behavior of the demented elder (Chenoweth & Spencer, 1986) in which caregivers become confined to the house because the elder requires constant supervision, yet friends no longer visit them, and they are deprived from the other sources of social contacts previously obtained through employment, volunteer work, or leisure activities.

The ability to generalize the findings is limited by the nonrandom, predominately middle-class nature of the sample. Although the measures of perceived stress and social support had high internal consistency reliability, further work with more developed measures is needed to validate these findings. Because social support was strongly related to the psychological well-being of these caregivers, additional research is needed to explore factors that contribute to satisfaction with social support. Knowledge of these factors might shed light on how support facilitates coping with the demands of providing care for a mentally impaired family member over a long period of time.

The findings of this study are helpful to practicing clinicians because they give credibility to planning intervention strategies that offer tangible assistance and emotional support to the caregiver, perhaps through members of the caregiver's own network. In addition to enhancing the psychological well-being of caregivers, focusing attention on the needs of caregivers has the potential to decrease additional problems, such as caregiver illness or elder abuse.

References

Archbold, P. G. (1982). An analysis of parent caring by women. *Home Health Care Services Quarterly, 3*(2), 5–25.

Cantor, M. H. (1983). Strain among caregivers: A study of experience in the United States. *The Gerontologist, 23,* 597–604

Chenoweth, B., & Spencer, B. (1986). Dementia: The experience of family caregivers. *The Gerontologist, 26,* 267–272.

Clark, N. M., & Rakowski, W. (1983). Family caregivers of older adults: Improving helping skills. *The Gerontologist, 23,* 637–642.

Cohen, J., & Cohen, P. (1975). *Applied multiple regression/correlation analysis for the behavioral sciences.* New York: John Wiley & Sons, Inc.

Derogatis, L. R. (1977). *SCL–90: Administration, scoring & procedures manual.* Baltimore: Johns Hopkins University.

Doty, P., Liu, K., & Wiener, J. (1985). Special report: An overview of long-term care. *Health Care Financing Review, 6*(3), 69–78.

Fengler, A. P., & Goodrich, N. (1979). Wives of elderly disabled men: the hidden patients. *The Gerontologist, 19,* 175–183.

Fiore, J., Becker, J., & Coppel, D. B. (1983). Social network interactions: A buffer or a stress. *American Journal of Community Psychology, 11,* 423–439.

Fiore, J., Becker, J., & Cox, G. B. (1986). Social support as a multifaceted concept: Examination of important dimensions for adjustment. *American Journal of Community Psychology, 14,* 93–111.

George, L.K., & Gwyther, L. P. (1986). Caregiver well-being: A multidimensional examination of family caregivers of demented adults. *The Gerontologist, 26,* 253–259.

Gilhooly, M. L. M. (1984). The impact of caregiving on care-givers: Factors associated with the psychological well-being of people supporting a dementing relative in the community. *British Journal of Medical Psychology, 57,* 35–44.

House, J. (1981). *Work stress and social support.* Reading, MA: Addison–Wesley Publishing Co.

Jones, D. A., & Vetter, N. J. (1984). A survey of those who care for the elderly at home: Their problems and their needs. *Social Science Medicine, 19,* 511–514.

McNair, D. M., Lorr, M., & Droppleman, L. F. (1971). *POMS manual for Profile of Mood States.* San Diego: Educational and Industrial Testing Service.

Montgomery, J. V., Gonyea, J. G., Hooyman, N. R. (1985). Caregiving and the experience of subjective and objective burden. *Family Relations, 34,* 19–26.

Poulshock, S. W., & Deimling, G. T. (1984). Families caring for elders in residence: Issues in the measurement of burden. *Journal of Gerontology, 39,* 230–239.

Pratt, C. C., Schmall, V. L., Wright, S., & Cleland, M. (1985). Burden and coping strategies of caregivers to Alzheimer's patients. *Family Relations, 34,* 27–33.

Robinson, B. C. (1983). Validation of a caregiver strain index. *Journal of Gerontology, 38,* 344–348.

Scott, J. P., Roberto, K. A., & Hutton, J. T. (1986). Families of Alzheimer's victims: Family support to the caregivers. *Journal of the American Geriatrics Society, 34,* 348–354.

Stoller, E. P. (1983). Parental caregiving by adult children. *Journal of Marriage and the Family, 45,* 851–858.

Verran, J. A., & Ferketich, S. L. (1987). Testing linear model assumptions: Residual analysis. *Nursing Research, 36,* 127–130.

Worchester, M. I., & Quayhagen, M. P. (1983). Correlates of caregiving satisfaction: Prerequisites to elder home care. *Research in Nursing & Health, 6,* 61–67.

Zarit, S. H., Reever, K. E., & Bach–Peterson, J. (1980). Relatives of the impaired elderly: Correlates of feelings of burden. *The Gerontologist, 20,* 649–655.

Zarit, S. H., Todd, P. A., & Zarit, J. M. (1986). Subjective burden of husbands and wives as caregivers: A longitudinal study. *The Gerontologist, 26,* 260–266.

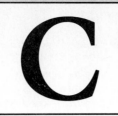

COMPARISONS OF RECTAL, FEMORAL, AXILLARY, AND SKIN-TO-MATTRESS TEMPERATURES IN STABLE NEONATES*

Mariamma T. Kunnel, Cecille O'Brien, Barbara Hazard Munro, and Barbara Medoff-Cooper

The purpose of this study was to compare four sites for temperature recording in the neonate: rectum, femoral, axilla, and skin-to-mattress. Simultaneous measurements were made at the four sites in 99 stable, term neonates. Temperatures were recorded each minute for 15 minutes. The optimal temperatures (highest temperature recorded minus 0.2°F) did not vary across the four sites, but there were significant differences in the mean times required to achieve optimal temperature and in the optimal placement times (time required for 90% of the subjects to reach optimal temperature). The rectal site required significantly less time than the other sites (M = 2.66 minutes, optimal placement time = 5 minutes). The femoral and axillary sites required significantly more time than rectal and significantly less time than skin-to-mattress (M = 6 minutes, optimal placement time = 11 minutes). The skin-to-mattress site required significantly more time than the other sites (M = 8.5 minutes, optimal placement time = 13 minutes).

Accurate monitoring of neonatal temperature is essential to provide information about the adjustment of the neonate to extrauterine life. The standard practice in many nurseries has been to use rectal measurements because they are believed to correlate most closely with deep body temperature and to require less time to obtain an accurate reading. There are, however, serious contraindications to the use of rectal thermometers. The risk of rectal

Accepted for publication October 7, 1987.

Mariamma T. Kunnel, RN, is a Level III nurse at the Hospital of the University of Pennsylvania, Philadelphia.

Cecille O'Brien, RN,C, is a Level III nurse at the Hospital of the University of Pennsylvania, Philadelphia.

Barbara Hazard Munro, PhD, RN, is an associate professor at the School of Nursing, University of Pennsylvania, and a research facilitator in the Division of Nursing, Hospital of the University of Pennsylvania, Philadelphia.

Barbara Medoff-Cooper, PhD, RN, is an associate professor at the School of Nursing, University of Pennsylvania, and a clinical specialist in the Department of Obstetrics/Neonatal Nursing, Hospital of the University of Pennsylvania, Philadelphia.

perforation associated with rectal temperature taking is increased in the neonate because the neonate's colon acutely changes from an anterior to posterior angle at a depth of 3 centimeters (Merentstein, 1970). Although rectal perforation is a rare event, it is a most serious one. Greenbaum, Carson, Kincannon, and O'Laughlin (1969) found a 70% mortality rate with rectal perforation in a group of full-term infants.

Because of the risks associated with rectal temperature taking, it is essential that alternate methods be tested for accuracy and efficiency. Previous studies have failed to provide the empirical data necessary to establish the most clinically satisfactory alternative site and the optimal time for measurement of the temperature.

The purpose of this study was to determine (a) if accurate temperature recordings could be made at alternative sites and (b) optimal thermometer placement time at the sites. Definitions for optimal and maximal temperatures and placement times were adopted from Nichols, Ruskin, Glor, and Kelly (1966). Maximal temperature is the highest reading of the thermometer during the testing period. Optimal temperature equals the time required for 90% of the subjects to reach optimal temperatures.

Relevant Literature

Adaptation to extrauterine life involves a severe biologic adjustment, including the need to respond to a radical alteration in environmental temperature (Stern, 1980). Although it is now known that the newborn has the attributes of a homoiotherm, that is, ability to maintain a remarkable constant deep body temperature, this mechanism can be overwhelmed by extremes of cold or heat stress. During extrauterine transition, the range of environmental temperatures over which the infant can operate successfully is quite restricted, compared to the adult. The infant is at a definite disadvantage with a relatively large surface area, poor thermal insulation, and a small mass to act as a heat sink (Scopes, 1981).

Once past the extrauterine adjustment period, there are additional concerns about changes in body temperature for the newborn infant. A fall in temperature may be a sign of severe and important underlying systemic disease. This alteration may be the first and only definite sign of sepsis of the newborn, which is a medical complication most effectively managed if detected in the early stages of development (Scopes, 1981).

Given the importance of evaluating body temperature in the newborn period, establishing the most reliable and safe site and the optimal measurement time are essential for appropriate nursing care. Research in this area has been sparse, and studies have been flawed by poor design, limited numbers of subjects, and lack of clear definitions.

Studies have provided inconclusive findings concerning sites and measurement time. Haddock, Vincent, and Merrow (1986) in their study of 30 healthy full-term infants between 24 and 72 hours of age found that 90% of the infants reached optimal axillary temperature within 5 minutes; 87% reached optimal rectal temperature within 2 minutes and all by 4 minutes. None of the infants showed a difference of as much as one degree between maximal rectal and maximal axillary temperature. There did not seem to be a fixed temperature for the newborns; maximal temperature varied as frequently as all other physiologic measurements. In the study, the two methods of temperature measurement were not measured simultaneously, rather one following the other.

In contrast, Mayfield, Bhatia, Nakamura, Rios, and Bell (1984) simultaneously evaluated core, rectal, axillary, and skin-to-mattress temperatures in 99 full-term infants. Core temperature was measured by placing a thermistor probe into the rectum to a depth of 5 cm. Skin-to-mattress temperature was measured by placing the thermometer underneath the infant between the skin and surface of the mattress. The infants ranged in age from 1 to 10 days. The mean stabilization times for all four sites were between 3 to 5 minutes with 90% stabilization within 5 minutes. There

were no significant differences in the accuracy or time for stabilization of temperature in the four methods.

These findings were not corroborated by Schiffman (1982) who found significant differences between axillary and rectal temperatures if compared minute by minute in a sample of 46 full-term infants. Axillary temperature never reached stabilization during the 10-minute observation period. Despite the differences between sites in the minute-by-minute temperatures, there was a significant positive correlation between axillary and rectal temperatures, with a range from .76 at 1 minute to .92 at 10 minutes. The measurements in this study were not conducted simultaneously.

Because of conflicting findings, failure to reach maximal temperature in the allotted time, and lack of simultaneous measures, studies to date have not provided data for the establishment of optimal site and time for measurement of neonatal temperature. The only current recommendation has been from the American Academy of Pediatrics (1983) for a 3-minute placement of axillary temperature. This recommendation applies to a general pediatric population and is not specific to neonates.

Method

Design: To control for individual characteristics of the neonates that might affect temperature, a repeated measures design was used in which the subjects served as their own controls. Rectal, femoral, axillary, and skin-to-mattress temperatures were taken simultaneously on each subject over a 15-minute period.

Sample: After obtaining informed parental consent, a convenience sample based on subject and data collector availability was used. Ninety-nine full-term neonates (38–40.5 weeks gestation, $M = 39.7$, $SD = 1.02$) of normal weight (2,750–4,000 grams, $M = 3,191$, $SD = 299$) who were admitted to normal newborn nurseries directly from the delivery room of the Hospital of the University of Pennsylvania were included in the study. Study subjects were stable, 1 to 4 days old, and with no known abnormalities. The sample included 62 females and 37 males. Eighty-nine were black, 7 white, and 3 Oriental. Eighty-two were bottle-fed and 17 breast-fed. The neonates were resting or pacified in open bassinets. Twenty slept through the entire data collection period, 25 were awake and quiet, and the rest displayed a mixture of behaviors from sleep to crying. Data were collected from September through December 1985. During that time, the nursery room temperature varied between 72° and 84° Fahrenheit ($M = 77°$, $SD = 2°$).

Instruments: Four identical mercury in glass thermometers were used for the simultaneous monitoring of the neonates' rectal, femoral, axillary, and skin-to-mattress temperatures. Prior to data collection, the accuracy of these thermometers was checked by immersing them in a temperature-controlled circulating water bath and then checking the readings against the National Bureau of Standards (NBS) thermometer. Thermometers which varied 0.2 °F from the NBS thermometer reading were discarded. The thermometers were cleansed with soap and water and kept in alcohol between subjects. The alcohol solution was changed every third day as recommended by the infectious disease control department. Thermometers were retested after data collection was completed and found to be accurate, according to the NBS thermometer.

Procedure: Once determination was made that the newborn met the physical criteria, the procedure, risks, and benefits of the study were explained to the mother in lay terms. The mother was given time to consider whether to participate. If she agreed, the consent form was signed, and a time was set so the mother could observe the procedure if she chose.

Prior to testing, neonates' diapers and shirts were changed as necessary. During the procedure, neonates lay on their sides wearing a shirt with one sleeve removed and the diaper opened. The mercury was shaken down below 94 °F in each thermometer before placement. *Axillary temperature* was measured by placing the thermometer in the center of the axilla,

holding the arm securely over the thermometer, and then adjusting the thermometer for visibility. *Skin-to-mattress temperature* was measured by placing the thermometer underneath the neonate between the skin and surface of the mattress, between the levels of the fourth and the tenth thoracic vertebrae. *Rectal temperature* was measured by inserting a lubricated thermometer into the rectum no more than 2 cms. *Femoral temperature* was measured by placing the thermometer in the inguinal fold. All thermometers were left in place for 15 minutes. The temperature readings were recorded at all four sites each minute for 15 minutes. The nurse securing the axillary thermometer recorded temperature readings at the axilla and skin-to-mattress sites first. Then she recorded her colleague's temperature readings at the femoral and the rectal sites as they were reported each minute.

Prior to data collection, staff nurses were asked to participate in this study. Thirteen staff nurses with an average of 6 years of neonatal experience in the Hospital of the University of Pennsylvania neonatal nurseries responded. Each collector received a written description of the study criteria and procedure. Each data collector was observed by an investigator during one to five procedures to insure proper compliance with the protocol and interrater reliability of the temperature recordings. The interrater reliability of the temperature readings was further established by randomly checking 60% of the final readings in the following way: Thermometers were removed at the end of the test (15th minute) from the subject, reread by the nurse, then exchanged with a colleague, who also read the thermometer. Ninety-eight percent were 100% accurate. The 2% that varied did by only ±0.1 °F.

A flow sheet was used to record data. The data collected included identification of neonate, sex, race, gestational age, birth weight, age in hours at the time of test, temperatures at the four sites, time of last feeding, activity of the neonate during the procedure, placement times, room temperature, and names of data collectors.

Table 1 Optimal Temperatures Across Sites

Site	Optimal temperature (SD)
Skin-to-mattress	98.11 (.49)
Femoral	98.25 (.42)
Axillary	98.34 (.43)
Rectal	98.60 (.39)

Table 2 Repeated Measures Analysis of Variance on Time to Optimal Temperature

Source of variation	SS	df	MS	F	p
Between subjects	801.49	98	8.18		
Within subjects	4397.75	297	14.81		
Between measures	1725.66	3	575.22	63.29	.000
Residual	2672.09	294	9.09		
Total	5199.24	395	13.16		

Results

The optimal temperatures (highest temperature recorded minus 0.2 °F) did not differ meaningfully across the four sites (see Table 1).

The amount of time necessary to register optimal temperatures varied markedly across the sites. The average amount of time required to achieve optimal temperature varied from a low of 2.66 minutes at the rectal site to a high of 8.52 minutes at the skin-to-mattress site.

Repeated measures analysis of variance was used to compare these mean times (see Table 2). The mean times at the four sites differed significantly, $F = 63.29$, $p = .000$. Paired t tests were used to test for differences among the four mean times. To protect against an inflated risk of Type I error due to multiple comparisons among means, the Bonferroni correction was used, which resulted in a probability level of .008 being considered significant. The results demonstrated that the average amount of time required to record the optimal temperature at the rectal site (2.66 minutes, $SD = 2.2$) was significantly less than the time required at any of the other three sites. The skin-to-mattress site required significantly more time (8.52 minutes, $SD = 3.4$) than any of the other three sites. The time required at the femoral (5.88 minutes, $SD = 3.0$) and the axillary (6.14 minutes, $SD = 3.2$) sites did not differ significantly; these two sites required significantly more time than the rectal site, and significantly less time than the skin-to-mattress site.

Optimal placement time has been defined as the time required for the optimal temperature to be recorded for 90% of the subjects. These figures are: rectal, 5 minutes; axillary, 11 minutes; femoral, 11 minutes; skin-to-mattress, 13 minutes. The results indicate, therefore, that although accurate recordings can be made at all four sites, the time required to do so differs substantially.

Discussion

Simultaneous recording of temperature at four sites in 99 neonates indicated that although the optimal temperatures recorded did not vary across the sites, the time required to obtain the recordings did vary significantly. The lack of meaningful difference in optimal temperature for the four measurement sites is similar to the findings by Mayfield et al. (1984); however, the second finding of difference in the mean time required to reach optimal temperature is not in agreement with the Mayfield et al. study. The mean amount of time ranged from 2.66 minutes for the rectal site to 8.52 minutes for the skin-to-mattress site. These measurement times are much longer than the reported 3 to 5 minutes for mean stabilization time at core, rectal, axillary, and skin-to-mattress sites reported by Mayfield et al. The amount of time required for 90% of the infants to reach optimal temperatures (optimal placement time) ranged from 5 minutes at the rectal site to 13 minutes at the skin-to-mattress site. Mayfield et al. reported 90% stabilization within 5 minutes.

Both the mean and the optimal placement times are much shorter at the rectal site, but given the safety factors, it is the least desirable site. Of the remaining three sites, femoral and axillary\sites are the most efficient routes for optimal temperature measurement with minimal concerns for safety. Skin-to-mattress, with mean time of 8.52 minutes and an optimal placement time of 13 minutes, would be the least likely choice of clinicians. A possible explanation for the great difference between the skin-to-mattress temperature site and the axillary and femoral sites may be related to the occasional repositioning of the infant. Wet shirts or diapers were changed prior to measurement of the temperature, but during this process the infant may have experienced some conductive heat loss from neonate to the mattress. In addition, the anatomy of some neonates was such that during respiration their bodies would lift off the skin-to-mattress thermometer which also would contribute to conductive heat loss.

These results indicate that temperature measured at a variety of sites provides the clinician with reliable data. Axillary and femoral sites seem to be the best choices for use in the newborn nursery based on time to achieve optimal temperature and on safety. The results of this research indicate that the thermometer must be in place 6 minutes on the average and 11 minutes to be sure that 90% of the infants measured have reached their optimal temperature. Therefore, it is recommended that placement time be increased to achieve a more reliable measurement.

References

American Academy of Pediatrics. (1983). *Standards and recommendations for hospital care of newborn infants.* Elk Grove Village, IL: American Academy of Pediatrics.

Greenbaum, E., Carson, M., Kincannon, W., & O'Laughlin, B. (1969). Rectal thermometer-induced pneumoperitoneum in the newborn. *Pediatrics, 44,* 539–542.

Haddock, B., Vincent, P., & Merrow, D. (1986). Axillary and rectal temperatures of full-term neonates: Are they different? *Neonatal Network, 4,* 36–40.

Mayfield, S., Bhatia, J., Nakamura, K., Rios, G., & Bell, E. (1984). Temperature measurement in term and pre-term neonates. *Journal of Pediatrics, 104,* 2712–2715.

Merenstein, G. (1970). Rectal perforation by thermometer. *Lancet, 1,* 1007.

Nichols, G., Ruskin, M., Glor, B., & Kelly, W. (1966). Oral, axillary and rectal temperature determination and relationships. *Nursing Research, 17,* 312–320.

Schiffman R. (1982). Temperature monitoring in the neonate: A comparison of axillary and rectal temperatures. *Nursing Research, 31,* 274–277.

Scopes J. (1981). Thermoregulation in the newborn. In G. Averty (Ed.), *Neonatology: Pathophysiology and management of the newborn* (pp. 177–181). Philadelphia: J. B. Lippincott.

Stern, L. (1980). Temperature regulation in the premature and full-term infant. In M. Rathi & S. Kumir (Eds.) *Perinatal medicine: Clinical and biochemical aspects* (vol. 1, pp. 563–596). New York: Hemisphere Publishing Corp.

Index

A

Abstraction, definition of, 92
Advances in Nursing Sciences, 9
After-only design, 152
After-only nonequivalent control group design, 155-156
AJN; *see American Journal of Nursing*
Alpha, 316
Alternate form reliability, 257, 261
American Journal of Nursing, 7, 366
American Nurses' Association
    Commission on Nursing Research of, 5
    Committee on Research and Studies of, 8
    First Nursing Research Conference of, 9
American Nurses' Association Human Rights Guidelines for Nurses, 53
ANA; *see* American Nurses' Association
Analysis
    factor, construct validity established with, 254
    power, sample size estimated using, 281
Analysis of covariance test, 322
Analysis of variance test, 320, 322, 326
ANCOVA; *see* Analysis of covariance test
Animals, experimentation on, legal and ethical aspects of, 51-52
Annual Review of Nursing Research, 10
Anonymity, definition of, 45
ANOVA; *see* Analysis of variance test
Applied Nursing Research, 10
Article, research, personal judgment in preparing, 382
Assent, versus consent, in pediatric research, 48
Assumptions
    definition of, 32
    scientific approach to research guided by, 32

B

Bibliography card, 81
Biomedical Computer Programs, 339
BMD; *see* Biomedical Computer Programs

C

Causal-comparative studies, 170
Central processing unit, 330
Chance error; *see* Random error
Change, resistance to, and utilization of nursing research in practice, 364-365, 370-371
Chi-square test, 320, 322, 326
CINAHL; *see Computerized Index of Nursing and Allied Health Literature*
Clinical nurse researchers, 368
Close-ended items, 235, 236
CNRs; *see* Clinical nurse researchers
Code of Federal Regulations, research governed by, 40, 43
Coefficients
    correlation, 321- 322
    phi, 322
Collaboration
    interdisciplinary, nursing research in practice and, 369-370
    intradisciplinary, nursing research in practice and, 369
Commission on Nursing Research of American Nurses' Association, 5
Committee on Nursing and Nursing Education, 6
Committee on Public Health Nursing of National League of Nursing Education, 7
Committee on Research and Studies, American Nurses' Association, 8
Communication
    between nursing researchers and practicing nurses, 363-364, 369-370
    of research findings to nursing profession, 363, 366-367
Computer hardware, 330, 342
Computer language, 332
Computer software, 331, 332-333, 342
Computerized Index of Nursing and Allied Health Literature, 82
Computers; *see also* Data processing; Microcomputers
    guidelines for analyzing use of, in research studies, 342

Page numbers followed by t indicate tables.

Computers—cont'd
  mainframe
    editing system of, 331
    versus microcomputers, 334t
  operating system of, 331
  overview of, 330-331
  personal, 331
  in research, 329-342
  research process and, 334-342
  types of, 331-332, 342
Concealment by observer, 233
Concept(s)
  defining, 98-99
  definition of, 97, 105
  interrelationships between, identifying,
    97-98
  operationalization of, 100, 105
  purpose of, in theoretical framework, 103
  selection of, in developing theoretical frame-
    work, 97
Conceptualization, purpose of, in qualitative re-
    search, 184
Conclusions, research, critiquing, 384t
Confidentiality, definition of, 45
Consent, informed, 39-41, 46-47
  guidelines for, 44-45
  waiving, 49
Consistency
  in data collection, 230
  internal, of measurement instruments, 257-
    259
Constancy in data collection, 134-135
Constant comparative method, data analysis us-
    ing, 192
Constant error; *see* Systematic error
Construct replication, 372
Construct(s)
  definition of, 92
    instrument development and, 20
  validity of, 252-254
Content analysis, 236
Content validity, 250-251
Contrasted-groups, construct validity established
    with, 254
Control
  definition of, 129, 133
  in experimental research, 149
  in research design, 129, 143
    over tested variables, 133-136
  in scientific approach to research, 29
Correlation coefficients, 321-322
Correlation(s), 304
  between variables, 321

Correlation(s)—cont'd
  item to total, homogeneity assessed with,
    257-258
  Spearman rank order, 322
Correlational studies, 168-170
  advantages and disadvantages of, 169
Covariance, analysis of, 322
CPU; *see* Central processing unit
Criteria, eligibility, 269, 287
Criticism in historical research, 215-216
Cronbach's alpha, homogeneity assessed with,
    259, 260
Cross-sectional studies, 172-173
Cumulative Index Medicus, 82
*Cumulative Index to Nursing and Allied Health
    Literature*, 336
Curve, normal, 300

D
Data
  analysis of; *see* Data analysis
  available, 238-239, 244-245
  collection of; *see* Data collection
  descriptive, qualitative research and, 186
  organization of, computers used for, 339-340
  qualitative, purposes of, 183-184
  sources for, 215
  summarizing, 307
  synthesis of, research report and, 216-217
Data analysis
  computers used for, 339-340
  critiquing, 384t
  descriptive, 291-307; *see also* Descriptive sta-
    tistics
  in grounded theory, 192
  in historical research, 215-216
  inferential, 311-327
Data bases, 335
  computerized, 81
Data collection
  biological, 230-232
  computers used for, 336-337
  consistency in, 230
  constancy in, 134-135
  in historical research, 215
  with interviews and questionnaires, 235-238,
    244
  methods for, 227-245
    critiquing, 241-243
    selection of, 229
  objective, 227
  observational, 232-235, 244
    critiquing, 241-242

Data collection—cont'd
  physiological, 230-232
  subjective, 227
Data processing; *see also* Computers
  in nursing research, 333-334
Definition(s)
  conceptual, 99-100
    in hypothesis statement, 121
    operationalization of, 105
  critiquing, 383t
  operational, 100
    in hypothesis statement, 121
    of variables, 229-230
Degrees of freedom, 318
Delimitations, 269-270, 287
Descriptions, narrative, qualitative research and,
    186
Descriptive statistics
  critiquing, 304-306
  definition of, 292, 312
  presentation of, 292-293
  purpose of, 307
  tests of relationships between variables and,
    321
Descriptive studies; *see* Study(ies), ex post
    facto
Design
  after-only, 152
  after-only nonequivalent control group, 155-
    156
  definition of, 128
  nonequivalent control group, 155
  one-group pretest-posttest, 156-157
  preexperimental, 156
  research; *see* Research design(s)
  Solomon four-group, 151-152
  time series, 157-158
Determinism, 32
Developmental studies, 172-175
Deviation, standard, 303, 307
df; *see* Degrees of freedom
Distribution
  frequency, 295, 296t, 307
  leptokurtic, 301
  modality of, 297, 307
  nonsymmetrical, 307
  normal, 300-301
  platykurtic, 301
  sampling, 314-316; *see also* Inferential statis-
    tics
    of means, 300, 307, 315, 326
  skewness of, 300-301
  symmetrical, 301

Dock, L., 6
Driving forces, change facilitated by, 370-371

E
Education, nursing
  nursing research and, 6, 362, 365-366
  reforms in, 6
Education and Professional Position of Nurses, 6
Educational Resources Information Center, 82
Elderly, vulnerable, research and, 48-49
Element(s), 287
  definition of, 270
  random selection of, 275
Eligibility, criteria for, 269, 287
Empiricism in scientific approach to research, 30
Equivalence of measurement instruments, 259-
    261
ERIC; *see* Educational Resources Information
    Center
Error
  chance, 249
  constant, 249
  measurement, 249
  random, 249
  sampling, 314
  standard, of the mean, 315
  systematic, 249
  type I, 316, 326
  type II, 316, 326
  types of, in statistical inference, 316-318
Error variance, 249
Ethnography, 187-190
  definition of, 188
Evaluation, definition of, 221
Ex post facto studies, 170-171; *see also* Research
    design(s), quasiexperimental
Experience, definition of, in phenomenology,
    194
Experiment(s)
  definition of, 149
  field, 152
  laboratory, 152-153
Experimental design; *see* Research design(s),
    experimental
Experimentation, quality assurance and, 158-
    159
Explanatory studies, 170
External criticism, 215-216

F
Face validity, 251
Factor analysis, construct validity established
    with, 254

Facts in surveys, 168
Federal Register, 44
Figures in research reports, 350
Findings
 definition of, 346
 research; *see* Research findings
First Nursing Research Conference, 9
Formative evaluation, 221
Framework, theoretical; *see* Theoretical framework
Frequency distribution, 295, 296t, 307
Funds
 for conduct and utilization of nursing research, 364, 370
 for evaluation of utilization of research in clinical setting, 376-377

G

Garbage In, Garbage Out axiom, 339
Generalization, 26, 353-354
 in scientific approach to research, 30
GIGO axiom; *see* Garbage In, Garbage Out axiom
Goldmark Report, reforms in nursing education and, 6
Grounded theory method, 185, 190-193
 critiquing, 204
 data analysis in, 192
 purposes of, 190-191
 qualitative research and, 184
Groups, control and experimental, 135

H

Hardware, computer, 330, 342
Hawthorne effect, 154
History
 definition of, 212
 internal validity affected by, 137
History of Nursing, 6
Homogeneity, 134
 of measurement instruments, 257-259
Human rights, protection of, evidence of, 287
Human Rights Guidelines for Nurses, American Nurses' Association, 53
Hypothesis testing, 96
 construct validity established by, 252, 253t
 inferential statistics and, 313-314, 326
Hypothesis(es), 98, 109-124
 characteristics of, 111-118
 consistency of, with defined theory base, 113-114
 critiquing, 120-123, 124, 383t
 definition of, 110-111

Hypothesis(es) — cont'd
 directional
  advantages to, 116-117
  definition of, 115
 nondirectional, definition of, 115
 null, 313; *see also* Hypothesis(es), statistical
 purpose of, 123
  in theoretical framework, 103-104
 relationship of research design with, 118-119, 122
 scientific, 313; *see also* Hypothesis(es), research
 statistical
  examples of, 119t
  versus research, 117-118
 testability of, 113, 122
 testing, 96
 wording, 114-115, 116-117t

I

Illustration, purpose of, in qualitative research, 183
Illustrations in research reports, 350
Improved Standards for the Laboratory Animals' Act, 51-52
Indexes, literature, 81
 commonly used in nursing research, 82
Inference, negative, principles of, 313
Inferential statistics, 292, 312-313; *see also* Distribution, sampling; Sampling, random
 commonly used, 318-319
 definition of, 312
 example of use and critique of, 325-326
 results of, critiquing, 323-326, 327
Informants, key, 187, 189
Information
 background, 204-205
 exchange of, 193
 storage of, by computers, 331
Informed consent, 39-41, 46-47
 guidelines for, 44-45
 waiving, 49
Institutional Animal Care and Use Committee, 51
Institutional review boards, 43-44, 54
Instrumentation
 internal validity affected by, 138
 purpose of, in qualitative research, 183
Instruments, measurement; *see* Measurement instruments
Interference, definition of, 365
Internal criticism, 216
International Nursing Index, 82

Interpersonal Conflict Scale, 257
Interrater reliability, equivalence tested with, 259-261
Interrelationship studies, 168-175, 177-178
Interval width, 295
Intervention by observer, 233
Interviewing key informants in qualitative research, 187
Interviews
    data collection by, 235-238, 244
        critiquing, 241-243
    in phenomenological study, 196
Intuition
    definition of, 23
    as source of knowledge, 23-24
IRBs; *see* Institutional review boards
Items; *see* Questions

J
Journal of Nursing Research, 8
Journal of Obstetric, Gynecologic, and Neonatal Nursing, 382
Journals, nursing, publication goals of, 382
Judgment, personal, in preparing research article, 382

K
Kendall's tau, 322
Knowledge
    experiential, qualitative research and, 200-201
    intuition as source of, 23-24
    logical reasoning as source of, 25-27
    nursing
        development of, 103
        impact of philosophy and science on development of, 22-23
    scientific approach to, 27-32
    sources of, 23-32, 33
    tradition and authority as source of, 25
    trial-and-error as source of, 24-25
Known groups, construct validity established with, 254
KR-20 coefficient; *see* Kuder-Richardson coefficient
Kuder-Richardson coefficient, homogeneity assessed with, 258-259
Kurtosis, 301, 307

L
Laboratory Animal Welfare Act, 51
Language, computer, 332
Level of significance, 316-317
Likert scale, 235-236, 259

Limitations of research study, 347
Literature
    conceptual, definition of, 78
    data-based, definition of, 78
    indexes to, 81
        used in nursing research, 82
    related, identification of, 81
    review of; *see* Literature review
    scientific, research problems generated by, 61-62t
Literature review, 78-87
    computers used for, 335-336
    conducting, 80-83
    critiquing, 85-87, 383t
    definition of, 78, 87
    evaluation of, in theoretical framework, 104
    goals of, 78-80
    organization of, 83-84
    purpose of, 85-86, 87, 98
    weak, 86t
Longitudinal studies, 172-173
Lysaught Report, 9

M
Mainframes, 331
    statistical programs for, 339
Manipulation in experimental research, 149
Mann-Whitney U test, 320
Manuscripts, research, guidelines for preparation of, 386
Maturation, internal validity affected by, 137-138
Mean(s), 299-300, 307
    sampling distribution of, 300, 315, 326
    standard error of, 315
Measurement instruments
    critiquing, 384t
    equivalence of, 259-261
        definition of, 255
    homogeneity of, 257-259
        definition of, 255
    new, construction of, 239-240
    reliability of, 255-261
        definition of, 263
    reliability and validity of, 247-263
    stability of, 256-257
        definition of, 255
    validity of, 250-254
        definition of, 263
Measurement(s)
    biological, 230-232
    definition of, 293
    error in, 249

Measurement(s) — cont'd
  interval, 294-295
  levels of, 307
    in descriptive statistics, 293-295
  nominal, 293
  ordinal, 293-294
  physiological, 230-232, 244
    critiquing, 241-242
  ratio, 295
  reliability of, 255
Measures of central tendency, 292, 297-300,
    307
Median, 299, 307
Median test, 320
Medical devices, testing, Food and Drug Ad-
    ministration guidelines for, 41-42
MEDLINE, 335-336
Memory
  computer, 330
  random access, 330
  read only, 330
Mental Measurement Yearbook, 337
Methodology, definition of, 217
Microcomputers, 331
  operating and editing systems of, 331-332
  statistical programs for, 339-340
  versus mainframe computers, for data process-
    ing, 334t
Modal percentage, 302
Modality of distribution, 297, 307
Mode, 297, 299, 307
Model, conceptual
  definition of, 102
  in nursing, 102-103, 105
Modem, 332
Mortality, internal validity affected by, 138-139
Multidimensional Health Locus of Control
    Scale, 257
Multiple regression, 322-323

N

National Center for Nursing Research, 10
National Commission for Study of Nursing and
    Nursing Education Report, 9
National League for Nursing, 8
National League of Nursing Education, Com-
    mittee on Public Health Nursing of, 7
National Research Act, 43, 53, 54
NCNR; *see* National Center for Nursing Re-
    search
Negative inference, principles of, 313
Nightingale, F., 6
NLN; *see* National League for Nursing

NLNE; *see* National League of Nursing Educa-
    tion
Nonequivalent control group design, 155
Normal curve, 300
Normal distribution, 300-301
Nuremberg Code, 39
Nurse Practice Act of 1943, 7
Nurse researchers, clinical, 368
Nurse(s)
  with associate degrees, nursing research
    and, 10
  with baccalaureate degrees, nursing research
    and, 10-12, 15
  as consumer of research, 5
  with doctorate degrees, nursing research by,
    12, 15
  educational preparation of, utilization of nurs-
    ing research by, 362, 365, 366
  with master's degrees, nursing research by,
    12, 15
  as researcher and patient advocate, 52-53
Nursing
  master's and doctoral programs in, growth
    of, 9
  systematic ways of acquiring knowledge in,
    29t
Nursing education
  nursing research and, 6
  reforms in, 6
  types of, delineation of research activities by,
    10-13
Nursing for the Future, 7
Nursing journals, publication goals of, 382
Nursing models
  conceptual, 105
  contribution of, to research, 102-103
Nursing and Nursing Education in the United
    States Landmark Study, 6
Nursing practice
  development of, based on theory, 9
  gap between nursing research and,
    361-371
  nursing research for scientific validation of,
    13-16
Nursing research, 16
  applied, definition of, 13t
  assessing relevance of, to clinical setting, 374-
    377
  basic, definition of, 13t
  climate for, 363, 367-368
  clinical, definition of, 13t; *see also* Nursing re-
    search, practice-related
  conferences on, 367

Nursing research—cont'd
  consumer of, versus nursing researcher, 360-361
  contribution of nursing models to, 102-103
  critiquing application of, to clinical practice, 384t
  data processing in, 333-334
  early course on, 7
  evaluation of, in clinical setting, 377-378
  feasibility of applying, to clinical setting, 374-375
  future of, 17
  future directions of, 13-16
  gap between clinical practice and, 361-371
  historical evolution of, 6-10, 16
  international code of ethics for, 41
  knowledge base created by, evaluation of, 371-373
  literature indexes used in, 82
  in the mid- and late-nineteenth century, 6
  in the 1980's, 10
  practice-related
    after 1950, 7-9
    before 1950, 6-7
    in 1960's, 8-9
  priorities in, 15
    reorganizaton of, 8-9
  risks of applying, to clinical setting, 373
  role of baccalaureate nursing graduate in, 10-12, 15, 16
  role of doctoral nursing graduate in, 12, 15, 16
  role of master's nursing graduate in, 12, 15, 16
  roles and issues in, 1-56
  roles of nurses in, 10-13
  in the twentieth century, 6-9
  types of, 13t
  utilization of, 359-378
    criteria for, 371-374
    and educational preparation of nurses, 362, 365-366
    financial support for, 364, 370
    organizational resources and, 363-364, 367-370
    resistance to change and, 364-365, 370-371
Nursing research committee, 368-369
Nursing Research Index, 82
Nursing Research journal, 382
Nursing service administrator, utilization of research findings and, 367-368
Nursing Studies Index, 82

Nursing theory, definition of, 102
Nutting, A., 6

O

Observation
  data collection by, 232-235, 244
  participant, in grounded theory method, 191-192
  structured, 234
  types of, 233-234
  unstructured, 234
Observer, role of, in observational data collection, 233-234, 244
One-group pretest-posttest design, 156-157
Open-ended items, 235, 236
Operationalization
  of concepts, 100, 105
  definition of, 227
  of variables, computers used for, 337
Ordered steps, 28-29
Orlando, I.J., 9

P

p value, 321
Parallel form reliability, 257, 261
Parameter, definition of, 312
Participants, observation of, in grounded theory method, 191-192
PCs; *see* Computers, personal
Pearson product moment correlation coefficient, 321
Pearson r test, 321
Peplau, H., 9
Percentile, 303
Phenomenology, 194-199
Philosopher, 22
Philosophy, 22
Population, 269-270
  accessible, 270, 287
  definition of, 269, 287
  parameter for, 312
  random selection of, 284
  representativeness of, 287
    in sample, 284-285
  specification of
    in problem statement, 67
    in sample, 283-284
  target, 270, 287
  vulnerable, 45, 48-50
Pound seizure laws, 51
Power analysis, sample size estimated using, 281
Practice, nursing; *see* Nursing practice
Prediction studies, 171-172

Primary sources, 215
  literature review and, 83
Probability, 314-316
Probability value, 321
Problem
  defining, 63
  identification of, computers used for, 334-335
Problem statement(s), 59-74
  characteristics of, 65
  components of, and related criteria, 68t
  critiquing, 71-73, 383t
  in declarative form, 66t
  differentiation of, from statement of purpose, 70
  examples of unrefined and refined, 69-70t
  final, 65-70
  formulating, 60, 73
  in interrogative form, 66t
  refining, 63-64
Process consent, 202
Product testing, 41-42
Program, computer, 332
Propositions in theoretical framework, 93
Prospective studies, 174-175
Psychological Abstracts, 82
Psychometrics, 217
Public Law 99-158, 10
Purposes, definition of, 92

Q

Quality assurance, experimentation and, 158-159
Quasiexperimental design; *see* Research
    design(s), quasiexperimental
Questionnaires, data collection using, 235-238,
    244
  critiquing, 241-243
Questions
  case study, 200-201
  close-ended, 235, 236
    examples of, 237
  ethnographic, 188-190
  grounded theory, 191-193
  in historical research, 214
  open-ended, 235, 236
    examples of, 237
  phenomenological, and research process, 194-
    199
  process, in qualitative research, 186
  research, 119-120, 122-123, 124
    critiquing, 204, 383t

R

RAM; *see* Memory, random access
Random error, 249

Randomization, 135-136, 149
Range
  definition of, 302
  semiquartile, 302-303
Rationale, theoretical, 105
  formulating, 99-100
Reactivity
  external validity affected by, 140
  in observational data collection, 233
Reality and causality, assumptions about, in sci-
    entific approach to research, 32
Reasoning
  deductive, 27
    definition of, 26
  inductive, 26
    definition of, 25-26
    qualitative research and, 186-187
  logical, as source of knowledge, 25-27
Recommendations, 354-355, 356
  critiquing, 384t
Records as source of data, 238-239, 244-245
  critiquing, 243
Regression, multiple, 322-323
Relationship statement, 112
Reliability
  critiquing, 261-263, 384t
  interrater, 259-261
  of measurement instruments, 255-261
    definition of, 255, 263
  parallel or alternate form, 257, 261
  split-half, homogeneity assessed with, 258
  testing, 255-256
  test-retest, 256
Reliability coefficient, interpretation of, 255
Replication
  construct, 372
  of research findings in clinical setting, 362,
    371-372
Report, research; *see* Research report
Research; *see also* Research study; Study(ies)
  additional types of, 211-224
  on animals, legal and ethical aspects of, 51-52
  approach to, critiquing, 384t
  computers used in, 329-342
  definition of, 5, 16
  design of; *see* Research design(s)
  ethical and legal considerations in, 38-41
  ethnographic; *see* Ethnography
  evaluating methodology of, 24-25
  evaluative, 218, 221-224
    critiquing, 222, 223
  grounded theory process of; *see* Grounded
    theory method

Research—cont'd
historical, 212-217, 223
  critiquing, 222, 223
  problem identification in, 213-214
on humans, federal guidelines for, 43-45
  reviewing, 50-51
legal and ethical issues in, 37-54
as the link between theory, education, and
    practice, 5
methodological, 217-218, 223
  considerations in development of tools for,
    219-220t
  critiquing, 222, 223
nurses as consumers of, 5
nursing; *see* Nursing research
pediatric, assent versus consent in, 48
phenomenological, 194-199; *see also* Phenom-
    enology
  styles of, 196t
process of
  components of, 32, 33f
  computers for, 334-342
  evaluating, 381-412
  staff development programs on, 367
qualitative
  approaches to, 185-187
  case studies in, 199-201
  combined with quantitative approaches,
    203-204
  critiquing, 204-206
  definition of, 183
  ethical guidelines for, 201
  historical perspectives on, 184-185
  issues and problems in, 201-204
  orientation and structure of, 183
  purposes of, 183-184
  reliability and validity of, 203
qualitative approaches to, 181-207
qualitative tradition in, 182-187
quantitative, combined with qualitative ap-
    proaches, 203-204
role of, in nursing, 3-17
role of intuition in, 23
scientific, definition of, 28
scientific approach to, 21-35
significance of, in nursing, 4-5
special legal and ethical considerations in, 45,
    48-50
survey, 167-168, 177, 235
unauthorized, 42
unethical conduct of, 49
versus clinical evaluation, 41
versus clinical evaluation of research, 377-378

Research base
clinical merit of, 374
definition of, 362
Research design(s), 125-143
accuracy of, 130-131
control of, flexibility in, 136
control over tested variables in, 133-136
critiquing, 141-143, 384t
economy of, 131, 132t
experimental, 136, 148
  advantages and disadvantages of,
    153-154
  properties of, 149-150
  true, 149-153, 150-151, 161
experimental and quasiexperimental, 147-161
  critiquing, 159-161
exploratory, 136
feasibility of, 131, 132t
nonexperimental, 165-178
  causality in, 175
  critiquing, 176-177
nonexperimental versus experimental, 177
purpose of, 129-130, 143
quasiexperimental, 148, 154-158, 161; *see also*
    Study(ies), ex post facto
  advantages and disadvantages of, 158
relationship of hypothesis to, 118-119, 122
three concepts of, 129
types of, 136, 150-152
Research findings
analysis of, 345-357
assessing relevance of, to clinical setting, 374-
    377
communication of
  computers used for, 341-342
  to nursing profession, 363, 366-367
cost-effectiveness of applying, to clinical set-
    ting, 375
feasibility of applying, to clinical setting, 374-
    375
gap between dissemination and use of, in
    practice, 378
implementation of, clinical control of nurses
    over, 374
replication of, in clinical setting, 362, 371-
    372
utilization of, clinical evaluation of, 375-377
Research manuscripts, guidelines for preparation
    of, for publication, 386
Research in Nursing and Health, 9
Research population; *see* Population
Research problem
  conceptualization of, objectivity in, 130

Research problem — cont'd
  definition of, 70
  feasibility of, 64, 73
  generating, 60-62
  refinement of, 73
  significance to nursing of, 64
  testability of, specified in problem statement,
    67-68
Research report; *see also* Research study
  results section in, 347-351
    critiquing, 355-356
  synthesis of data in, 216-217
Research study; *see also* Research report
  analyzing use of computers in, guidelines for,
    342
  critique of, sample of, 386-400, 400-413
  evaluating, 381-412
  generalizability of, 355-356
  inferential statistics used in, 312-313
  limitations of, 347
  purpose of, 70
  results of; *see* Results
  scientific merit of, evaluation of, 373
  section on results of, in research report, 347-
    351
  theoretical framework in, purpose of, 97
  theoretical framework used as guide in, 93-96
  validity of, 142-143
Researchers, nursing, versus nursing research
    consumer, 360-361
Researcher-subject relationships, 199
Results
  analyzing, computers used for, 340
  critiquing, 355-356
  discussion of, 351-355
  external validity of, 139-141
  internal validity of, 137-139
  section on, in research report, 347-351
  validity of, 136-141
Retrospective studies, 174; *see also* Ex post facto
    studies
Richards, L., 6-7
ROM; *see* Memory, read only

S

SD; *see* Standard deviation
Sample(s)
  critiquing, 283-287, 288, 383t
  definition of, 270, 287
  representative, 271
  selection of, computers used for, 337-339
  size of, 280-282, 288
    evaluation of, 286

Sample(s) — cont'd
  types of, 271-280
Sampling, 267-288
  cluster, 278-279
  concepts in, 269-271
  convenience, 272-273
  criteria for, 283-287, 288
  criteria for evaluating, 285
  definition of, 267, 270, 287
  homogeneous, 134
  multistage, 278
  nonprobability, 271-274, 285,
    287-288
  probability, 271, 275-280, 284, 288
  procedures used for, 282-283
  purpose of, 270-271
  purposive, 274
  quota, 273
  random, 284, 288; *see also* Inferential statistics
    simple, 275-277
    stratified, 277-278
  strategies for, 272t
  suitability of, to research design, 285-286
  systematic, 279-280
  theoretical, 192
Sampling distribution of the means, 300, 307,
    315, 326
Sampling error, 314
Sampling unit, 270, 287
Scale; *see also* Measurement instruments
  definition of, 235
  Interpersonal Conflict, 257
  Likert, 235-236, 259
  Multidimensional Health Locus of Control,
    257
  reliable, attributes of, 255
  unidimensional, 257
Scatter plot, 304, 307
Scholarly Inquiry for Nursing Practice, 10
Science, 22
  philosophy of, 22-23
  systematic ways of acquiring knowledge in,
    29t
Science Citation Index, 82
Scientific approach, 33
  components of, 28-32
  to knowledge, 27-32
Scientific literature; *see also* Literature
  review of, refining problem statement and,
    63-64
Scientist, 22
Secondary sources, 215
  literature review and, 83

Selection
  bias in, internal validity impacted by, 139
  external validity affected by, 140
  random, of elements, 275
Sensitization, purpose of, in qualitative research, 183-184
Settings, natural, qualitative research and, 185-186
Sign test, 320, 327
Signed ranks test for related groups, 320, 327
Significance
  level of, in statistical inference, 316-317
  practical versus statistical, 317-318
  statistical, 326
    tests of, 318-323
  statistical versus practical, 317-318
Skew, 307
  distribution described in terms of, 300-301
Social desirability, 236
Social Science Citation Index, 82
Social sciences, systematic ways of acquiring knowledge in, 29t
Software, computer, 331, 332-333, 342
Solomon four-group design, 151-152
Sources for data, 215
Spearman-Brown formula, 258
SPSSX; *see* Statistical Package for the Social Sciences
Standard deviation, 303, 307
Statement
  declarative, in hypothesis, 112, 121
  definition of, 212
  hypothesis, conceptual and operational definitions in, 121
  problem; *see* Problem statement
  relationship, 112
Statistical inference, type I and type II errors in, 316-318
Statistical Package for the Social Sciences, 333-334, 339
Statistical significance, 326
  practical versus, 317-318
  tests of, 318-323
Statistics
  advanced, 322-323
  definition of, 312
  descriptive; *see* Descriptive statistics
  inferential; *see* Inferential statistics
  parametric versus nonparametric, 318
  sample, 312
  summary, 297
  t, 319-320
Steward, I., 7

Study(ies); *see also* Research; Research design(s); Research study
  case, in qualitative research, 199-201
  causal-comparative, 170
  correlational, 136, 168-170
    advantages and disadvantages of, 169
  cross-sectional, 172-173
  descriptive, 170
  developmental, 172-175
  ex post facto, 170-171; *see also* Research design(s), quasiexperimental; Study(ies), retrospective
  explanatory; *see* Study(ies), ex post facto
  interrelationship, 168-175, 177-178
  longitudinal, 172-173
  prediction, 171-172
  prospective, 174-175
  retrospective, 174
  survey, 167-168
Subjectivity in qualitative research, 185
Summative evaluation, 221
Survey studies, 167-168
Surveys, descriptive, 167
Systematic, definition of, 92
Systematic error, 249

T
t test, 326
Tables in research reports, 350
Terminal, 331
  remote, 332
Test scores, variability in, 249
Test(s)
  chi-square, 320, 322, 326
  of difference, 319-321
  of difference or association, 319t
  Mann-Whitney U, 320
  median, 320
  nonparametric, 318
  parametric, 318
  Pearson r, 321, 327
  of relationships, 321-322
  sign, 320, 327
  signed ranks, for related groups, 320, 327
  Student t, 319-320
  t, 326
Testability
  of hypothesis, 113, 122
  of research problem, 67-68
Testing
  external validity affected by, 140-141
  hypothesis
    construct validity established by, 252, 253t

Testing — cont'd
  hypothesis — cont'd
    in inferential statistics, 326
    inferential statistics used in, 313-314
  internal validity affected by, 138
Test-retest reliability, instrument stability estimated with, 256
Theoretical framework, 91-105; *see also* Theory(ies)
  associated with grounded theory, 190
  critiquing, 103-104, 105
  definition of, 92-93
  development of, 97-99
  purpose of, in research study, 97
  used as a guide in research study, 93-96
Theory(ies); *see also* Theoretical framework
  base in, 113-114
  borrowed versus new, 100-101
  definition of, 30, 92, 105
  importance of, 104
  and method, relationship between, 32-33
  nursing
    definition of, 102
    research problems generated by, 62t
  probability, 314-316
  role of, in research, 33-34
  scientific approach to research and, 30-32
Time series design, 157-158
Time-sharing, 331
Tools
  development of, for methodological research, 219-220t
  measurement; *see* Measurement instruments
Trial-and-error as source of knowledge, 24-25
Triangulation of qualitative and quantitative research, 203

U

U.S. Cadet Nurses Corps, 7

V

Validity
  concurrent, 251
  construct, 252-254
    multitrait-multimethod establishment of, 253-254
  content, 250-251
  convergent, construct validity established by, 252
  criterion-related, 251-252
  critiquing, 261-263, 384t
  determination of, 142-143

Validity — cont'd
  divergent, construct validity established by, 253
  external
    critiquing, 384t
    factors affecting, 139-141
  face, 251
  internal
    critiquing, 384t
    threats to, 137-139
  of measurement instruments, 250-254
    definition of, 263
  predictive, 251
Variability, measures of, 307
  interpreting, 302-304
  range of, 302
Variable(s), 100
  antecedent, 150
  attitude, in surveys, 167-168
  correlation of, 304, 321
  definition of, 65
  dependent, 66-67, 148
  extraneous
    control of, 133
    definition of, 133
  in hypothesis, 121
  independent, 65-66, 148
    manipulation of, 135
  interrelationship between, correlational study of, 168-170
  intervening, 150
  measuring, 227-230
    computers used for, 337
  nature of relationship of, 112
  operational definition of, 229-230
  operationalization of, computers used for, 337
  opinion, in surveys, 167-168
  relationships between, tests of, 321-322
Variance
  analysis of, 320, 322, 326
  error, 249

W

Walter Reed Army Institute of Research, 8
Western Journal of Nursing Research, 9
Wiedenbach, E., 9
Wilcoxon matched-pairs, 320, 327

Z

Z score, 303-304, 307

EFFECTIVE PATIENT CARE

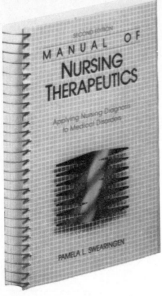

MANUAL OF NURSING THERAPEUTICS: APPLYING NURSING DIAGNOSES TO MEDICAL DISORDERS
2nd Edition
Pamela L. Swearingen, R.N.
April 1990
ISBN 0-8016-5847-0

Completely revised and updated with more than 185 medical-surgical disorders, this clinical reference is designed to help nursing students and staff effectively plan and evaluate care of the adult medical-surgical patient.

- Disorders are discussed in a consistent and easy-to-use format that includes definition; assessment; diagnostic tests; medical management; nursing diagnoses and intervention; and patient/family teaching and discharge planning.

- Clinical experts from various practice settings have contributed to this authoritative manual to provide a comprehensive scope of experience and knowledge.

- Content is organized by body systems to facilitate thorough and effective patient care.

- Extensive appendices provide information on common patient care considerations, nursing diagnoses, abbreviations used in the manual, and heart and breath sounds.

  To order ask your bookstore manager or call toll-free 1-800-221-7700, ext. 15A. We look forward to hearing from you.